ANNUAL EDITIONS

Nutrition
Twelfth Edition

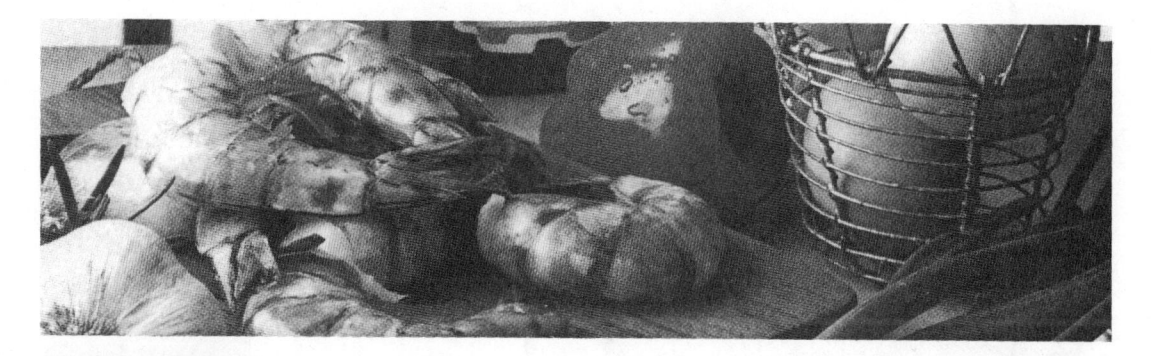

00/01

EDITOR

Charlotte C. Cook-Fuller
Towson University

Charlotte Cook-Fuller has a Ph.D. in community health education and graduate and undergraduate degrees in nutrition. She has worked for several years in public health services and has also been involved with the federally funded WIC (Women, Infants, and Children) program. Now as a professor, she teaches nutrition within both professional and consumer contexts, as well as courses for health education students. She has coauthored a nutrition curriculum for grades K–12 and is currently involved in a multidisciplinary effort to provide strategies to public school teachers for teaching about global issues such as hunger.

Editorial Consultant

Stephen Barrett, M.D.
Editor, *Nutrition Forum*

Dushkin/McGraw-Hill
Sluice Dock, Guilford, Connecticut 06437

Visit us on the Internet
http://www.dushkin.com/annualeditions/

S0-FNS-725

Credits

1. Trends Today and Tomorrow
Unit photo—© 2000 by Cleo Freelance Photography.
2. Nutrients
Unit photo—© 2000 by PhotoDisc, Inc.
3. Through the Life Span: Diet and Disease
Unit photo—© 2000 by Cleo Freelance Photography.
4. Fat and Weight Control
Unit photo—© 2000 by Cleo Freelance Photography.
5. Food Safety
Unit photo—Courtesy of Dushkin/McGraw-Hill.
6. Health Claims
Unit photo—Courtesy of Dushkin/McGraw-Hill.
7. World Hunger and Malnutrition
Unit photo—United Nations photo.

Copyright

Cataloging in Publication Data
Main entry under title: Annual editions: Nutrition. 2000/2001.
 1. Nutrition—Periodicals. 2. Diet—Periodicals. I. Cook-Fuller, Charlotte C., comp. II. Title: Nutrition.
ISBN 0–07–236568–4   613.2'.05   91–641611   ISSN 1055–6990

© 2000 by Dushkin/McGraw-Hill, Guilford, CT 06437, A Division of The McGraw-Hill Companies.

Copyright law prohibits the reproduction, storage, or transmission in any form by any means of any portion of this publication without the express written permission of Dushkin/McGraw-Hill, and of the copyright holder (if different) of the part of the publication to be reproduced. The Guidelines for Classroom Copying endorsed by Congress explicitly state that unauthorized copying may not be used to create, to replace, or to substitute for anthologies, compilations, or collective works.

Annual Editions® is a Registered Trademark of Dushkin/McGraw-Hill, A Division of The McGraw-Hill Companies.

Twelfth Edition

Cover image © 2000 PhotoDisc, Inc.

Printed in the United States of America   234567890BAHBAH543210   Printed on Recycled Paper

Members of the Advisory Board are instrumental in the final selection of articles for each edition of ANNUAL EDITIONS. Their review of articles for content, level, currentness, and appropriateness provides critical direction to the editor and staff. We think that you will find their careful consideration well reflected in this volume.

EDITORS

Charlotte C. Cook-Fuller
Towson University

with Stephen Barrett, M.D.
Editor, Nutrition Forum

ADVISORY BOARD

Becky Alejandre
American River College

John S. Braubitz
Cayuga Community College

Valencia Browning
Eastern Illinois University

Georgia W. Crews
South Dakota State University

Patricia Erickson
Skyline College

Sarah T. Hawkins
Indiana State University

Suzanne Hendrich
Iowa State University

David H. Hyde
University of Maryland
College Park

Dorothea J. Klimis
University of Maine
Orono

Manfred Kroger
Pennsylvania State University
University Park

Rebecca M. Mullis
University of Georgia

Gretchen Myers-Hill
Michigan State University

M. Zafar Nomani
West Virginia University

Thomas M. Richard
Keene State College

Karen J. Schmitz
Madonna University

Donna R. Seibels
Samford University

Diana M. Spillman
Miami University

Danielle Torisky
James Madison University

Linda Elaine Wendt
University of Wisconsin
Eau Claire

Royal E. Wohl
Washburn University

EDITORIAL STAFF

Ian A. Nielsen, Publisher
Roberta Monaco, Senior Developmental Editor
Dorothy Fink, Associate Developmental Editor
Addie Raucci, Senior Administrative Editor
Cheryl Greenleaf, Permissions Editor
Joseph Offredi, Permissions/Editorial Assistant
Diane Barker, Proofreader
Lisa Holmes-Doebrick, Senior Program Coordinator

PRODUCTION STAFF

Brenda S. Filley, Production Manager
Charles Vitelli, Designer
Lara M. Johnson, Design/Advertising Coordinator
Laura Levine, Graphics
Mike Campbell, Graphics
Tom Goddard, Graphics
Eldis Lima, Graphics
Juliana Arbo, Typesetting Supervisor
Marie Lazauskas, Typesetter
Kathleen D'Amico, Typesetter
Karen Roberts, Typesetter
Larry Killian, Copier Coordinator

To the Reader

In publishing ANNUAL EDITIONS we recognize the enormous role played by the magazines, newspapers, and journals of the public press in providing current, first-rate educational information in a broad spectrum of interest areas. Many of these articles are appropriate for students, researchers, and professionals seeking accurate, current material to help bridge the gap between principles and theories and the real world. These articles, however, become more useful for study when those of lasting value are carefully collected, organized, indexed, and reproduced in a low-cost format, which provides easy and permanent access when the material is needed. That is the role played by ANNUAL EDITIONS.

New to ANNUAL EDITIONS is the inclusion of related World Wide Web sites. These sites have been selected by our editorial staff to represent some of the best resources found on the World Wide Web today. Through our carefully developed topic guide, we have linked these Web resources to the articles covered in this ANNUAL EDITIONS reader. We think that you will find this volume useful, and we hope that you will take a moment to visit us on the Web at **http://www.dushkin.com** to tell us what you think.

You may agree with Pudd'nhead Wilson (a character created by Mark Twain) who said, "The only way to keep your health is to eat what you don't want, drink what you don't like, and do what you'd rather not." Nutritionists would argue that you can't achieve or maintain good health on a diet of soft drinks and vending machine foods. But you might be surprised to learn that many of your favorite foods can fit into a good diet. In making food choices, remember that variety and moderation are two key words that will assist you in achieving positive health outcomes and avoiding the negative results of excesses or deficiencies.

An array of resources is available to help you make decisions, including popular publications, the news media, scientific journals, and people from many educational backgrounds. Your dilemma is to select reliable sources that will supply factual information based on science rather than exaggerations based on bias. It is important to avoid overreacting to nutrition-and-food-related news items or promotional materials, especially if they sound sensational or have shock value. The exaggeration and the myth are what much of the public grasps and, in large measure, reacts to. My challenge to you is to use this *Annual Editions: Nutrition 00/01*, preferably with a standard nutrition text, as an invitation to learning. Become a discriminating learner. Compare what you hear and read to the accepted body of knowledge. If this volume provides you with useful information, challenges your thinking, broadens your understanding, or motivates you to take some useful action, it will have fulfilled its purpose.

While this entire volume is essentially one of current events and current thinking, the first unit focuses on trends that give a preview of the future and that relate to characteristics of today's food consumer, the food industry, and views of foods and food components. The next three units are devoted to nutrients, diet and disease, and weight control. All are topics which directly relate to our health, and the dynamic state of knowledge on these subjects requires each of us to be constantly learning and adjusting. Units on food safety and health claims follow, areas in which consumers are especially vulnerable to media and promotional hype and misinformation. The last unit addresses hunger and malnutrition as social and political issues. This unit is intended primarily as a forum for global concerns, but it has become abundantly clear that hunger is also a national issue.

Although the units in this book are distinct, many of the articles have broader significance. The *topic guide* will help you to find other articles on a given subject. Also, *World Wide Web* sites can be used to further explore topics. These sites are cross-referenced by number in the topic guide. You also will find that many of the articles contain at least some element of controversy, the origin of which may be incomplete knowledge, questionable policy, pseudoscience, or competing needs. Sometimes these are difficult issues to resolve, and frequently any resolution creates further dilemmas. But creatively solving problems is our challenge. We take the world as it is and use it as the foundation for tomorrow's discoveries and solutions.

Annual Editions: Nutrition 00/01 is an anthology, and any anthology can be improved, including this one. You can influence the content of future editions by returning the postage-paid article rating form on the last page of this book with your comments and suggestions.

Charlotte C. Cook-Fuller
Charlotte C. Cook-Fuller
Editor

Contents

To the Reader　　　　　　　　　　　　　　　　iv
Topic Guide　　　　　　　　　　　　　　　　　2
⊙ Selected World Wide Web Sites　　　　　　　4

Overview　　　　　　　　　　　　　　　　　6

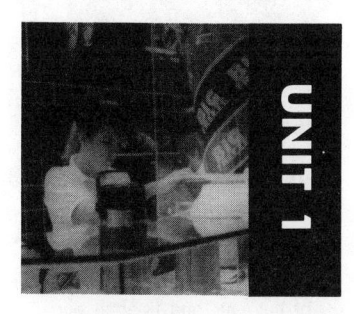

UNIT 1
Trends Today and Tomorrow

Ten articles examine the eating patterns of people today. Some of the topics considered include nutrients in our diet, eating trends, food labeling, and self-service outlets.

1. **Millennium: Food and Nutrition,** Jack Raso, *Priorities,* Volume 10, Numbers 2–3, 1998.　　　8
   The authors of this collection of essays comment on **current trends and developments** in the field of nutrition that they believe will have significant **impact** on the United States during the years ahead.

2. **Nutrient Requirements Get a Makeover: The Evolution of the Recommended Dietary Allowances,** *Food Insight,* September/October 1998.　　　13
   The **Recommended Dietary Allowances (RDAs)** were conceived in 1941 to establish nutrient amounts that would **prevent deficiency diseases.** Currently a **more comprehensive view** establishes average requirements, adequate intake, and tolerable upper intake levels.

3. **Staking a Claim to Good Health,** Paula Kurtzweil, *FDA Consumer,* November/December 1998.　　　16
   Health claims on **food labels** alert consumers to the protective effects of foods in reducing **disease risk.** Currently 10 such claims can be scientifically supported and are authorized by the FDA.

4. **Are Fruits and Vegetables Less Nutritious Today?** *University of California, Berkeley Wellness Letter,* May 1998.　　　20
   A **common fallacy,** which is that our **produce** is grown on poor soil, fuels concern about the **nutrient content** of fruits and vegetables.

5. **The Freshness Fallacy,** Minna Morse, *Health,* March 1998.　　　21
   It is a commonly held belief that **fresh produce** is superior to **frozen and canned fruits and vegetables.** Nevertheless, research supports the concept that fresh equals frozen equals canned.

6. **The New Foods: Functional or Dysfunctional?** *Consumer Reports on Health,* June 1999.　　　23
   As long as a specific disease is not mentioned and the benefit comes from the food's nutrients, Congress allows **"structure and function" claims** on food labels. **Ambiguities** over what this means has led to a proliferation of food items on grocery shelves.

7. **The Curse of Frankenfood: Genetically Modified Crops Stir Up Controversy at Home and Abroad,** Phillip J. Longman, *U.S. News & World Report,* July 26, 1999.　　　27
   Genetically modified crops are commonplace in our food supply. Paradoxically, they have both resolved some problems of crop production and raised **health and environmental issues** that are international in scope.

8. **Low-Calorie Sweeteners,** *Mayo Clinic Health Letter,* August 1999.　　　30
   Four **low-calorie sweeteners** are **FDA-**approved. Although consumers may be unlikely to consume unsafe amounts of low-calorie sweeteners, they may be lured into making **poor food choices.**

9. **It's Crunch Time for P&G's Olestra,** Pamela Sherrid, *U.S. News & World Report,* May 31, 1999.　　　32
   The synthetic fat **olestra** has achieved some acceptance but remains highly **controversial.** Food activists have persistently opposed its use. Consumers and food producers are wary of the label warning required by the FDA.

10. **Supermarket Psych-Out,** *Tufts University Health & Nutrition Letter,* January 1999.　　　33
    Great effort goes into **influencing your buying decisions** in the **grocery store.** Colors, shapes, and sizes of products, even the display signs, are carefully crafted to increase your purchases.

The concepts in bold italics are developed in the article. For further expansion please refer to the Topic Guide, the Glossary, and the Index.

v

UNIT 2

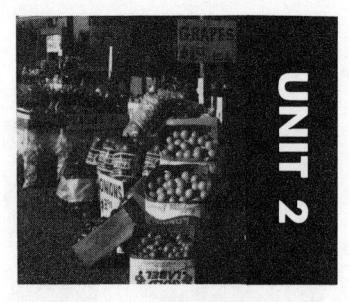

Nutrients

Ten articles discuss the importance of nutrients and fiber in our diet. Topics include dietary standards, carbohydrates, fiber, vitamins, supplements, and minerals.

Overview 36

11. **Fats: The Good, the Bad, the Trans,** George Blackburn, *Health News,* July 25, 1999. 38
    Fats are required for good *health,* but the wrong kinds of fat can be harmful. In previous years we committed to margarine rather than butter to avoid saturated fat. Now we find that the *trans fatty acids* in margarine (and other processed foods) are just as harmful to health as is saturated fat.

12. **Should You Be Eating *More* Fat and *Fewer* Carbohydrates?** *Tufts University Health & Nutrition Letter,* February 1999. 40
    Emerging information about *heart disease* indicates that more *fat* as opposed to *carbohydrates* may be advisable for those with *syndrome X.* A discussion of these findings and approaches to achieving heart health provides useful guidelines.

13. **Sugar: What's the Harm?** *Consumer Reports on Health,* May 1999. 43
    In the popular view, *sugar* causes hyperactivity and even crime, but on these charges it remains guiltless. Some argue that it predisposes one to diabetes and heart attacks. At best, sugar provides only empty calories.

14. **Vitamin C: Foods Yes, Pills No,** *Consumer Reports on Health,* November 1998. 47
    Controversies about safe and healthy amounts of *vitamin C* have continued over the years. This new discussion supports more than the current RDA amounts—but only from food sources. Protection against colds is refuted.

15. **The Best D-Fense,** *University of California, Berkeley Wellness Letter,* December 1998. 50
    Research that links *vitamin D* with *cancer protection* is on the cutting edge, but vitamin D is critical for *strong bones.* Supplied both by food and by exposure of the skin to sunlight, it is still possible to get too little. *Guidelines* are provided.

16. **Can Vitamin E Prevent Heart Disease?** Beth Fontenot, *Nutrition Forum,* July/August 1999. 52
    Many physicians recommend *vitamin E supplements* to protect against *heart and other diseases.* However, relevant studies report conflicting results or undesirable effects. The debate continues.

17. **A Disease of Too Much Iron,** Vincent J. Felitti, *Health News,* January 5, 1999. 54
    While most of us are concerned about getting enough *iron* in our diets, a number of people with hereditary *hemochromatosis* absorb far too much. The excess iron is deposited in body tissues, leading to severe medical problems. Early detection is the key to preventing damage.

18. **National Academy of Sciences Introduces New Calcium Recommendations,** Luann Soliah, *Journal of Family and Consumer Sciences,* Volume 91, Number 1, 1999. 56
    As expected, the *National Academy of Sciences* has released new and higher *recommendations for calcium* intake to promote bone health and guard against osteoporosis. A discussion of the new guidelines and information on calcium food sources and supplements is provided.

19. **Fiber: Strands of Protection,** *Consumer Reports on Health,* August 1999. 61
    Fiber, although not a nutrient, is known to be *important to good health.* Studies have repeatedly shown that high fiber diets benefit the *heart,* reduce *blood pressure,* and maintain lower *insulin levels.* But studies related to the prevention of *colon cancer* have had conflicting results.

The concepts in bold italics are developed in the article. For further expansion please refer to the Topic Guide, the Glossary, and the Index.

20. **Food for Thought about Dietary Supplements,** 66
Paul R. Thomas, *Nutrition Today,* March/April 1996.
Billions of dollars are spent yearly on **dietary supplements.** Paul Thomas, who used them extensively, has since decided that a good dose of skepticism about supplement use is healthy. He believes that there is **no scientific support** for **routine supplement use.**

Overview 74

21. **Disease-Fighting Foods? (Many Are Overhyped. But All Offer Important Lessons about Good Nutrition),** *Consumer Reports on Health,* March 1999. 76
Miracle foods do not exist, but foods do contain active **ingredients that are protective** to the body. The cumulative protective effect of these chemicals adds further credence to the recommendation to eat a **wide variety of foods** daily.

22. **"Mediterranean Diet" Reduces Risk of Second Heart Attack,** *The Cleveland Clinic Heart Advisor,* July 1999. 78
The **Mediterranean Diet** has been promoted as **heart-healthy** for some time. This is not a low-fat diet, but it does rely on **unsaturated oils** and more **omega-3 fatty acids** than most of us get.

23. **Homocysteine: "The New Cholesterol"?** *The Cleveland Clinic Heart Advisor,* February 1999. 80
In the continued search to understand the etiology of **heart disease, homocysteine** has emerged as a possible key player. The current questions are whether or not low levels of **folic acid** and **B-6** might be causative, and if cardiac disease can be reduced by reducing homocysteine levels.

24. **Soy: Cause for Joy?** Jack Raso and Ruth Kava, *Priorities,* Volume 11, Number 1, 1999. 83
Soybeans contain an unusually high concentration of **isoflavones,** plant estrogens considered **protective** against diseases such as **coronary heart disease, cancer, and osteoporosis.** Soy products can be a good addition to the diet, but more research is needed to identify the risks of high intakes.

25. **False Alarms about Food,** *Consumer Reports on Health,* February 1999. 86
While **true allergies** exist, their incidence is greatly exaggerated. This article addresses **misconceptions** related to the frequence and seriousness of allergy occurrence, as well as lactose intolerance and monosodium glutamate reactions.

26. **Questions and Answers about Cancer, Diet and Fats,** *International Food Information Council,* May 27, 1999. 90
It is difficult to identify clear cause-and-effect relationships between **diet and cancer.** So far the strongest recommendations that can be supported indicate a **well-balanced diet** emphasizing fruits and vegetables, whole grains, and beans.

27. **How to Grow a Healthy Child,** *Dairy Council Digest,* November/December 1998. 92
Children's failure to eat **recommended diets** and the rise in **overweight** among the nation's youth trigger concern. Good childhood diets can protect against poor **early development** and later **osteoporosis.** Providing an environment for making healthy food selections is key.

28. **A Focus on Nutrition for the Elderly: It's Time to Take a Closer Look,** *Nutrition Insights,* July 1999. 97
Natural body changes due to aging, as well as chronic diseases, can alter the nutrient needs of the **elderly.** A comparison of what older people actually eat to the **Healthy Eating Index** provides a picture of their overall **diet quality.**

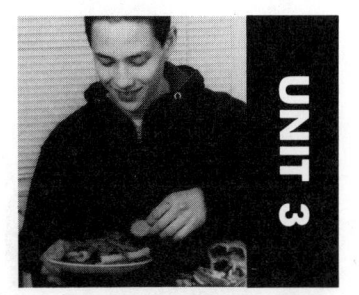

UNIT 3

Through the Life Span: Diet and Disease

Ten articles examine our health as it is affected by diet throughout our lives. Some topics include the links between diet and disease, cholesterol, and eating habits.

The concepts in bold italics are developed in the article. For further expansion please refer to the Topic Guide, the Glossary, and the Index.

29. **Physical Activity and Nutrition: A Winning Combination for Health,** Dairy Council Digest, May/June 1998. 99

Avoiding and delaying disease requires a healthy lifestyle that includes *exercise* as well as a *good diet.*

30. **Alcohol and Health: Straight Talk on the Medical Headlines,** Charles H. Hennekens, Health News, March 31, 1998. 104

The news about *alcohol and health* is another example of *mixed reviews.* Although moderate and heavy drinking may be involved in several *chronic diseases,* alcohol offers some protection from *heart disease.*

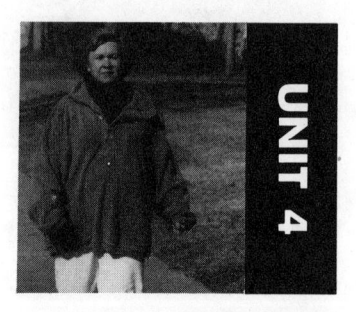

UNIT 4

Fat and Weight Control

Nine articles examine weight management. Topics include the relationship between dieting and exercise, the effects of various diet plans, and the relationship between being overweight and fit.

Overview 106

31. **Weight Control: Challenges and Solutions,** Dairy Council Digest, May/June 1999. 108

More than half of the adult population and a growing percentage of children are now categorized as either overweight or obese. Lack of *exercise* remains the primary key. Various *treatment and management approaches* are suggested.

32. **Childhood Obesity and Family SES Racial Differences,** Patricia B. Crawford, Allison Drury, and Sheila Stern, Healthy Weight Journal, May/June 1999. 113

Previous studies have shown *correlations between childhood obesity and socioeconomic status,* but newer studies find that this is not true for African American girls. *Weight similarities* between *white and African American girls* are associated with other variables of family structure.

33. **NIH Guidelines: An Evaluation,** Frances M. Berg, Healthy Weight Journal, March/April 1999. 115

This article *challenges the newest obesity guidelines* established by the National Heart, Lung, and Blood Institute (NHLBI). It points out fallacies related to *health risks* and reminds us that weight-loss methods are often ineffective and are themselves associated with health risks.

34. **The Great Weight Debate,** Consumer Reports on Health, January 1999. 119

This article acknowledges the *controversy* about weight, emphasizes the *health risks* of obesity, and points out that the *location of body fat* has significance. *Guidelines* for determining one's need to lose weight are offered.

35. **Exploding the Myth: Weight Loss Makes You Healthier,** Paul Ernsberger, Healthy Weight Journal, January/February 1999. 122

While *weight loss* is recommended to *ameliorate or cure a variety of conditions and diseases,* its ability to do so is *greatly exaggerated.* The benefits may be short-term only, but the *lifestyle changes* that accompany weight loss may be beneficial.

36. **Simplifying the Advice for Slimming Down,** Tufts University Health & Nutrition Letter, April 1999. 125

Once one has decided to lose weight, *choosing an appropriate weight loss plan* can be very difficult. *Guidelines* for selecting a safe plan and making it successful are offered.

37. **The History of Dieting and Its Effectiveness,** Wayne C. Miller, Healthy Weight Journal, March/April 1997. 128

Many *dieting schemes* have been tried with undesirable or temporary results. New approaches are often individualized but are expensive and may not be *safe* or *effective.*

The concepts in bold italics are developed in the article. For further expansion please refer to the Topic Guide, the Glossary, and the Index.

38. **Dieting Disorder,** David Rosen, *Health News,* May 10, 1999. — **131**

The reason why 5 million Americans suffer from **eating disorders** is still unclear, but a recent study confirms that **severe dieting is a stronger predictor.** This and recognizing other risk factors can be useful in early intervention.

39. **The Effects of Starvation on Behavior: Implications for Dieting and Eating Disorders,** David M. Garner, *Healthy Weight Journal,* September/October 1998. — **133**

During **starvation,** the **physical and psychological changes** experienced are virtually identical to the behaviors of those with **anorexia nervosa.** This article addresses the misconceptions that willpower alone can control body weight and that emotional disturbance leads to binge eating.

UNIT 5
Food Safety

Nine articles discuss the safety of food. Topics include food-borne illness, pesticide residues, naturally occurring toxins, and food preservatives.

Overview — **138**

40. **Food Safety: Don't Get Burned,** *Consumer Reports on Health,* July 1999. — **140**

Answers to **common misconceptions** about **food handling practices** include cooking temperatures, freezing, and cutting boards.

41. **Audits International's Home Food Safety Survey,** *Audits International,* 1999. — **143**

Issues of **food safety** are relevant to **food handling** at **home** as well as in commercial establishments. Only a quarter of **survey participants** prepared food acceptably, although they knew they were being observed.

42. **Avoiding Cross-Contamination in the Home,** *Institute of Food Science & Technology,* May 25, 1999. — **150**

Cross-contamination of food is preventable and would significantly reduce the incidence of **food-borne illness.** Using proper methods for food preparation and storage is essential.

43. **Why You Need a Kitchen Thermometer,** *Tufts University Health & Nutrition Letter,* June 1998. — **153**

Only the **thermometer** can tell you when your **food is safe.** To ensure that it has cooked enough, follow these tips.

44. **Campylobacter: Low-Profile Bug Is Food Poisoning Leader,** Audrey Hingley, *FDA Consumer,* September/October 1999. — **155**

The number-one cause of **food-borne illness** in the United States, **Campylobacter** is a resident of gastrointestinal tracts and is often found in raw **poultry.** Concern about **antibiotic resistance** in humans raises issues regarding the use of antibiotics in animals.

45. **E. Coli O157:H7—How Dangerous Has It Become?** *Nutrition & the M.D.,* September 1998. — **158**

The extreme **virulence** of **E. Coli O157:H7** means that we must eliminate it from food. Although the original **source** appears to be cattle, this organism has shown up in fresh produce as well.

46. **A Crackdown on Bad Eggs,** Amanda Spake, *U.S. News & World Report,* July 12, 1999. — **160**

The General Accounting Office estimates that hundreds of cases of **salmonellosis** occur yearly from **eggs.** New federal **storage standards** may help, but other problems must be addressed.

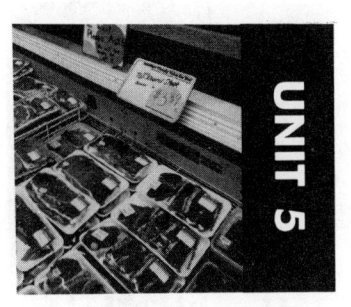

The concepts in bold italics are developed in the article. For further expansion please refer to the Topic Guide, the Glossary, and the Index.

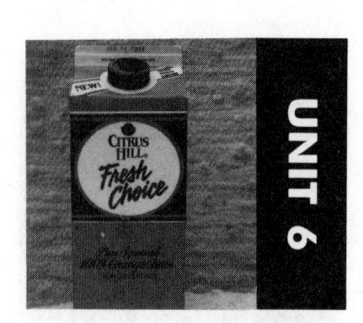

47. **Irradiation: A Safe Measure for Safer Food,** John **162**
Henkel, *FDA Consumer,* May/June 1998.
Increased concern about the **safety of food** has resulted in **FDA approval** of irradiation for red meat. Over a period of 40 years, the FDA has found **irradiation** to be a safe and effective process and allows its use with a variety of other food products.

48. **Questions Keep Sprouting about Sprouts,** Paula **167**
Kurtzweil, *FDA Consumer,* January/February 1999.
Increasingly, **food-borne illness** is linked to eating various kinds of **sprouts.** The seeds appear to be the source of the bacteria, making the solution difficult.

UNIT 6

Health Claims

Ten articles examine some of the health claims made by today's "specialists." Topics include quacks, fad diets, and nutrition myths and misinformation.

Overview **170**

49. **Twenty-Five Ways to Spot Quacks and Vitamin** **172**
Pushers, Stephen Barrett and Victor Herbert, *Quackwatch,* August 21, 1999.
Irresponsible promoters of practices and gimmicks that are either **useless or harmful** abound. The savvy consumer will find **useful clues** in this article that will help identify such promoters.

50. **Yet Another Study—Should You Pay Attention?** **179**
Tufts University Health & Nutrition Letter, September 1998.
A person reading reports of current health research will know that the evidence presented is often frightening and so contradictory that **finding truth** is difficult. However, knowing what different **types of studies are capable of proving** is key.

51. **Alternative Medicine—The Risks of Untested and** **182**
Unregulated Remedies, Marcia Angell and Jerome P. Kassirer, *The New England Journal of Medicine,* September 17, 1998.
Many **alternative therapies** are closely connected to nutrition in that they include the use of **herbals** and other dietary remedies. These therapies have simultaneously become both more popular and more controversial.

52. **The Mouse That Roared: Health Scares on the** **186**
Internet, *Food Insight,* May/June 1999.
Like information elsewhere, some **Internet sources** are **reliable,** and some initiate and promote **myths** that aren't always obvious. Learning how to choose sites is the first step in protection.

53. **Uprooting Herbal Myths,** *Consumer Reports on Health,* **189**
October 1998.
Myths and misconceptions about **herbs** are common. Chemicals in herbs act as drugs, some of which help while others actually do harm. Their sale and use is **unregulated.**

54. **Herbal Weight Loss Tea: Beware the Unknown** **192**
Brew, *Healthy Weight Journal,* November/December 1998.
Teas touted to promote **weight loss** can produce **risky** electrolyte imbalances, even causing death. This is another example of "let the buyer beware."

55. **5 Nutrition Topics That Are Not All They're Cracked** **195**
Up to Be, *Tufts University Health & Nutrition Letter,* Special Supplement, 1999.
Separating hype from fact on five popular topics is the purpose of this article. Even the fear of dehydration has found a large following.

56. **Pyruvate: Just the Facts,** Joseph P. Cannon, *Nutrition* **197**
Forum, September/October 1998.
Although **pyruvate studies** have been published in reputable journals, potential users should first know the **inside story.** The supportive evidence is sketchy and provided primarily by one researcher.

57. **Are Health Food Stores Better Bets than Traditional Supermarkets?** *Tufts University Health & Nutrition Letter*, May 1999. 200
To many consumers it is logical to assume that the most wholesome foods are the **organic produce** and **food supplements** available in **health food stores.** Check again; it may not be true, and the "nutrition expert" on board may not be very knowledgeable either.

58. **The Unethical Behavior of Pharmacists,** Stephen Barrett, *Nutrition Forum*, January/February 1998. 203
Pharmacists generally avoid the **ethical dilemma** that pits selling products to make a **profit** against selling **unproven herbals, homeopathic remedies, and excessive supplements.** By ignoring their obligation recommend and dispense such products responsibly, pharmacists contribute to misuse.

UNIT 7

World Hunger and Malnutrition

Five articles discuss the world's food supply. Topics include global malnutrition, water quality, agriculture, and famine.

Overview 206

59. **FAO Releases Annual State of Food and Agriculture Report Showing Worldwide Number of Hungry People Rising Slightly,** *Food and Agriculture Organization of the United Nations*, 1998. 208
Although progress has been made in **reducing hunger and malnutrition** in **developing countries,** the numbers of undernourished and hungry people continue to escalate. The failure to reduce **poverty** is the primary cause. Rapidly expanding cities are of special concern for the future.

60. **Special Programme for Food Security at the Food and Agriculture Organization,** *Journal of Family and Consumer Sciences*, Volume 91, Number 1, 1999. 212
Fears that **food security** cannot be achieved in developing countries are due to rapid **population expansion.** A program to **improve crop production** by small farmers has been proposed by the Food and Agriculture Organization (FAO) and approved by the World Food Summit.

61. **Starvation Syndrome in Africa,** Frances M. Berg, *Healthy Weight Journal*, September/October 1998. 214
What happened to the Ik in Africa illustrates how far-reaching the **effects of starvation** can be. Appalling as it seems, **humanity erodes** into mere survival, and acts of cruelty and unconcern become the norm.

62. **How to Measure Malnutrition,** *Healthy Weight Journal*, September/October 1998. 216
Standards for measuring starvation using body mass index (BMI) and guidelines for assessing **protein-calorie malnutrition** are provided.

63. **Hunger and Food Insecurity,** Katherine L. Cason, *Journal of Family and Consumer Sciences*, Volume 91, Number 1, 1999. 217
Problems **of poverty, hunger, and food insecurity** have not been resolved in the United States. Victims from all ages and ethnic groups fail to grow, are anemic, or risk diseases. They become hostile and insecure. The purposes and resources of **federal nutrition programs** are identified, and recommendations are made.

Glossary 222
Index 225
Article Review Form 228
Article Rating Form 229

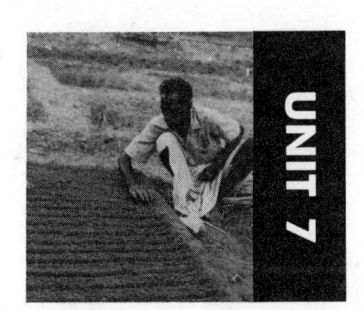

The concepts in bold italics are developed in the article. For further expansion please refer to the Topic Guide, the Glossary, and the Index.

1

Topic Guide

This topic guide suggests how the selections and World Wide Web sites found in the next section of this book relate to topics of traditional concern to students and professionals involved with the study of nutrition. It is useful for locating interrelated articles and Web sites for reading and research. The guide is arranged alphabetically according to topic.

The relevant Web sites, which are numbered and annotated on pages 4 and 5, are easily identified by the Web icon (◎) under the topic articles. By linking the articles and the Web sites by topic, this ANNUAL EDITIONS reader becomes a powerful learning and research tool.

TOPIC AREA	TREATED IN	TOPIC AREA	TREATED IN
Alcohol	30. Alcohol and Health ◎ 6, 13, 17		22. "Mediterranean Diet" Reduces Risk of Second Heart Attack 23. Homocysteine: "The New Cholesterol"? 24. Soy: Cause for Joy? 25. False Alarms about Food 26. Questions and Answers about Cancer, Diet and Fats 27. How to Grow a Healthy Child ◎ 1, 2, 5, 7, 9, 11, 12, 13, 14, 15, 16, 17, 27, 32, 35, 36, 37
Attitudes/ Knowledge	5. Freshness Fallacy 8. Low-Calorie Sweeteners 41. Audits International's Home Food Safety Survey 52. Mouse That Roared 53. Uprooting Herbal Myths 55. 5 Nutrition Topics That Are Not All They're Cracked Up to Be 57. Are Health Food Stores Better Bets than Traditional Supermarkets? 58. Unethical Behavior of Pharmacists ◎ 1, 2, 5, 7, 9, 10, 11, 32, 33, 34		
		Eating Disorders	37. History of Dieting and Its Effectiveness 38. Dieting Disorder 39. Effects of Starvation on Behavior ◎ 6, 17, 23, 25
Carbohydrates	12. Should You Be Eating More Fat and Fewer Carbohydrates? 13. Sugar: What's the Harm? ◎ 1, 2, 10, 11, 12, 23, 26	Elderly	28. Focus on Nutrition for the Elderly 29. Physical Activity and Nutrition 35. Exploding the Myth: Weight Loss Makes You Healthier ◎ 11, 20
Cancer	15. Best D-Fense 19. Fiber: Strands of Protection 24. Soy: Cause for Joy? 26. Questions and Answers about Cancer, Diet and Fats 29. Physical Activity and Nutrition ◎ 6, 13, 14	Fats/Substitutes	9. It's Crunch Time for P&G's Olestra 12. Should You Be Eating More Fat and Fewer Carbohydrates? 22. "Mediterranean Diet" Reduces Risk of Second Heart Attack ◎ 2, 11, 12, 24, 26
Children/Infants	27. How to Grow a Healthy Child 32. Childhood Obesity and Family SES Racial Differences ◎ 10, 16, 18, 19, 21	Fiber	19. Fiber: Strands of Protection ◎ 2, 11, 12
		Food Allergies	25. False Alarms about Food ◎ 16
Controversies	7. Curse of Frankenfood 9. It's Crunch Time for P&G's Olestra 12. Should You Be Eating More Fat and Fewer Carbohydrates? 13. Sugar: What's the Harm? 33. NIH Guidelines: An Evaluation 51. Alternative Medicine ◎ 1, 2, 8, 9, 11, 12, 13	Food Safety	7. Curse of Frankenfood 41. Audits International's Home Food Safety Survey 43. Why You Need a Kitchen Thermometer 44. Campylobacter 46. Crackdown on Bad Eggs 47. Irradiation 48. Questions Keep Sprouting about Sprouts ◎ 27, 28, 29, 30, 31
Coronary Heart Disease	11. Fats: The Good, the Bad, the Trans 12. Should You Be Eating More Fat and Fewer Carbohydrates? 22. "Mediterranean Diet" Reduces Risk of Second Heart Attack 23. Homocysteine: "The New Cholesterol"? 24. Soy: Cause for Joy? 29. Physical Activity and Nutrition ◎ 6, 15, 17, 32	Food Supply	4. Are Fruits and Vegetables Less Nutritious Today? 6. New Foods: Functional or Dysfunctional? 7. Curse of Frankenfood 10. Supermarket Psych-Out 59. FAO Releases Annual State of Food and Agriculture Report 60. Special Programme for Food Security at the Food and Agricultural Organization 61. Starvation Syndrome in Africa ◎ 3, 5, 36, 37
Diet/Disease	3. Staking a Claim to Good Health 11. Fats: The Good, the Bad, the Trans 12. Should You Be Eating More Fat and Fewer Carbohydrates? 13. Sugar: What's the Harm? 14. Vitamin C: Foods Yes, Pills No 16. Can Vitamin E Prevent Heart Disease? 18. National Academy of Sciences Introduces New Calcium Recommendations 19. Fiber: Strands of Protection 21. Disease-Fighting Foods?	Food-Borne Illness	40. Food Safety: Don't Get Burned 41. Audits International's Home Food Safety Survey 42. Avoiding Cross-Contamination in the Home 43. Why You Need a Kitchen Thermometer 44. Campylobacter

TOPIC AREA	TREATED IN	TOPIC AREA	TREATED IN
Food-Borne Illness (cont.)	45. E. Coli 0157:H7—How Dangerous Has It Become? 47. Irradiation 48. Questions Keep Sprouting about Sprouts **27, 28, 29, 30, 31**		52. Mouse That Roared 53. Uprooting Herbal Myths 55. 5 Nutrition Topics That Are Not All They're Cracked Up to Be 57. Are Health Food Stores Better Bets than Traditional Supermarkets? **2, 11, 12, 32, 33, 34**
Guidelines/Recommendations	2. Nutrient Requirements Get a Makeover 3. Staking a Claim to Good Health 8. Low-Calorie Sweeteners 11. Fats: The Good, the Bad, the Trans 12. Should You Be Eating *More* Fat and *Fewer* Carbohydrates? 14. Vitamin C: Foods Yes, Pills No 15. Best D-Fense 17. Disease of Too Much Iron 21. Disease-Fighting Foods? 22. "Mediterranean Diet" Reduces Risk of Second Heart Attack 28. Focus on Nutrition for the Elderly 29. Physical Activity and Nutrition 34. Great Weight Debate 36. Simplifying the Advice for Slimming Down 40. Food Safety: Don't Get Burned 41. Audits International's Home Food Safety Survey 42. Avoiding Cross-Contamination in the Home 43. Why You Need a Kitchen Thermometer 44. Campylobacter 46. Crackdown on Bad Eggs 48. Questions Keep Sprouting about Sprouts 50. Yet Another Study—Should You Pay Attention? 52. Mouse That Roared 53. Uprooting Herbal Myths 62. How to Measure Malnutrition **1, 2, 6, 9, 11**	**Nutrition Trends**	1. Millennium: Food and Nutrition **2, 11**
		Physical Activity	31. Weight Control: Challenges and Solutions **26, 32**
		Risk/Benefit	13. Sugar: What's the Harm? 14. Vitamin C: Foods Yes, Pills No 16. Can Vitamin E Prevent Heart Disease? 33. NIH Guidelines: An Evaluation 34. Great Weight Debate 35. Exploding the Myth: Weight Loss Makes You Healthier **1, 2, 3, 4, 5, 8**
		Sugar/Substitutes	8. Low-Calorie Sweeteners **2, 10, 11**
		Supplements	6. New Foods: Functional or Dysfunctional? 15. Best D-Fense 16. Can Vitamin E Prevent Heart Disease? 18. National Academy of Sciences Introduces New Calcium Recommendations 20. Food for Thought about Dietary Supplements **2, 5, 9, 11, 12, 13**
		Vitamins	5. Freshness Fallacy 14. Vitamin C: Foods Yes, Pills No 15. Best D-Fense **2, 10, 11, 12, 13**
Herbals	51. Alternative Medicine 53. Uprooting Herbal Myths 54. Herbal Weight Loss Tea 58. Unethical Behavior of Pharmacists **5, 9, 22, 32, 33, 34**	**Weight/Weight Control/Obesity**	13. Sugar: What's the Harm? 27. How to Grow a Healthy Child 29. Physical Activity and Nutrition 31. Weight Control: Challenges and Solutions 32. Childhood Obesity and Family SES Racial Differences 33. NIH Guidelines: An Evaluation 34. Great Weight Debate 35. Exploding the Myth: Weight Loss Makes You Healthier 36. Simplifying the Advice for Slimming Down 37. History of Dieting and Its Effectiveness 38. Dieting Disorder 54. Herbal Weight Loss Tea 56. Pyruvate: Just the Facts **2, 17, 23, 24, 25, 26**
Hunger/Malnutrition	37. History of Dieting and Its Effectiveness 39. Effects of Starvation on Behavior 59. FAO Releases Annual State of Food and Agriculture Report 61. Starvation Syndrome in Africa 62. How to Measure Malnutrition 63. Hunger and Food Insecurity **35, 36, 37**		
Labeling	3. Staking a Claim to Good Health		
Minerals	17. Disease of Too Much Iron 18. National Academy of Sciences Introduces New Calcium Recommendations **2, 10, 11, 12, 13**		
Myths/Misinformation	4. Are Fruits and Vegetables Less Nutritious Today? 5. Freshness Fallacy 25. False Alarms about Food 49. Twenty-Five Ways to Spot Quacks		

AE: Nutrition

The following World Wide Web sites have been carefully researched and selected to support the articles found in this reader. If you are interested in learning more about specific topics found in this book, these Web sites are a good place to start. The sites are cross-referenced by number and appear in the topic guide on the previous two pages. Also, you can link to these Web sites through our DUSHKIN ONLINE support site at *http://www.dushkin.com/online/*.

The following sites were available at the time of publication. Visit our Web site—we update DUSHKIN ONLINE regularly to reflect any changes.

General Sources

1. American Dietetic Association
http://www.eatright.org
This consumer link to nutrition and health includes resources, news, marketplace, search for a dietician, government information, and a gateway to related sites. The site includes a tip of the day and special features.

2. The Blonz Guide to Nutrition
http://www.blonz.com
The categories in this valuable site report news in the fields of nutrition, food science, foods, fitness, and health. There is also a selection of search engines and links.

3. Food Marketing Institute
http://www.fmi.org
FMI, a nonprofit association of grocery retailers, is committed to maintaining and improving a system of distribution of grocery products that is responsive to the changing needs and wants of customers.

4. Institute of Food Technologists
http://www.ift.org
This site of the Society for Food Science and Technology is full of important information and news about every aspect of the food products that come to market.

5. International Food Information Council Foundation
http://ificinfo.health.org
IFIC's purpose is to be the link between science and communications by offering the latest scientific information on food safety, nutrition, and health in a form that is understandable and useful for opinion leaders and consumers to access.

6. U.S. National Institutes of Health
http://www.nih.gov
Consult this site for links to extensive health information and scientific resources. Comprised of 24 separate institutes, centers, and divisions, the NIH is one of eight health agencies of the Public Health Service, which, in turn, is part of the U.S. Department of Health and Human Services.

Trends Today and Tomorrow

7. Food Science and Human Nutrition Extension
http://www.exnet.iastate.edu/Pages/families/fshn/
This extensive Iowa State University site links to latest news and reports, consumer publications, food safety information, and many other useful nutrition-related sites.

8. Food Surveys Research Group
http://www.barc.usda.gov/bhnrc/foodsurvey/home.htm
Visit this site of Beltsville Human Nutrition Research Center Food Surveys research group first, and then click on USDA to keep up with nutritional news and information.

9. U.S. Food and Drug Administration
http://www.fda.gov/default.htm
This is the home page of the FDA, which describes itself as the United States' "foremost consumer protection agency." Visit this site and its links to learn about food safety, food and nutrition labeling, and other topics of importance.

Nutrients

10. Dole 5 A Day: Nutrition, Fruits & Vegetables
http://www.dole5aday.com
The Dole Food Company, a founding member of the National 5 A Day for Better Health Program, offers this site that is designed to entice children into taking an interest in proper nutrition.

11. Food and Nutrition Information Center
http://www.nal.usda.gov/fnic/
Use this site to find dietary and nutrition information provided by various USDA agencies and to find links to food and nutrition resources on the Internet.

12. Nutrient Data Laboratory
http://www.nal.usda.gov/fnic/foodcomp/
This USDA Agricultural Research Service site provides information about the USDA Nutrient Database. Search here for answers to FAQs, a glossary of terms, facts about food composition, and useful links.

13. U.S. National Library of Medicine
http://www.nlm.nih.gov
This huge site permits you to search a number of databases and electronic information sources such as MEDLINE, learn about research projects, keep up on nutrition-related news, and peruse the national network of medical libraries.

Through the Life Span: Diet and Disease

14. American Cancer Society
http://www.cancer.org/frames.html
Open this site and its various links to learn the concerns and lifestyle advice of the American Cancer Society. It provides information on tobacco, alternative therapies, other Web resources, and more.

15. American Heart Association
http://www.americanheart.org
The AHA offers this site to provide the most comprehensive information on heart disease and stroke as well as late-breaking news. The site presents facts on warning signs, a reference guide, and explanations of diseases and treatments.

16. The Food Allergy Network
http://www.foodallergy.org
This site, which welcomes consumers, health professionals, and reporters, includes product alerts and updates, information about food allergies, daily tips, and links to other sites.

17. Go Ask Alice! from Columbia University Health Services
http://www.goaskalice.columbia.edu
This interactive site provides discussion and insight into a number of issues of interest to college-age people and those younger and older. Many questions about physical and emo-

tional well-being, fitness and nutrition, and alcohol, nicotine, and other drugs are answered.

18. Heinz Infant & Toddler Nutrition
http://www.heinzbaby.com

This site includes an educational section full of nutritional information and meal-planning guides for parents and caregivers, as well as articles and reviews by leading pediatricians and nutritionists.

19. LaLeche League International
http://www.lalecheleague.org

This site provides important information to mothers who are contemplating breast feeding. There are links to other sites.

20. National Osteoporosis Foundation
http://www.nof.org

The NOF has a mission of reducing the widespread prevalence of osteoporosis. It contains information about causes, prevention, detection, and treatment.

21. Nutrition for Kids: 24 Carrot Press
http://www.nutritionforkids.com

This Web site of 24 Carrot Press publishes material that takes a positive, fun approach to the more serious issues that affect children, including poor eating habits, obesity, and inactivity. Their site includes How to Teach Nutrition to Kids, Activity Guide, stickers, *Feeding Kids Newsletter*, and links.

22. Vegetarian Resource Group
http://www.vrg.org

The VRG offers information on everything of interest to vegans, vegetarians, and others.

Fat and Weight Control

23. American Anorexia Bulimia Association
http://www.aabainc.org/home.html

The AABA is a nonprofit organization of concerned people dedicated to the prevention and treatment of eating disorders. It offers many services, including help lines, referral networks, school outreach, support groups, and prevention programs.

24. Calorie Control Council
http://www.caloriecontrol.org

The Calorie Control Council's Web site offers information on cutting calories, achieving and maintaining healthy weight, and low-calorie, reduced-fat foods and beverages.

25. Eating Disorders: Body Image Betrayal
http://www.geocities.com/HotSprings/5704/edlist.htm

This extensive collection of links leads to information on compulsive eating, bulimia, anorexia, and other disorders.

26. Shape Up America!
http://www.shapeup.org

At the Shape Up America! Web site you will find the latest information about safe weight management, healthy eating, and physical fitness. Links include Support Center, Cyberkitchen, Media Center, Fitness Center, and BMI Center.

Food Safety

27. Centers for Disease Control and Prevention
http://www.cdc.gov

The CDC offers this home page, from which you can learn information about travelers' health, data and statistics related to disease control and prevention, general nutritional and health information, publications, and more.

28. FDA Center for Food Safety and Applied Nutrition
http://vm.cfsan.fda.gov

This informative site leads to other sites that will tell you everything you might want to know about food safety and what government agencies are doing to ensure it.

29. Food Safety Information from North Carolina
http://www.ces.ncsu.edu/depts/foodsci/agentinfo/

This site from the Cooperative Extension Service at North Carolina State University has a database designed to promote food safety education via the Internet.

30. Food Safety Project
http://www.exnet.iastate.edu/Pages/families/fs/

The goal of this project is to develop educational materials that help the public to minimize the risk of food-borne illness. The site contains food safety lessons, 10 steps to a safe kitchen, consumer control points, and food law.

31. USDA Food Safety and Inspection Service
http://www.fsis.usda.gov

The FSIS, part of the U.S. Department of Agriculture, is the government agency "responsible for ensuring that the nation's commercial supply of meat, poultry, and egg products is safe, wholesome, and correctly labeled and packaged."

Health Claims

32. Diet, Health & Fitness
http://www.ftc.gov/bcp/menu-health.htm

This site of the Federal Trade Commission on the Web offers consumer education rules and acts, which include a wide range of subjects, from aging parents, to buying exercise equipment, to fraudulent health claims, to virtual health "treatments."

33. National Council against Health Fraud
http://www.ncahf.org

The NCAHF does business as the National Council for Reliable Health Information. At its Web page it offers links to other related sites, including Dr. Terry Polevoy's "Healthwatcher Net."

34. QuackWatch
http://www.quackwatch.com

Quackwatch Inc., a nonprofit corporation, provides this consumer guide to examine health fraud. Data for intelligent decision making on health topics are also presented.

World Hunger and Malnutrition

35. Population Reference Bureau
http://www.prb.org

This is a key source for global population information—a good place to pursue data on nutrition problems worldwide.

36. World Health Organization
http://www.who.ch

This home page of the World Health Organization will provide you with links to a wealth of statistical and analytical information about health and nutrition around the world.

37. WWW Virtual Library: Demography & Population Studies
http://demography.anu.edu.au/VirtualLibrary/

A multitude of important links to information about global poverty and hunger can be found here.

We highly recommend that you review our Web site for expanded information and our other product lines. We are continually updating and adding links to our Web site in order to offer you the most usable and useful information that will support and expand the value of your Annual Editions. You can reach us at:
http://www.dushkin.com/annualeditions/.

Unit 1

Unit Selections

1. **Millennium: Food and Nutrition,** Jack Raso
2. **Nutrient Requirements Get a Makeover: The Evolution of the Recommended Dietary Allowances,** Food Insight
3. **Staking a Claim to Good Health,** Paula Kurtzweil
4. **Are Fruits and Vegetables Less Nutritious Today?** University of California, Berkeley Wellness Letter
5. **The Freshness Fallacy,** Minna Morse
6. **The New Foods: Functional or Dysfunctional?** Consumer Reports on Health
7. **The Curse of Frankenfood: Genetically Modified Crops Stir Up Controversy at Home and Abroad,** Phillip J. Longman
8. **Low-Calorie Sweeteners,** Mayo Clinic Health Letter
9. **It's Crunch Time for P&G's Olestra,** Pamela Sherrid
10. **Supermarket Psych-Out,** Tufts University Health & Nutrition Letter

Key Points to Consider

❖ Which of the trends and developments predicted in the article, "Millenium, Food and Nutrition," do you believe are accurate? Why?

❖ What current consumer trends in the food industry will and will not support healthier lifestyles?

❖ Is the philosophical change that has occurred with the change from RDAs to DRIs a good one? Defend your answer.

❖ What demands do you think your generation will place on the food industry two or three decades from now? Why?

❖ What do you see as the issues related to the use of functional foods and those produced from genetically modified crops? How would you decide whether or not to buy them?

❖ Take a trip to the grocery store and try to identify the extent to which you are influenced by marketing techniques.

❖ Does change always equal progress? Why or why not? Give examples from the nutrition field.

DUSHKIN ONLINE Links   www.dushkin.com/online/

7. **Food Science and Human Nutrition Extension**
   http://www.exnet.iastate.edu/Pages/families/fshn/
8. **Food Surveys Research Group**
   http://www.barc.usda.gov/bhnrc/foodsurvey/home.htm
9. **U.S. Food and Drug Administration**
   http://www.fda.gov/default.htm

These sites are annotated on pages 4 and 5.

Trends Today and Tomorrow

> It is change, continuing change, inevitable change, that is the dominant factor in society today. No sensible decision can be made any longer without taking into account not only the world as it is, but the world as it will be.
>
> —Isaac Asimov, 1981

The average consumer is a phantom, constantly reshaping and reemerging under the influences of the food industry, the media, activist organizations, and whatever health headlines are currently most persuasive. For the sake of heart health, we have been persuaded first to switch from animal fats to vegetable oils and margarine, then to avoid tropical oils, and now to beware of trans-fatty acids produced in the manufacture of solid margarine. Americans are constantly bombarded by health and nutrition messages and admonitions, many of which are misleading and contradictory. As more and more people access the Internet, this problem may be exacerbated rather than lessened.

American consumers still believe in good and bad foods, unaware that it is the total diet and not single foods that counts. Food consumption studies indicate that we are closer to the goal of at least five fruits and vegetables daily, having increased our average yearly consumption by 81 pounds of vegetables and 57 pounds of fruit. At the same time, however, we are eating more cheese and fats/oils and drinking more beer but less milk.

Market trends indicate that consumers are increasingly less likely to prepare their food and more willing to spend for ready-to-eat, great tasting, and easily accessible meals. These meals are very likely to be picked up at supermarkets, where nearly half of all current culinary school graduates are employed and where diversity has expanded to include gourmet, ethnic, and organic options.

Consumers' beliefs and behaviors are not always consistent. The Food Marketing Institute says consumers find that their cravings are not satisfied with fat-free foods. Consumption of a spartan meal followed by an exceptionally rich dessert is not uncommon. Olestra, a synthetic fat, was supposed to fill the desire for a gratifying, rich texture and taste in foods without the higher calories of real fat. But an article in this unit verifies what we all suspected: although olestra is selling reasonably well, Procter and Gamble is not pleased.

With a renewed focus on calories rather than on fat alone, interest in low-calorie sweeteners is likely to continue. Another article in this unit describes the FDA-approved sweeteners, all of which are safe for most people. However, saccharin and aspartame must carry warnings on their labels, and the FDA has established maximum daily intakes over a lifetime that it considers to be safe and prudent.

The first article in this unit contains a selection of responses from professionals to a question concerning the trends and developments they expect to see in food and nutrition as we enter a new millennium.

A consumer who wants established guidelines to assist in making food choices should have no difficulty finding them. The next article chronicles the origin and development of the familiar Recommended Dietary Allowances (RDAs), now called DRIs for Dietary Reference Intakes. The DRIs mirror a shift in philosophical emphasis from that of preventing deficiencies to that of preventing chronic diseases. Food labels, the topic of the next article, also provide guidance, which can be utilized to make decisions while shopping. Not only do labels include a panel of nutrition facts, but health claims alert consumers to the role certain foods can play in reducing some disease risks. These health claims are carefully controlled by the FDA (Food and Drug Administration) and are authorized only when scientific experts agree that the claims can be validated. More general guidelines can be found in a list published every 5 years by the U.S. Departments of Agriculture and Health and Human Services. These guidelines are being updated in 2000 and may include, for the first time, a message on food-borne illness.

The next two articles discuss plant products and may dispel common misinformation. In recognition of strong supporting evidence, the FDA has agreed to allow canned fruits and vegetables, as well as fresh and frozen ones, to be sold as "healthy." In fact, nutritionally speaking, fresh equals frozen equals canned. Furthermore, and contrary to common belief, it is not the vitamin content of a crop that suffers from being grown on depleted soil but rather the size of the crop produced. Common sense tells us that farmers cannot afford this lack of productivity and must replenish their soil. The nutrient values of plants will vary by climate, and the genetic potential of different varieties.

Two articles follow that address issues of a highly controversial nature. One article discusses functional foods, a $15 billion industry. Urged on by baby boomers now reaching the years when aches and pains emerge, the food industry is producing many food products that resemble medicines. Marketers have moved beyond the original concept of fortification of specific products with a limited set of nutrients to adding herbals and other substances claimed to provide health benefits to almost any food. Thus, one wonders, do potato chips or sodas or margarines that have been "doctored" become really healthy after all? Confusing and misleading, some authorities will argue.

In another controversial issue, genetically altered crops are stirring up a heap of trouble for the U.S. food industry. Europeans are particularly afraid of bioengineered foods, and the result is real and threatened trade wars. Once again activist organizations such as Greenpeace have made headlines, with the result that both Gerber and Heinz apparently have decided not to use genetically modified ingredients in their baby food. In actuality, many of the foods we eat contain some genetic modification.

By reading "Supermarket Psych-Out," you may be able to turn the tables when you shop because you will better understand how you are being programmed to buy certain items. Color, shape, size—all are carefully orchestrated to reach the buyer where he/she is vulnerable. Even signs that limit how much of a sale item you may purchase are found to increase total sales.

In summary, it seems safe to predict that an emphasis on the relationship of food to disease will continue and that the food industry will persevere in capitalizing on this information to market new products. But, consuming vitamins, minerals, and other chemicals from foods, rather than from supplements or functional foods, has the added advantage of being absorbed in amounts that are protective without being harmful.

Article 1

Millennium

For this issue I asked hundreds of scientists, educators, and other professionals in diverse fields—including all members of the ACSH Board of Scientific and Policy Advisors—to submit essays on trends and prospective developments in their respective areas of expertise and/or interest. Below are some of the contributions I received. Almost without exception, the opinions offered in the essays I received did not factor in my deciding whether to publish any particular submission.

Such opinions are not necessarily mine or ACSH's. And, as always, responses to published items would be welcome.

I have categorized each composition below broadly and somewhat arbitrarily and have alphabetized the essays within subcategories according to surnames. Thanks to all those who submitted essays!*

—Jack Raso

Food and Nutrition

Biotechnology and Food Safety

In the 21st century even high-tech food producers will have serious production problems, but access to vast information will make these manageable. With further research such access will enable the efficient, environmentally safe feeding of a U.S. population of 270 million people—an increase of which by 125 million is expected in 50 years.

The battle to control plant and animal diseases and foodborne human diseases will continue. As we learn to control *Eschericia coli* 0157:H7 (beef), *Campylobacter jejuni* (poultry), *Salmonella typhimurium* DT 104 (cattle, pigs, sheep, and poultry), and bovine spongiform encephalopathy ("mad cow disease") and other pathogens that are currently troublesome, new drug-resistant organisms will appear. The emergence of such pathogens on the farm will be the subject of much research into origins, new drugs, and control measures. Biotechnology—especially recombinant DNA technology, better known as genetic engineering—will be most useful in this battle; and, despite some current opposition to it, the public will come to perceive the need for biotech and to appreciate its benefits.

The food industry will continue to create science-based, healthful food products, herbal beverages, and "nutraceuticals." Consumers of the future will probably

---

*Editor's Note: These selections have been chosen from a longer article in Priorities, *Volume 10, Numbers 2 & 3, 1998.*

Reprinted with permission from *Priorities*, Vol. 10, Nos. 2-3, 1998, pp. 19-39. © 1998 by the American Council on Science and Health, Inc., 1995 Broadway, 2nd Floor, New York NY 10023-5860

care less whether a food is "natural" or "organic" than do today's consumers, provided the product is safe, convenient, and appetizing. Means of controlling pathogens during food processing will include irradiation by accelerated electron beams or gamma rays, pulsed electric-field technology, ultra-high pressure, ozone treatment, microwaves, and new "bacter-viricides." In sterile packages, foods thus processed will be safely storable at room temperature for many months longer than are conventionally processed foods.

Future nutrition scientists will emphasize molecular and cellular biology. Health professionals will be able to individualize diets according to both genetic makeup and medical history.

We will know more about the health effects of homocysteine, omega-3 and other fatty acids, *trans* fats, low-calorie fat replacers, and possible endocrine disrupters and of such nonnutrient phytochemicals as: allicin (a constituent of garlic); indoles and isothiocyantes (broccoli); phyto-estrogens (soy); lycopene (tomatoes); and quercetin (apples).

More research will be conducted on botanicals such as echinacea, ginseng, St. John's wort, saw palmetto, and ginkgo biloba. And the public's desire for more useful information on safety and efficacy will lead to a revising of the Dietary Supplement and Health Education Act of 1994 to require that supplement-label claims meet the evidential standards for FDA approval that today apply to label claims for conventional foods.

It will become obvious to the public that a widespread inability to make critical judgments on matters of science was responsible for the popularity of considering Alar, biotechnology, food additives, food irradiation, and pesticides major hazards in the U.S. The public will also become able to distinguish scientifically competent, ethical organizations such as ACSH from groups that try to benefit from the spread of misinformation.

A new federal agency—the U.S. Food Safety Agency—will be established to monitor the global food supply and to regulate food imports. Consequently, false public health alarms and the need for food-disparagement laws and related actions will diminish.

—HENRY A. DYMSZA, PH.D.
Professor Emeritus,
Department of Food Science and Nutrition,
University of Rhode Island

Body Weight

The most significant public health problem we face over the next several years is a pervasive and uniform increase in the average body weight of adults aged 18 to 70. Over the past decade the average, age-adjusted body weight of both female and male American adults has increased by about 10 pounds, and there has been no indication that this trend will not continue. As people continue to gain weight, an increase in the incidence of obesity-related diseases such as Type 2 diabetes mellitus and heart disease is likely.

This sudden increase in average body weight coincided with repetitious mass-media messages to the effect that dietary fat causes weight gain and chronic health problems. The public apparently inferred from this, erroneously, that calories from carbohydrates can be consumed ad lib without health consequences.

To reverse this trend, the biomedical community must emphasize caloric balance, not merely fat intake.

—JOHN B. ALLRED, PH.D.
Professor of Nutrition,
Department of Food Science and
Technology, The Ohio State University

Dietary Carcinogens and Selenium

The American Council on Science and Health has done much to dispel the fear that potential carcinogens in the diet may be dangerous at any level. At low levels many potential carcinogens—natural and synthetic—are perfectly harmless. Centuries ago Paracelsus said: "The dose makes the poison." It is the amount of a potential carcinogen, as well as its nature, that determines whether it can cause cancer.

The trace element selenium illustrates Paracelsus's adage well. Selenium was regarded primarily as an American-West livestock poison before the discovery that in minute quantities it is an essential nutrient for humans. But later it was pronounced, mistakenly, a carcinogen. Under the terms of the Delaney amendment to the Pure Food and Drug Law, this allegation meant that selenium could not legally be added to feed or to foods deficient in the element. More recently, however, it has been found that, far from being an active carcinogen, selenium has anticarcinogenic properties that afford significant relief of several forms of cancer. Additionally, it has recently been found that selenium can contribute to protection against certain types of viral infection.

It seems likely that other substances toxic at one dietary level will prove salutary at lower levels.

—JAMES E. OLDFIELD, PH.D.
Emeritus Professor of Animal Nutrition,
Department of Animal Sciences, Oregon State University

Dietary Supplements

With early baby boomers turning 50—and because human longevity is increasing at an unprecedented rate—the proportion of elderly people in the U.S. population will increase substantially in the next several decades. Such demographic information is viewed with interest by many people, not the least interested of whom are entrepreneurs—especially those eyeing a geriatric niche.

Thus into the marketplace has come a plethora of dietary supplements promoted to the elderly as enhancers of the length and quality of life. But, while the use of certain supplements may help some individuals with specific conditions or deficiencies, in many cases supplementation is questionable with regard to both safety and efficacy.

Although a prescription is not necessary for the purchase of most nutrient preparations, all dietary supplements should be treated as medicines. Many of the major ingredients of supplements have not undergone thorough or rigorous testing. Indeed, confirmatory data for many health-related claims concerning supplements may be totally absent. Moreover, drug-nutrient interactions are possible.

The National Institutes of Health is sponsoring basic research on a number of the more publicized dietary supplements. Within the next decade much more information on the potential utility and potential drawbacks of supplementation will become available. Dietary supplements are hardy products, and it is likely that they will continue to multiply.

—RUSSEL J. REITER, PH.D., D.MED.
*Professor of Neuroendocrinology,
Department of Cellular and Structural
Biology, University of Texas*

Fertilizers

One area that certainly causes us no end of trouble on the food production front is the way environmentalist ideologues attack us for using "synthetic" mineral fertilizers, especially nitrogenous fertilizers. In their antiscience and antitechnology fervor, they often lump fertilizers, bactericides, fungicides, herbicides, and insecticides as though all these agents were identical in terms of toxicity. They seem to forget that, unlike the active ingredients of the aforementioned "cidal" agents, the active ingredients of "synthetic" fertilizers—nitrogen, phosphorus, and potassium, for example—are essential nutrients for plants. Such categorizing befuddles the public.

The "greenies" also exaggerate the riskiness of subsoil water pollution from man-made nitrogenous fertilizers. Proven health effects do not justify the prevalence and diversity of published fears of nitrate from fertilizer leaking into groundwater. In many areas—particularly centers of beef, pork, and poultry production—considerable and increasing pollution of air and water is due to natural and organic material: animal manure. Yet most greenies urge using organic fertilizers as a "magic bullet" for soil infertility.

Certainly we should properly use manures and all crop residues to restore fertility to soils. But the amount of nitrogen available from these sources, even with the addition of nitrogen fixed in the nodules of legumes, is insufficient to produce enough food for today's 5.9 billion people—hence the demand for and current production of about 80 million nutrient tons of synthetic nitrogen annually.

We should never forget how a pseudoscientist—Lysenko—contributed to the destruction of the Soviet Union. Let us not gullibly believe that it cannot happen again in other countries, including the United States.

—NORMAN E. BORLAUG, PH.D.
*Nobel Laureate, Distinguished
Professor of International Agriculture,
Texas A&M University*

Food Irradiation

Except for thermal canning—a sterilization technology discovered in 1809—food irradiation was the first entirely new mode of preserving foods and controlling foodborne pathogens developed since the time of ancient Rome. The versatility of food irradiation is very impressive. But in 1958, when atomic weapons were a recent phenomenon and getting much coverage, America's legislators created the legal fiction that food irradiation is a "food additive" rather than a physical process. This categorization of food irradiation permitted very tight regulation of the new process.

Forty years of research into all aspects of food irradiation—including dietary-safety, nutrient-adequacy, chemical, and microbial aspects—have proved not only that irradiated foods lack radioactivity due to the process but also that they are in all ways at least as safe for consumer use as their nonirradiated counterparts.

Petitions against food irradiation and the time-consuming reviews they entail are delays that, annually, cause approximately 30 million cases of foodborne illness and 9,000 related deaths in the United States.

I predict—and hope—that within the next 10 to 20 years the preservative use of ionizing radiation will be categorized correctly—as a process such as freezing or pasteurization—and will become common as a means of improving the hygienic quality of foods available to American consumers. Two 1997 occurrences justify my optimism: The Food and Drug Administration approved an omnibus meat petition; and a World Health Organization panel concluded that there should be no toxicological dose limit for food irradiation—that only such variables as color, scent, taste, and texture figure in determining dose maximums for particular foods.

—EDWARD S. JOSEPHSON, PH.D.
*Adjunct Professor of Food Science and Nutrition,
University of Rhode Island*

Food Safety

Authorities point to increases in year-round consumption of fresh fruits and vegetables and to increases in dining out as contributors to rises in "reported" incidents of foodborne illness. What enables such consumption is food importation, and foods are usually imported from developing regions, where surveillance may be inadequate in terms of food safety. With favorable weather conditions and low labor costs, food importation will continue to increase.

But through education and good management the highest sanitation standards can be brought to bear to make imported produce equal in overall quality to domestically grown products. In the United States, employee education, good management, and regulatory supervision are effective deterrents to behaviors that can lead to outbreaks of food poisoning. Most operators of chain restaurants and foodservice organizations—and even many operators of independent restaurants, which are often small—are aware of what must be done to prevent foodborne illness and act accordingly. But the application of additional strategies is desirable.

Using microprocessors to control food-preparation and handling processes in places where food is served has great potential for minimizing the possibility that human error will cause foodborne illness in customers. For example, a microprocessor-controlled freezing machine for dispensing soft ice cream was introduced commercially a few years ago. Properly sanitizing the previously available ice-cream-dispensing machines requires disassembling them daily. Because this is tedious and usually scheduled for the end of the workday, to expect constant adequate diligence would be unreasonable. Microbiological trouble was an inevitable consequence.

The microprocessor in the new dispensing machine makes daily disassembly unnecessary. The freezer component is programmed to enter a heating cycle at the end of each workday: Essentially, its contents are re-pasteurized, then brought to a temperature slightly above freezing, and kept at that temperature until the machine is reactivated. Manual cleaning, which requires disassembly, is necessary only after 14 cycles—the program's limit. This fail-safe system almost eliminates the human element.

Many experts consider instances of food poisoning reported to government officials just the tip of the iceberg. The incidence of illness due to improper preparation or handling of food at home—most of which goes unrecorded—has not gotten attention commensurate with the seriousness of the problem.

There have been rumbles about high-tech companies foreseeing opportunities in controlling home kitchens. Considering such benefits as those of the microprocessor-controlled freezing machine, bringing home kitchens on-line would be a decidedly positive step toward improving food safety in the home.

—PHILIP G. KEENEY, PH.D.
Professor Emeritus,
Department of Food Science,
The Pennsylvania State University

Food Safety and Nitrites

A notion shared by consumers, politicians, and many government regulators—that complete food safety is achievable—is false and misleading. The degree of safety of any food depends on many factors, including the source of the food; the effects of manufacture-related processing on the food; how foodservice workers handle the food before sale; and finally—unquestionably the weakest link in the chain—how consumers handle it. It is because of many such variables that absolute food safety is unattainable. A further complication is that consumers differ in how susceptible they are to food toxicants—those that are natural parts of food, those that are contaminants (natural and man-made), and those that arise from microorganisms in food.

An example of the misbegotten views that unrealistic food-safety expectations can engender is that nitrites used in curing meat may turn into carcinogenic N-nitrosamines and therefore must be eliminated from the curing process. A 1997 Council for Agricultural Science and Technology (CAST) report and a 1981 National Research Council (NRC) report address the issue of nitrites in cured-meat products. A conclusion of both reports is that the protection against botulism afforded by nitrites is more important than their possible carcinogenicity. In any case, in a 1975 article J. W. White pointed out that the nitrates naturally present in plant products turn into more nitrite in the human digestive tract than would wind up there as a result of eating cured meats.

This leads me to propose that we should pursue food safety on the basis of cost-benefit analyses rather than as a quest for absolute food safety.

—ALBERT M. PEARSON, PH.D.
Professor Emeritus,
Department of Animal Sciences,
Oregon State University

Public Health Nutrition

Among many important trends and developments in public health and clinical nutrition, I'd like to call attention to three that interrelate: (1) increasing recognition of the importance of the genetic makeup of individuals (or "biochemical individuality," if you will) in formulating dietary recommendations for decreasing the risk of heart disease and other chronic diseases; (2) the public's interest in the intricacies of nutrition and health; and (3) the increasing availability of information and misinformation on the Internet related to food, nutrition, and health.

The public diet recommendations of reputable organizations have had a long history of changes. Early on, diets high in polyunsaturates were recommended; later, low-fat diets. Recently, the American Heart Association acknowledged that low-fat diets may increase heart-disease risk for some patients. Clearly, we need to view global diet recommendations through the lens of genetic propensities and susceptibilities.

Recent searches of the World Wide Web with the search engine AltaVista for certain nutrition-related words and phrases yielded the following figures.

Word(s) or phrase	Approximate number of "hits" (matches)
nutrition	410,000
nutrition and science	105,000
herbs and health	55,000

Only a third of the more than 400,000 "hits" for "nutrition" referred to science—and most of those that did were not sources of nutrition information but rather curriculum, course, or meeting descriptions.

I submit the following observations.

• When one offers dietary advice for decreasing the risk of heart disease and other chronic diseases, one must offer individualized advice.

• The number of people who consider food groups and dietary guidelines inadequate as tools for improving health nutritionally is increasing. Progressively, many such people are turning to the Internet as an important source of information on nutrition and health—but, also increasingly, much on-line health-related material consists of misinformation or even disinformation.

• Responsible nutrition-and-health authorities and organizations must use the Internet as a means of influencing the increasing number of consumers interested in the technicalities of public health nutrition.

—RICHARD G. JANSEN, PH.D.
Professor and Chairman Emeritus,
Department of Food Science and Human Nutrition,
Colorado State University

Article 2

Nutrient Requirements Get a Makeover:

The Evolution of the Recommended Dietary Allowances

Ever wonder how much of the essential vitamins and minerals, like folate, vitamin A or calcium, you really need to eat every day to be healthy? For more than 50 years, the Food and Nutrition Board of the National Academy of Sciences has been reviewing nutrition research and defining nutrient requirements for healthy people. Until recently, one set of nutrient intake levels reigned supreme: the Recommended Dietary Allowances or RDA.

History of the RDAs

When the RDAs were created in 1941, their primary goal was to prevent diseases caused by nutrient deficiencies. They were originally intended to evaluate and plan for the nutritional adequacy of *groups,* for example, the armed forces and children in school lunch programs, rather than to determine *individuals'* nutrient needs.

But, because the RDAs were essentially the only nutrient values available, they began to be used in ways other than the intended use. Health professionals often used RDAs to size-up the diets of their individual patients or clients. Statistically speaking, RDAs would prevent deficiency diseases in 97 percent of a population, but there was no scientific basis that RDAs would meet the needs of a single person.

It was evident that the RDAs were not addressing individual needs, and new science needed to be included. Therefore, the Food and Nutrition Board sought to redefine nutrient requirements and develop specific nutrient recommendations for individuals, as well as for groups. Along with these changes, concepts such as tolerable upper intakes and adequate intakes emerged to better meet individuals' needs.

Further, the new RDAs were set with prevention of chronic disease in mind. Sandra Schlicker, Ph.D., Senior Staff Officer with the Food and Nutrition Board, explained that the new RDAs will still prevent nutrient deficiencies, but they are now set with an additional purpose. "For the first time, the RDAs are no longer focused only on preventing deficiency diseases such as scurvy or beriberi. Now they are also aimed at reducing the risk of diet-related chronic conditions such as heart disease, diabetes, hypertension and osteoporosis."

How RDAs became DRIs

In 1993, the Food and Nutrition Board put the RDA revision process into motion by holding a symposium and asking for scientific and public comment on how the RDAs should be revised. Utilizing feedback from

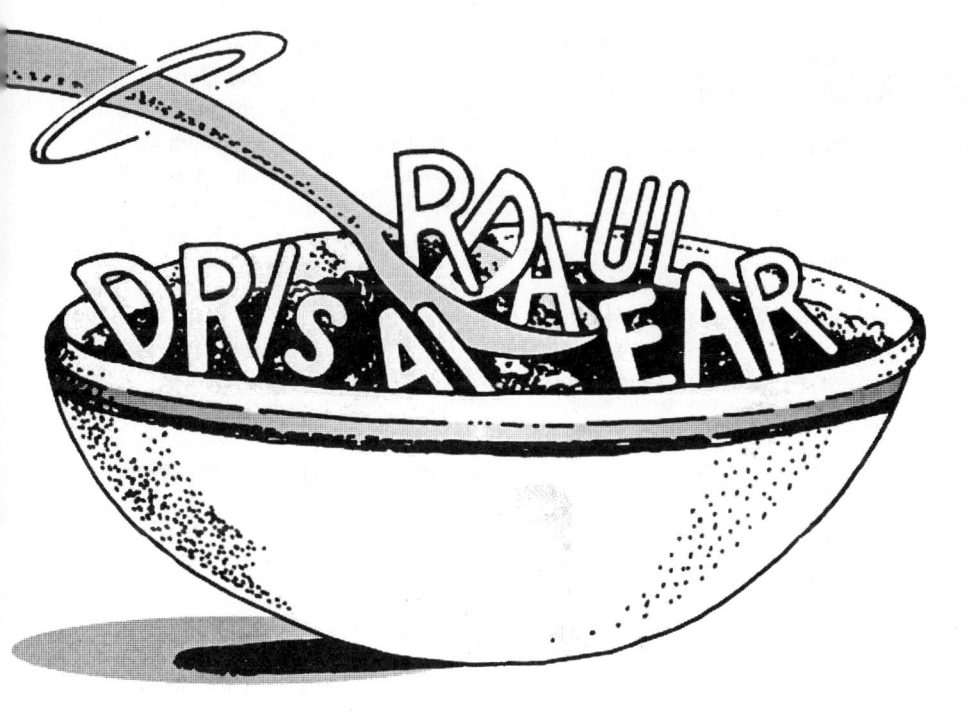

From *Food Insight,* September/October 1998, pp. 1, 4-5. Reprinted with permission from the International Food Information Council Foundation.

1 ❖ TRENDS TODAY AND TOMORROW

RDA/DRI Time Line

1941: First edition of the Recommended Dietary Allowances (RDAs) published.

1941-1989: RDAs periodically updated and revised based on cumulative scientific data. 10th edition published in 1989.

1993: The Food and Nutrition Board (FNB) held symposium, "Should the Recommended Dietary Allowances Be Revised?" Based on comments and suggestions from this meeting, FNB proposed changes to the development process of RDAs.

1995: The Dietary Reference Intake (DRI) Committee announced that seven expert nutrient group panels would review major nutrients, vitamins, minerals, antioxidants, electrolytes, and other food components.

---

this conference and other sources, the Food and Nutrition Board developed an ambitious framework for revamping the old RDAs: rather than having a single group of scientists revise the existing set of RDAs, they had expert panels review nutrient categories in much more detail than had ever been done before.

Not only did the definition of RDAs change, but three new values were also created: the Estimated Average Requirement (EAR), the Adequate Intake (AI), and the Tolerable Upper Intake Level (UL). All four values are collectively known as Dietary Reference Intakes or DRIs.

The Food and Nutrition Board partnered with Health Canada, the Canadian government agency responsible for nutrition policy, and the two groups jointly appointed a Dietary Reference Intakes (DRI) Committee. Seven expert panels and two subcommittees assisted the DRI Committee. All members of the DRI Committee, the expert panels and the subcommittees are leaders in their fields of nutrition and food science.

The first report of the DRI Committee was released in 1997 and focused on calcium, vitamin D, phosphorus, magnesium and fluoride. The second report on thiamin, riboflavin, niacin, vitamin B6, folate, vitamin B12, pantothenic acid, biotin and choline was released in Spring 1998. Future reports will be published in the next few years. (See timeline for estimated report release dates.)

Extending the RDA Family: Meet the New Members

As a result of the DRI Committee's work to meet individuals' nutrient needs and incorporate current nutrition science, there are now four nutrient requirement values—the RDA, Estimated Average Requirement (EAR), Adequate Intake (AI), and Tolerable Upper Intake Level (UL). The new RDAs are based on Estimated Average Requirements. The Estimated Average Requirement is the amount of a nutrient that will meet the needs of at least 50 percent of healthy people and is typically based on strong research evidence.

However, sometimes an Estimated Average Requirement cannot be accurately determined for a nutrient (e.g., vitamin D, fluoride, pantothenic acid) because the available scientific research is not conclusive. If this is the case, an Adequate Intake is estimated. Although Adequate Intakes are less precise than RDAs, they are still intended to meet or exceed the nutritive needs of nearly all healthy people.

There is more that is new to the nutrient value family. Tolerable Upper Intake Levels for some vitamins and minerals have been established for the first time. The Tolerable Upper Intake Level is the highest amount of a nutrient that can be safely consumed on a daily basis. Past editions of the RDAs have addressed toxicity levels of certain vitamins and minerals but have never clearly defined safe upper intake levels. At this time, Tolerable Upper Intake Levels cannot be established for all nutrients because of incomplete scientific information.

Appropriate Uses of the DRIs

DRIs—the compilation of RDAs, Estimated Average Requirements, Adequate Intakes, and the Tolerable Upper Intake Levels—can be used to evaluate or plan diets for individuals as well as groups. Practitioners who

---

DEFINITIONS

Dietary Reference Intakes (DRIs): The new standards for nutrient recommendations that can be used to plan and assess diets for healthy people. Think of Dietary Reference Intakes as the umbrella term that includes the following values:

- *Estimated Average Requirement (EAR):* A nutrient intake value that is estimated to meet the requirement of half the healthy individuals in a group. It is used to assess nutritional adequacy of intakes of population groups. In addition, EARs are used to calculate RDAs.

- *Recommended Dietary Allowance (RDA):* This value is a goal for individuals, and is based upon the EAR. It is the daily dietary intake level that is sufficient to meet the nutrient requirement of 97–98% of all healthy individuals in a group. If an EAR cannot be set, no RDA value can be proposed.

- *Adequate Intake (AI):* This is used when a RDA cannot be determined. A recommended daily intake level based on an observed or experimentally determined approximation of nutrient intake for a group (or groups) of healthy people.

- *Tolerable Upper Intake Level (UL):* The highest level of daily nutrient intake that is likely to pose no risks of adverse heath effects to almost all individuals in the general population. As intake increases above the UL, the risk of adverse effects increases.

2. Nutrient Requirements Get a Makeover

1997: First DRI report issued on calcium, phosphorus, magnesium, vitamin D, and fluoride.

1998: Second DRI report issued on thiamin, riboflavin, niacin, vitamin B6, folate, vitamin B12, pantothenic acid, biotin, and choline.

1999: Estimated release date of report on vitamins C and E, beta carotene, and other selected antioxidants.

2000-2003: Estimated release dates for reports on trace elements (e.g., selenium, zinc), vitamins A and K; electrolytes and fluids; energy and macronutrients; and other food components (e.g., phytoestrogens, fiber, and phytochemicals found in foods such as garlic or tea).

work with individual clients should use the new RDAs and Adequate Intakes as goals for optimal intake. People who eat less than the RDA/Adequate Intakes or exceed the Tolerable Upper Intake Level for a particular nutrient may be at nutritional risk. However, clinical, biochemical and or anthropometric data are required to accurately assess an individual's nutritional status. For groups, the Estimated Average Requirement can be used to set goals for nutrient intake and to measure the prevalence of poor nutrient intake.

To help practitioners and others learn how to use the new DRIs in their work settings, the Food and Nutrition Board appointed a Uses and Interpretations Subcommittee to develop a "user's manual." Committee chair Suzanne Murphy, Ph.D., R.D., Adjunct Associate Professor of Nutrition at the University of California at Davis, believes that the guide will help health professionals, nutrition policy planners, and others use the DRIs to their full advantage. "The process of developing the DRIs has been very thorough and represents a huge step forward for assessing the nutrient requirements of Americans. Now we want to make sure that health professionals and others know how to correctly use these new numbers." Dr. Murphy's goal is that the manual, which will be published within a few years, "be practical and easy to read. We hope that nutrition professionals and policy makers will be able to use it as a first reference before using the DRIs."

For More Information

Updates on the DRI process are available on the National Academy of Sciences web site (www2.nas.edu/fnb). The site features information about the committee, expert panels and subcommittees. The DRI reports on calcium and the B vitamins can also be accessed. To order copies of the reports, call the National Academy Press at 800-624-6242.

DIETARY REFERENCE INTAKES:
Selected Recommended Levels for Individual Intakes

Nutrient	Old RDA or ESADDI[1] (ages 25–50 yrs) Male	Female	New RDA or AI[2] (31 to 50 yrs) Male	Female
Calcium (mg)	800	800	1,000*	1,000*
Phosphorus (mg)	800	800	700	700
Magnesium (mg)	350	280	420	320
Vitamin D (µg)[3]	5	5	5*	5*
Fluoride (µg)	1.5-4.0[§]	1.5-4.0[§]	4*	3*
Thiamin (mg)	1.5	1.1	1.2	1.1
Riboflavin (mg)	1.7	1.3	1.3	1.1
Niacin (mg)	19	15	16	14
Vitamin B$_6$ (mg)	2.0	1.6	1.3	1.3
Folate (µg)	200	180	400	400
Vitamin B$_{12}$ (µg)	2.0	2.0	2.4	2.4
Pantothenic Acid (mg)	4-7[§]	4-7[§]	5*	5*
Biotin (µg)	30-100[§]	30-100[§]	30*	30*
Choline (µg)	not determined	not determined	550*	425*

(mg=milligrams µg=micrograms)

[1] RDAs and Estimated Safe and Adequate Daily Dietary Intake (ESADDI) published by the Food and Nutrition Board in 1989.
[2] RDA and Adequate Intake (AI) values from the 1997 and 1998 DRI reports.
[3] Vitamin D as cholecalciferol = 400 IU of vitamin D.
[§] ESADDI value.
*AI value.

Article 3

Staking a CLAIM to Good Health

FDA and Science Stand Behind Health Claims On Foods

by Paula Kurtzweil

HEALTH CLAIMS authorized by the Food and Drug Administration are one of several ways food labels can win the attention of health-conscious consumers.

These claims alert shoppers to a product's health potential by stating that certain foods or food substances—as part of an overall healthy diet—may reduce the risk of certain diseases. Examples include folic acid in breakfast cereals, fiber in fruits and vegetables, calcium in dairy products, and calcium or folic acid in some dietary supplements. But food and food substances can qualify for health claims only if they meet FDA requirements.

"Health claims are not your fad-of-the-week," says Jim Hoadley, Ph.D., a senior regulatory scientist in FDA's Office of Food Labeling. Instead, he says, for health claims to be used, there needs to be sufficient scientific agreement among qualified experts that the claims are factual and truthful.

FDA initially authorized seven health claims in 1993 as part of the 1990 Nutrition Labeling and Education Act (NLEA). Since 1993, FDA has authorized three more.

Under NLEA, companies petition FDA to consider new health claims through rule-making. However, this process may require more than a year to complete because of the necessary scientific review and the need to issue a proposed rule to allow for public comment. And, in an effort to speed more of this kind of information to consumers, the Food and Drug Administration Modernization Act of 1997 includes a provision that is intended to expedite the process that establishes the scientific basis for health claims.

Although food manufacturers may use health claims to market their products, the intended purpose of health claims is to benefit consumers by providing information on healthful eating patterns that may help reduce the risk of heart disease, cancer, osteoporosis, high blood pressure, dental cavities, or certain birth defects.

What Is a Health Claim?

Health claims are among the various types of claims allowed in food labeling. They show a relationship between a nutrient or other substances in a food and a disease or health-related condition. They can be used on conventional foods or dietary supplements.

They differ from the more common claims that highlight a food's nutritional content, such as "low fat," "high fiber," and "low calorie."

Health claims are different from so-called "structure/function" claims, which also may appear on conventional food or dietary supplement

From *FDA Consumer*, November/December 1998, pp. 16-21. Reprinted by permission of *FDA Consumer*, the magazine of the U.S. Food and Drug Administration.

3. Staking a Claim to Good Health

Interest in health claims is likely to remain high, and newer claims are likely to hit food labels within the foreseeable future.

labels. Manufacturers may make statements about a food substance's effect on the structure or function of the body—for example, "calcium builds strong bones." Unlike health claims, structure/function claims do not deal with disease risk reduction. Also, FDA does not pre-approve or authorize structure/function claims. Rather, when the manufacturer uses a structure/function claim, the company is responsible for making sure that the claim is truthful and not misleading.

Health claims can include implied claims, which indirectly assert a diet-disease relationship. Implied claims may appear in brand names (such as "Heart Healthy"), symbols (such as a heart-shaped logo), and vignettes when used with specific nutrient information. However, all labels bearing implied claims must also bear the full health claim.

Public Confidence

Health claims became a hot issue in the 1980s, when food marketing strategies began reflecting increased recognition of the role of nutrition in promoting health. At that time, some of the claims used were considered misleading, and many consumers began to doubt their truthfulness. NLEA's intent, in part, was to rein in exaggerated claims by reinforcing FDA's authority to regulate health claims and to require that claims be supported by sufficient scientific evidence.

According to an FDA study, consumer confidence in health claims grew in the months following implementation of NLEA. Thirty-one percent of consumers contacted by phone in November 1995—17 months after implementation of NLEA—said they believed health claims were accurate, compared with 25 percent in March 1994, two months before NLEA went into effect. And fewer respondents—39 percent in 1995 compared with 47 percent in 1994—agreed with the statement "Claims are more like advertising than anything else."

FDA's phone survey also indicated more consumers were using health claims to make more informed food choices: 25 percent in 1995 said they were using health claims, compared with 20 percent in March 1994.

According to Brenda Derby, a statistician in the consumer studies branch of FDA's Center for Food Safety and Applied Nutrition, a 1996 FDA label-reading study of more than 1,400 grocery shoppers found that, in general, the effectiveness of health claims is similar to that of nutrient claims and had no greater effect than nutrient claims alone in influencing shoppers' purchasing decisions. Health claims are most effective when they provide consumers with new information, the study found.

Expediting New Claims

A provision in the Food and Drug Administration Modernization Act of 1997 can speed up the process. The new law allows companies to notify FDA of their intent to use a new health claim based on an authoritative statement of one or more federal scientific bodies. It gives FDA 120 days to respond. If the agency does not act to prohibit or modify the claim within that time, the claim can be used.

In a guidance document for industry, FDA earlier this year established interim criteria for determining the adequacy of health claims submitted under the new procedure. Under these criteria, which will remain in place until FDA publishes final regulations, the authoritative statement, which is the basis for the health claim, must:

- come from a federal scientific body (for example, the National Institutes of Health, national Centers for Disease Control and Prevention, U.S. Department of Agriculture, or National Academy of Sciences)
- be published by the scientific body and be currently in effect
- state a relationship between a nutrient and a disease or health-related condition
- not be a statement made individually by an employee of a federal scientific body but rather reflect a consensus within the scientific body
- be based on the scientific body's deliberative review of the scientific evidence.

FDA said it would consult with the scientific body when appropriate to determine whether a statement is an authoritative one.

With the new alternative approach for determining the scientific basis for a health claim, interest in health claims is likely to remain high, and newer claims are likely to hit food labels within the foreseeable future.

"This is a new frontier for industry," says Anna Matz, a spokeswoman for the Grocery Manufacturers of America. "A lot of [consumers] are looking for solid information about the products they buy. Health claims are a perfect way to provide this information."

Paula Kurtzweil is a member of FDA's public affairs staff.

According to an FDA study, consumer confidence in health claims grew in the months following implementation of NLEA.

Authorized Health Claims

Here are the FDA-authorized health claims and some specifics on their use.

Calcium and osteoporosis

Low calcium intake is one risk factor for osteoporosis, a condition of lowered bone mass, or density. Lifelong adequate calcium intake helps maintain bone health by increasing as much as genetically possible the amount of bone formed in the teens and early adult life and by helping to slow the rate of bone loss that occurs later in life.

Typical Foods: Low-fat and skim milks, yogurts, tofu, calcium-fortified citrus drinks, and some calcium supplements.

Requirements: Food or supplement must be "high" in calcium and must not contain more phosphorus than calcium. Claims must cite other risk factors; state the need for regular exercise and a healthful diet; explain that adequate calcium early in life helps reduce fracture risk later by increasing as much as genetically possible a person's peak bone mass; and indicate that those at greatest risk of developing osteoporosis later in life are white and Asian teenage and young adult women, who are in their bone-forming years. Claims for products with more than 400 mg of calcium per day must state that a daily intake over 2,000 mg offers no added known benefit to bone health.

Sample Claim: "Regular exercise and a healthy diet with enough calcium helps teen and young adult white and Asian women maintain good bone health and may reduce their high risk of osteoporosis later in life."

Sodium and hypertension (high blood pressure)

Hypertension is a risk factor for coronary heart disease and stroke deaths. The most common source of sodium is table salt. Diets low in sodium may help lower blood pressure and related risks in many people. Guidelines recommend daily sodium intakes of not more than 2,400 mg. Typical U.S. intakes are 3,000 to 6,000 mg.

Typical Foods: Unsalted tuna, salmon, fruits and vegetables, and low-fat milks, low-fat yogurts, cottage cheeses, sherbets, ice milk, cereal, flour, and pastas (not egg pastas).

Requirements: Foods must meet criteria for "low sodium." Claims must use "sodium" and "high blood pressure" in discussing the nutrient-disease link.

Sample Claim: "Diets low in sodium may reduce the risk of high blood pressure, a disease associated with many factors."

g = gram   mg = milligram   mcg = microgram

Dietary fat and cancer

Diets high in fat increase the risk of some types of cancer, such as cancers of the breast, colon and prostate. While scientists don't know how total fat intake affects cancer development, low-fat diets reduce the risk. Experts recommend that Americans consume 30 percent or less of daily calories as fat. Typical U.S. intakes are 37 percent.

Typical Foods: Fruits, vegetables, reduced-fat milk products, cereals, pastas, flours, and sherbets.

Requirements: Foods must meet criteria for "low fat." Fish and game meats must meet criteria for "extra lean." Claims may not mention specific types of fats and must use "total fat" or "fat" and "some types of cancer" or "some cancers" in discussing the nutrient-disease link.

Sample Claim: "Development of cancer depends on many factors. A diet low in total fat may reduce the risk of some cancers."

Dietary saturated fat and cholesterol and risk of coronary heart disease

Diets high in saturated fat and cholesterol increase total and low-density (bad) blood cholesterol levels and, thus, the risk of coronary heart disease. Diets low in saturated fat and cholesterol decrease the risk. Guidelines recommend that American diets contain less than 10 percent of calories from saturated fat and less than 300 mg cholesterol daily. The average American adult diet has 13 percent saturated fat and 300 to 400 mg cholesterol a day.

Typical Foods: Fruits, vegetables, skim and low-fat milks, cereals, whole-grain products, and pastas (not egg pastas).

Requirements: Foods must meet criteria for "low saturated fat," "low cholesterol," and "low fat." Fish and game meats must meet criteria for "extra lean." Claims must use "saturated fat and cholesterol" and "coronary heart disease" or "heart disease" in discussing the nutrient-disease link.

Sample Claim: "While many factors affect heart disease, diets low in saturated fat and cholesterol may reduce the risk of this disease."

Fiber-containing grain products, fruits, and vegetables and cancer

Diets low in fat and rich in fiber-containing grain products, fruits, and vegetables may reduce the risk of some types of cancer. The exact role of total dietary fiber, fiber components, and other nutrients and substances in these foods is not fully understood.

Typical Foods: Whole-grain breads and cereals, fruits, and vegetables.

Requirements: Foods must meet criteria for "low fat" and, without fortification, be a "good source" of dietary fiber. Claims must not specify types of fiber and must use "fiber," "dietary fiber," or "total dietary fiber" and "some types of cancer" or "some cancers" in discussing the nutrient-disease link.

Sample Claim: "Low-fat diets rich in fiber-containing grain products, fruits, and vegetables may reduce the risk of some types of cancer, a disease associated with many factors."

Fruits, vegetables, and grain products that contain fiber, particularly soluble fiber, and risk of coronary heart disease

Diets low in saturated fat and cholesterol and rich in fruits, vegetables, and grain products that contain fiber, particularly soluble fiber, may reduce the risk of coronary heart disease. (It is impossible to adequately distinguish the effects of fiber, including soluble fiber, from those of other food components.)

Typical Foods: Fruits, vegetables, and whole-grain breads and cereals.

Requirements: Foods must meet criteria for "low saturated fat," "low fat," and "low cholesterol." They must contain, without fortification, at least 0.6 g of soluble fiber per reference amount, and the soluble fiber content must be listed. Claims must use "fiber," "dietary fiber," "some types of dietary fiber," "some dietary fibers," or "some fibers" and "coronary heart disease" or "heart disease" in discussing the nutrient-disease link. The term "soluble fiber" may be added.

Sample Claim: "Diets low in saturated fat and cholesterol and rich in fruits, vegetables, and grain products that contain some types of dietary fiber, particularly soluble fiber, may reduce the risk of heart disease, a disease associated with many factors."

Fruits and vegetables and cancer

Diets low in fat and rich in fruits and vegetables may reduce the risk of some cancers. Fruits and vegetables are low-fat foods and may contain fiber or vitamin A (as beta-carotene) and vitamin C. (The effects of these vitamins cannot be adequately distinguished from those of other fruit or vegetable components.)

Typical Foods: Fruits and vegetables.

Requirements: Foods must meet criteria for "low fat" and, without fortification, be a "good source" of fiber, vitamin A, or vitamin C. Claims must characterize fruits and vegetables as foods that are low in fat and may contain dietary fiber, vitamin A, or vitamin C; characterize the food itself as a "good source" of one or more of these nutrients, which must be listed; refrain from specifying types of fatty acids; and use "total fat" or "fat," "some types of cancer" or "some cancers," and "fiber," "dietary fiber," or "total dietary fiber" in discussing the nutrient-disease link.

Sample Claim: "Low-fat diets rich in fruits and vegetables (foods that are low in fat and may contain dietary fiber, vitamin A, or vitamin C) may reduce the risk of some types of cancer, a disease associated with many factors. Broccoli is high in vitamins A and C, and it is a good source of dietary fiber."

Folate and neural tube birth defects

Defects of the neural tube (a structure that develops into the brain and spinal cord) occur within the first six weeks after conception, often before the pregnancy is known. The U.S. Public Health Service recommends that all women of childbearing age in the United States consume 0.4 mg (400 mcg) of folic acid daily to reduce their risk of having a baby affected with spina bifida or other neural tube defects.

Typical Foods: Enriched cereal grain products, some legumes (dried beans), peas, fresh leafy green vegetables, oranges, grapefruit, many berries, some dietary supplements, and fortified breakfast cereals.

Requirements: Foods must meet or exceed criteria for "good source" of folate—that is, at least 40 mcg of folic acid per serving (at least 10 percent of the Daily Value). A serving of food cannot contain more than 100 percent of the Daily Value for vitamin A and vitamin D because of their potential risk to fetuses. Claims must use "folate," "folic acid," or "folacin" and "neural tube defects," "birth defects spina bifida or anencephaly," "birth defects of the brain or spinal cord anencephaly or spina bifida," "spina bifida and anencephaly, birth defects of the brain or spinal cord," "birth defects of the brain and spinal cord," or "brain or spinal cord birth defects" in discussing the nutrient-disease link. Folic acid content must be listed on the Nutrition Facts panel.

Sample Claim: "Healthful diets with adequate folate may reduce a woman's risk of having a child with a brain or spinal cord birth defect."

Dietary sugar alcohol and dental caries (cavities)

Between-meal eating of foods high in sugar and starches may promote tooth decay. Sugarless candies made with certain sugar alcohols do not.

Typical Foods: Sugarless candy and gum.

Requirements: Foods must meet the criteria for "sugar free." The sugar alcohol must be xylitol, sorbitol, mannitol, maltitol, isomalt, lactitol, hydrogenated starch hydrolysates, hydrogenated glucose syrups, erythritol, or a combination of these. When the food contains a fermentable carbohydrate, such as sugar or flour, the food must not lower plaque pH in the mouth below 5.7 while it is being eaten or up to 30 minutes afterwards. Claims must use "sugar alcohol," "sugar alcohols," or the name(s) of the sugar alcohol present and "dental caries" or "tooth decay" in discussing the nutrient-disease link. Claims must state that the sugar alcohol present "does not promote," "may reduce the risk of," "is useful in not promoting," or "is expressly for not promoting" dental caries.

Sample Claim: Full claim: "Frequent between-meal consumption of foods high in sugars and starches promotes tooth decay. The sugar alcohols in this food do not promote tooth decay." Shortened claim (on small packages only): "Does not promote tooth decay."

Dietary soluble fiber, such as that found in whole oats and psyllium seed husk, and coronary heart disease

When included in a diet low in saturated fat and cholesterol, soluble fiber may affect blood lipid levels, such as cholesterol, and thus lower the risk of heart disease. However, because soluble dietary fibers constitute a family of very heterogeneous substances that vary greatly in their effect on the risk of heart disease, FDA has determined that sources of soluble fiber for this health claim need to be considered case-by-case. To date, FDA has reviewed and authorized two sources of soluble fiber eligible for this claim: whole oats and psyllium seed husk.

Typical Foods: Oatmeal cookies, muffins, breads and other foods made with rolled oats, oat bran or whole oat flour; hot and cold breakfast cereals containing whole oats or psyllium seed husk; and dietary supplements containing psyllium seed husk.

Requirements: Foods must meet criteria for "low saturated fat," "low cholesterol," and "low fat." Foods that contain whole oats must contain at least 0.75 g of soluble fiber per serving. Foods that contain psyllium seed husk must contain at least 1.7 g of soluble fiber per serving. The claim must specify the daily dietary intake of the soluble fiber source necessary to reduce the risk of heart disease and the contribution one serving of the product makes toward that intake level. Soluble fiber content must be stated in the nutrition label. Claims must use "soluble fiber" qualified by the name of the eligible source of soluble fiber and "heart disease" or "coronary heart disease" in discussing the nutrient-disease link. Because of the potential hazard of choking, foods containing dry or incompletely hydrated psyllium seed husk must carry a label statement telling consumers to drink adequate amounts of fluid, unless the manufacturer shows that a viscous adhesive mass is not formed when the food is exposed to fluid.

Sample Claim: "Diets low in saturated fat and cholesterol that include 3 g of soluble fiber from whole oats per day may reduce the risk of heart disease, One serving of this whole-oats product provides__ grams of this soluble fiber."

Article 4

Are fruits and vegetables less nutritious today?

Our readers often tell us they are concerned that the soil is mineral-depleted and that the produce they buy is not nutritious—understandable concerns, given the compost heap of misinformation that's out there. So we decided to dig into the subject.

As has been known for centuries, agriculture tends to wear out the soil. Erosion, as well as planting, depletes top soil. Replenishing the soil is what agriculture is all about, and always has been. Fertilizers, in some form, have been used by farmers since the beginnings of agriculture. The main goal is to replace minerals, especially trace minerals. Another goal is not to add too much fertilizer. There are many, many methods that improve and maintain soil quality: water management, erosion control, planting legumes to replace nitrogen in the soil, crop rotation, adding compost, manure, and chemical fertilizers, and otherwise boosting organic matter. Enormous expertise is brought to bear on these problems—they do not go unnoticed.

Indeed, the fertility of the soil here and in the rest of the world is a matter of intense concern to farmers, governments, international investors and thousands of scientists. The amount of nutrients in the soil controls crop development and agricultural yield. Will the soil of planet Earth produce enough food to keep up with population growth, particularly if people who now go hungry are also fed? Will there be enough to nourish everybody in the year 2010? 2050? The Food and Agriculture Organization of the United Nations and the World Bank study such questions, along with the USDA and our land-grant colleges, to name only a few of the interested parties. Predicting the future, even from solid scientific data, is always difficult. So far, however, predictions are optimistic, assuming that sound agricultural policies will be followed.

Each year, around the world, there are international conferences to discuss these issues.

The one essential fact

"Fruits, vegetables, and grains will not grow, cannot be sold, and will not be bought if they contain insufficient nutrition. If there's an inadequate amount of nutrients in the soil, plants may die because of insect infestation or disease, or cannot be sold because of poor appearance." These are the words of Dr. Gary Banuelos, a soil scientist with the USDA Research Service in Fresno, California, and they echo the conclusions of other experts. As any gardener knows, plants just won't grow properly in depleted soil. Vitamins in plants are created by the plants themselves. Minerals—such as phosphorus, potassium, iodine, calcium, copper, iron, selenium, fluoride, molybdenum, and zinc—must come from the soil. If the elements aren't there, the plant droops, fails to flower, and may die. *If the fruits and vegetables you buy look healthy, you can be certain they contain the nutrients they should.* According to Joanne Ikeda, a cooperative extension nutrition-education specialist at UC Berkeley, "The idea that the soil is being depleted of nutrients and thus our food doesn't contain nutrients is one of those myths we can't seem to eradicate, though I have certainly spent years trying."

Bottom line: *People who tell you that the soil is depleted and our food is no longer nutritious are unacquainted with the truth, or not telling it. They're usually trying to get you to take some sort of mineral supplements. Certainly, nutrients will vary from one batch of produce to another, depending on climate, handling, and other factors. But a varied, balanced diet will make up for this over the long term.*

Reprinted with permission from *University of California at Berkeley Wellness Letter*, May 1998, p. 1. © 1998 by Health Letter Associates. For information, call (800) 829–9170.

The Freshness Fallacy

Who says the veggies in the produce bin are better for you than the ones in the freezer?

By MINNA MORSE

I am, I confess, a frozen-vegetable devotee. From chopped spinach to green beans, asparagus to broccoli, veggies that have spent most of their lives in a freezer compartment are the mainstay of my diet. When company is coming I seek out fresh, but when I'm on my own, dinner is often a plate of frozen brussels sprouts, cooked in the microwave and topped with melted cheddar cheese.

For one thing, it's so easy. There's no chopping involved, no stringing or peeling, and thanks to the microwave, I've got only one dish to wash at the end of the meal. Besides, when I do buy fresh produce, much of it ends up going to waste.

The vast majority of Americans would probably think I'm crazy—or at least nutritionally deprived. According to a study by the Opinion Research Corporation in Princeton, New Jersey, 92 percent believe that fresh vegetables pack more vitamins and minerals than frozen. At the same time, however, they say they're too busy to prepare fresh vegetables, so they don't bother to eat many at all. Only 5 percent meet the daily recommended amount of five or more servings a day.

Fortunately, they're wrong (and I'm vindicated). In a recent study at the University of Illinois at Urbana, researchers compared the nutritional profiles of four fresh vegetables with their frozen counterparts. After almost one year of storage, the frozen samples had roughly the same amount of vitamin C—one of the least stable vitamins—as fresh green beans and corn at eight days, broccoli at 14 days, and carrots at 21 days.

This isn't the first time research has touted the nutritional benefit of frozen foods. But Barbara Klein, the food scientist who led the study, says most other analyses compared the results of separate studies—one on fresh, say, and another on frozen. In this one, however, researchers divided a large batch of vegetables into groups, then left some of each variety sitting on the shelf and sent some to the freezer. (A third group was canned, and it scored nearly as high as the frozen—even without the liquid that the vegetables had been canned in.)

"We pretty much knew what we were going to find," says Klein. "But we also knew about people's distrust of frozen vegetables. So we figured this would be a definitive way to prove the point and hopefully get folks to eat more veggies."

Why exactly aren't fresh carrots and corn much more nutritious than frozen? Because fresh isn't always what it seems. It turns out there are two primary ways to sap nutrients from a vegetable: by letting it sit around after it's been harvested and by cooking it.

Fresh vegetables suffer the most from the first part of this rule. From the time they're picked in the field to the moment you serve them for dinner, a good two weeks may have passed. During that stretch they can lose anywhere from 10 to 50 percent of some of their nutrients.

1 ❖ TRENDS TODAY AND TOMORROW

> ## Protecting Your Frozen Assets
>
> Not all frozen vegetables get the star treatment provided in commercial facilities: namely, airtight packaging and ultracold temperatures. But you can spot some signs of poor handling when shopping for frozen foods. And when freezing at home, you can take steps to ensure a professional outcome.
>
> **Check packages** for signs of water migration. At some point during their lifetime—in transit, perhaps, or waiting around at the grocery before its shelves are restocked—the vegetables may have partially thawed. The result: When they refreeze, the vegetables form ice crystals and can clump together, both of which lead to greater nutrient loss and softening in texture. (The same thing happens on a small scale every time your freezer goes through its self-defrosting cycle.) If you're looking at a bag of frozen peas, the vegetables should be loose or break apart easily; if it's a solid box of spinach, the greens should fill the package rather than bunching to one side.
>
> **Set your refrigerator** at zero, the temperature used in commercial facilities. (Your ice cream will come out too hard to serve, however, so remember to let it sit awhile after you take it out.) Vegetables can last up to six months at this temperature. If your freezer does not have a separate temperature control, it may be as much as ten degrees warmer than that, in which case your veggies will be good only for about three months.
>
> **When freezing** your own produce, make sure you pack it in an airtight container or a plastic bag. To squeeze air out of a filled bag, try this trick: Fill a bowl or basin with water. Dunk the loaded bag into the water almost up to the top, then seal. When you pull the bag out, the plastic will cling tightly to the contents. If you do a lot of freezing at home, consider buying a gadget that vacuum-seals plastic bags.

Case in point: Most of the green beans you buy in winter are grown in the Culiacán region on the west coast of Mexico. After those beans are harvested, they may be in transit for five or more days before they arrive at a grocery near you. There they might sit for another few days, and who knows what'll happen once you get them home? Sure, you planned on making three-bean salad the next night, but you worked late and didn't feel like cooking, and the night after that you're invited out for dinner. Before you know it, three more days have gone by.

Frozen vegetables, on the other hand, end up on ice within hours of being picked. By this count, in fact, they'd seem to be doing *better* than their fresh brothers and sisters. But before a vegetable is sent to the freezer, it's plunged into hot water for a minute or two. This process stabilizes the vegetable and helps preserve its color and texture, but for certain nutrients it can be just as bad as sitting around. The rate of vitamin loss varies depending on the vegetable, but in general, says Klein, fresh and frozen come out pretty even down the line.

And not just on vitamin C. Happily, most of the health goodies contained in a vegetable are a lot more stable than you might think. Fiber, beta-carotene, and all of its minerals are locked into the vegetable whatever treatment it receives.

The reason C is so vulnerable is that it oxidizes easily. When a plant is on the vine, its vitamins are protected. But as soon as it's picked, the cell walls start to break down, allowing oxygen to enter and come into contact with the vitamins. And oxygen alters the chemical structure of vitamin C, rendering it inactive. (Vitamin C also dissolves in water, but that's mainly a problem in cooking, not storage.) Folic acid is another easily oxidized vitamin, though according to Klein, it's a little less vulnerable than C because it binds to the plant's proteins, which help keep it intact.

Of course, no matter how vitamin-rich a frozen vegetable may be, there's still the issue of taste. How can a frozen stalk of broccoli possibly compare to fresh?

Well, it may not if you're talking about one that's freshly picked and steamed to perfection. And there's no doubt that the texture won't be quite up to snuff. But even a food professional like Arthur Schwartz, cookbook author and former restaurant critic for the *New York Daily News,* says that many frozen vegetables taste just fine, particularly when mixed into a casserole or stew. Carrots and onions are two exceptions: "Their taste begins to die as soon as you cut them."

Having had my frozen-veggie habit validated by a nutritionist *and* a restaurant critic, I decided it was time to see how much freshness really mattered to my foodie friends. I would throw a dinner party using almost exclusively frozen ingredients, but I wouldn't tell any of the guests about the menu.

I went all out. First, a vegetarian pâté made of pureed green beans and walnuts. Next, individual puff pastries filled with spinach and feta cheese. I even used corn kernels and broccoli florets in a pasta salad, where they couldn't hide beneath a sauce or a buttery crust. Finally, the pièce de résistance: angel food cake smothered with a scarlet sauce of pureed raspberries.

The forks clanked, the conversation bubbled, the chairs slid back. And I heard nothing but raves.

The new foods: Functional or dysfunctional?

Are 'nutraceuticals' foods, supplements, drugs—or baloney?

As you wander through your local food store, you may wonder whether you've stumbled into a drugstore by mistake. The soup aisle features Hain's *Kitchen Prescription Chicken Broth and Noodles with Echinacea* to "support your immune system" and *Chunky Tomato with St. John's Wort* to "give your mood a natural lift." The snack section has Robert's American Gourmet *Kava Kava Corn Chips* to "promote relaxation," and *Ginkgo Biloba Rings,* a potato-corn snack, to "increase memory and alertness." You see sodas, juices, drinks, gum candy, frozen desserts—all spiked with supposedly health-enhancing herbs. Even products from mainstream food-manufacturing giants like Kellogg, Procter & Gamble, and Tropicana are taking on a decidedly pharmaceutical cast these days, with specially added nutrients and special health claims against heart disease or osteoporosis, the brittle-bone disease.

Welcome to the weird new world of "nutraceuticals," or "functional foods," the hottest new terms in food marketing. Americans have been eating *fortified* foods since 1924, when manufacturers started adding iodine to salt to prevent the nutritional deficiency that causes goiters. But functional foods represent a new concept in several ways—and a triumph of marketing ingenuity. The various added ingredients are generally intended to treat or prevent either symptoms or diseases, not deficiency; many of them aren't normally found in foods at all; and most of them are added primarily to let the manufacturer make enticing health claims.

Such products are flooding the market due largely to relaxed and fuzzy rules governing what's allowed in foods and what their manufacturers can say about them. First, the Food and Drug Administration began to approve specific disease-fighting claims. Then Congress allowed manufacturers to make "structure and function" claims—" helps maintain healthy cholesterol levels," for example—without FDA approval, provided they don't actually mention a specific disease. But while that rule applies to all supplement manufacturers, *food* companies can make such unapproved claims only if the proposed benefit stems from the food's "nutritive value." Not even the FDA—let alone your average food manufacturer—knows exactly what that phrase means.

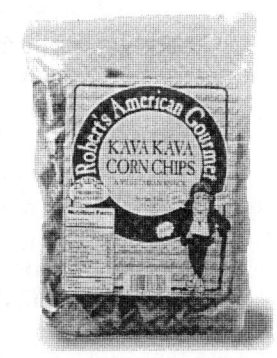

Some companies try to sidestep the morass and legitimize an unapproved claim by marketing their food as a dietary supplement. Others simply ignore the rules, in hopes that the overloaded FDA won't challenge them.

But even foods that bear FDA-approved health claims aren't necessarily healthful. And foods that carry unapproved claims—or that contain impressive-sounding special ingredients—may be nutritionally worthless, or worse.

Capitalizing on claims

The FDA opened the functional-food floodgates in 1993, when it ruled that products high in calcium, such as milk and yogurt, could sport labels claiming protection against osteoporosis. Seizing the opportunity, several manufacturers promptly started *adding* calcium—about 350 milligrams, a bit more than the amount in a glass of milk—to items that are not naturally rich in the mineral, such as *Tropicana Pure Premium* orange juice, Procter & Gamble's *Sunny Delight* orange beverage, and Kellogg's *Eggo Homestyle* frozen waffles. For a while, you could even buy *Pringle's Potato Chips* with extra calcium.

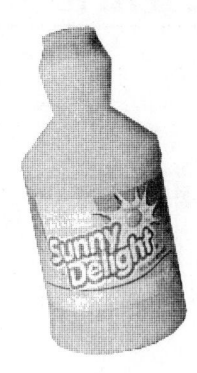

Most Americans, particularly women, don't get the recommended amounts of calcium: 1,200 milligrams a day for post-menopausal women if they take bone-bolstering drugs, and 1,500 milligrams if they don't; 1,000 milligrams for other adults up to age 50, then 1,200 milligrams from age 50 to 65 and 1,500 after 65. The best way to meet those recommendations is by eating a variety of healthful, calcium-rich foods, such as low-fat dairy products, dark-green leafy vegetables, beans, tofu prepared with calcium salts—and, yes, even calcium-fortified orange juice. Those foods, including OJ, are rich not only in calcium but also in numerous other nutrients, and they've all been linked to a variety of benefits beyond strong bones, such as reduced risk of coronary disease and cancer.

In contrast, calcium-fortified waffles (mainly refined flour) and orange drink (mainly sugar and water), have little to offer except calcium. If you can't get enough calcium from your diet, you'd be better off eating unrefined foods like whole-wheat products, or drinking 100 percent fruit juices, and taking a modest calcium supplement than consuming the nutritionally weak waffles or drink.

A slick ensemble

Kellogg's *Ensemble* product line, the first offering from the company's new functional-foods division, takes the nutraceuticals idea one step further: Unlike calcium, the psyllium husks that are added to these foods aren't found in the ordinary diet at all.

Kellogg laid the groundwork for introducing its new product line by convincing the FDA that the soluble fiber found in psyllium husks, like the soluble fiber in oats, reduces the blood-cholesterol level and thus should reduce the risk of developing coronary disease. After the FDA approved that health claim in February of last year, Kellogg quickly released its psyllium-fortified line, including frozen pasta entrees, dry pasta, breads, breakfast cereals, snacks, and desserts—many in packages emblazoned with a claim about cholesterol, heart disease, or heart health. All the products are sold at premium prices: For example, a 20-ounce loaf of *Ensemble Split-Top Sandwich Bread* costs $2.29, nearly twice as much as most other white breads, and slightly more than many whole-wheat breads.

It's true that the various *Ensemble* products are good sources of soluble fiber. So they're better than the same foods without the added fiber. But that's damningly faint praise. Like the calcium-containing waffles and orange drink, almost none of the *Ensemble* products offers much except the added ingredient: Nearly all the products are made from refined flour, several of them pack too much fat or salt to qualify for the health claim, and several are loaded with sugar. The three breakfast cereals are made from oat flour, another good source of soluble fiber, but even the cereals are moderately high in sugar.

> **Almost none of the Ensemble products offers much except the added ingredient.**

Instead of stocking up on those products, you can get all the fiber you need—and a host of other important nutrients as well—by eating the recommended 5 to 9 daily servings of produce and 6 to 11 servings of whole grains. Among many other things, those foods supply lots of *in*soluble fiber, which helps prevent constipation and possibly colon cancer as well.

Margarine medicine?

Two brand-new margarines contain added ingredients that, like soluble fiber, help reduce cholesterol levels. But those ingredients are even more obscure than psyllium, and the FDA hasn't yet allowed any health claim.

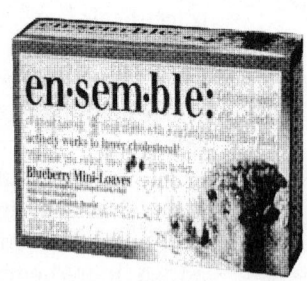

Regular margarine contains little saturated fat but lots of trans fat, which makes the spread roughly as bad for your cholesterol levels as butter (which is loaded with saturated fat). Several margarines, including

6. New Foods: Functional or Dysfunctional?

Lipton's *Take Control* and Johnson & Johnson's *Benecol*, are specially formulated to minimize or eliminate the trans fat. But *Take Control* also contains concentrated plant compounds called sterols, which help keep the cholesterol that the body produces or ingests from getting into the bloodstream, where it can contribute to clogged arteries. *Benecol* contains a similar-acting sterol derivative. Clinical trials have shown that consuming three pats of *Benecol* spread a day instead of other low-trans margarines can reduce the blood-cholesterol level by an average of 10 to 14 percent. *Take Control* may have a similar though slightly smaller benefit.

But for both margarines, the studies tested only modest amounts and lasted no longer than a year. Further, they still contain as much *total* fat and as many calories as the other margarines. So don't regard their potential benefits as license to indulge your fat tooth. These products, which cost several times more than regular spreads and some low-trans spreads, may be worth trying only if you have an elevated cholesterol level and don't mind the uncertainty about safety if you plan to use them for a long time.

Johnson & Johnson initially hoped to sell *Benecol* as a dietary supplement, but the FDA rejected that proposal. Whether the company will now try to peg a health claim on *Benecol's*

Foods in the medicine cabinet?

"The first medical food recommended by doctors for the dietary management of vascular disease." That's the claim on *HeartBar*, a $1.95 snack bar that debuted in January. *HeartBars* contain the amino acid L-arginine which, the company says, relieves angina, or heart-related chest pain, by dilating the coronary arteries.

If *HeartBar* were a drug, the Food and Drug Administration would require reams of evidence from the maker, Cooke Pharma, documenting its safety and effectiveness. If it were a dietary supplement or just a food, the FDA could prohibit claims about a specific disease (though the agency might allow more general claims—see story.) But Cooke has sidestepped those restraints by selling the bars as a "medical food," an obscure regulatory category for foods that treat diseases with clear nutritional requirements, such as malnutrition or intractable diarrhea.

The labels must state that such foods should be eaten only under a doctor's supervision. But they can be sold without a prescription (usually in drugstores), and manufacturers can make specific claims without FDA approval. In recent years, a few companies hoping to take advantage of that loophole have developed products for common diseases with less-definite nutritional links. And the FDA has started to reconsider how it deals with such foods. Here's the lowdown on the most common medical foods:

■ *HeartBar.* A growing body of evidence—mostly from animal research—does suggest that L-arginine can help relax the arteries. And a few clinical trials in humans have shown that it can relieve angina in at least some patients. But other trials have found no benefit. And there's no long-term evidence on L-arginine's safety or effectiveness. The bottom line: A serious problem like angina should be managed only with proven medications, not with a *possibly* helpful snack bar.

■ *NiteBite and Choice dm.* These chocolate-flavored snack bars are loaded with starch; that carbohydrate is meant to prevent the hypoglycemia, or low blood-sugar level, that afflicts some diabetic individuals, usually when they sleep or work out. But any carbohydrate-rich snack eaten shortly before bedtime or exercise can help prevent hypoglycemia. And sometimes the best way to avoid the problem is not by eating a snack but by adjusting the dosage or type of antidiabetic medication you take. Your doctor may suggest a safer, more effective option than downing starch bars (which cost $1.20 apiece).

■ *Cardia.* When this salt alternative hit the shelves two years ago it was marketed as a medical food, complete with a claim that it helps control hypertension. The manufacturer has now dropped that claim, in order to drop the accompanying warning about medical supervision. But the claim never amounted to much in the first place.

Some research does suggest that *Cardia*—which basically contains half the sodium of regular salt, plus potassium and magnesium—can reduce blood pressure in hypertensive people. But that effect is typically modest. Further, people who have kidney disease or take either an ACE inhibitor or a "potassium-sparing" diuretic should indeed check with a doctor first, since the potassium in *Cardia* theoretically may cause excessive potassium buildup. As for people with normal blood pressure, it's not clear whether they benefit even from salt restriction—and there's no evidence they'd benefit from *Cardia*.

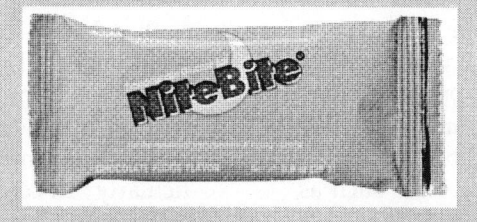

25

"nutritive value"—and how the FDA might react—remains to be seen.

Off the deep end

While the world of herbs is largely uncharted territory, there are at least trends toward standardized doses of the pills and extracts and toward warnings about risks. But the addition of herbs to *foods* is a step backward into the darkest jungle. Such products may be worthless or even harmful, for any of these reasons:

■ **The herb may not work.** Journey's *Tropical Herb Ginseng Soda* highlights its "Brazilian Suma ginseng." But the variety of ginseng thought to offer possible benefits is Asian Panax; Brazilian Suma isn't even real ginseng. And the herb added to Hain's *Chunky Tomato with St. John's Wort* consists of stems, while the active ingredient (which may indeed ease mild depression) appears to come mainly from the leaves and flowers.

■ **The amount is absurdly small.** A serving of that Hain's soup contains 98 milligrams of St. John's wort *stems*. The apparently effective dose of the leaves and flowers, on the other hand, is 20 to 30 times higher—and it's supposed to be taken three times a day for at least a month. *Peace Cereal Vanilla Almond Crisp,* described as "an herbal brain power cereal," contains some 2 milligrams of ginkgo-leaf extract, while the possibly effective dose is 120 to 240 milligrams—and any benefit from the herb is probably limited to people who have cognitive problems such as those in early-stage Alzheimer's disease.

■ **The herb may sometimes be unsafe.** If certain products do contain any significant doses, the herb might cause harm in some cases. For example, if Robert's American Gourmet *Kava Kava Corn Chips* actually contain much kava kava, pigging out on them theoretically might relax your muscles enough to precipitate a fall or an accident—particularly if you're drinking alcohol or taking another muscle-relaxing drug. SoBe's *Energy* drink contains yohimbe at what the maker calls "supplement" levels. If that's true, the herb may pose certain risks, especially for people who have diabetes or heart, liver, or kidney disease or who take antidepressants known as MAO inhibitors. And if the echinacea added to several functional foods constitutes a substantial dose, it might harm people who have autoimmune disorders such as rheumatoid arthritis. While many herbal *supplements* carry that warning, it's not on any of the echinacea-fortified *foods* that we've seen.

■ **Juiced-up junk is still junk.** The main ingredient in such products as Blue Sky's *Ginseng Creme Soda,* RJ Corr's *Ginseng Rush Natural Soda,* and Ben & Jerry's new *Tropic of Mango Frozen Smoothie* with echinacea—apart from an uncertain amount of an herb with uncertain benefits—is sugar.

Summing up

Most "functional foods" function mainly to boost manufacturers' profits, not to improve your health. Apart from calcium-fortified orange juice and possibly the *Ensemble* breakfast cereals and the two margarines for people with a high blood-cholesterol level, none of the functional foods makes good dietary sense. Adding a single healthful ingredient, like calcium or psyllium, does not turn a nutritional nonentity into a desirable food—particularly since you can get the same or equivalent ingredients from foods loaded with additional nutrients, often at a lower price. Dumping *herbs* into foods is even more dubious, since the herb or the dose may be ineffective or unsafe.

The curse of Frankenfood

Genetically modified crops stir up controversy at home and abroad

By Phillip J. Longman

In speeches and on his Web site, the Prince of Wales warns that he would never eat the stuff and proclaims that he won't stand for it being grown on his land. Former Beatle Paul McCartney, when he learned that traces could be found in his late wife Linda's vegetarian food line, reacted with the same fear and revulsion as do most Britons: He ordered the offending ingredient removed immediately. British newspapers now publish advice columns on how to avoid feeding the stuff accidentally to your pets, and protesters regularly vandalize farm fields where it is grown. Indeed, not only in Britain but throughout Europe, public fears are running so high that there is widespread resistance to any imported food—a situation that could provoke a major trade war with the United States.

Yet chances are, if you live on this side of the pond, you're only dimly aware of so-called genetically modified organisms, or "Frankenfood," as the British tabloids call it. And chances are, too, that you had some for breakfast. And lunch. And dinner. In the past five years, a revolution has occurred in the American diet. Since the last century, humans have crossbred plants to make them tastier or hardier or to give them some other desired quality. But with the advent of new gene-splicing technology researchers are now able to remove individual genes from one species and insert them into another. So, for example, a gene from a cat can be put into a dog, or a gene from a soil bacterium can be spliced into a tomato.

The ability to crossbreed diverse forms of life has had a profound impact on U.S. agriculture. The first genetically modified crop, the Flavr-Savr tomato, went into supermarkets five years ago. By 1998, 25 percent of corn, 38 percent of soybeans, and 45 percent of cotton grown in the United States were genetically altered, either to make the crops resistant to weedkillers or to produce their own pesticides.

And tofu, too. It is now virtually impossible for Americans to avoid eating genetically modified organisms, or GMOs, as they're often called. Bioengineered corn and soybeans in particular are used as ingredients in a wide range of processed food, from soft drinks and beer to breakfast cereal. They are also fed to farm animals. Even products found in health-food stores, such as tofu and canola oil, often contain genetically modified ingredients.

In many instances, food manufacturers themselves don't know which GMOs may lurk in their products. Pillsbury, for example, avers that its Green Giant brand sweet corn varieties are not genetically modified. But in a written statement, the company allows that "many of our products contain food ingredients derived from soy (soy oil, soy protein, soy sauce) and corn (corn starch, corn oil, high fructose corn syrup), all of which could have been produced using genetic modification. Since soy and corn are managed as commodity ingredients in the United States, it is possible that traditional and genetically modified products could become commingled during harvest, storage, and processing."

Some major food companies, such as Coca-Cola and PepsiCo, claim that any GMOs they use as raw material are eliminated in the production process. But that's open to dispute. John Fagan, chairman and chief scientific officer at Genetic ID, which does genetic testing for the food industry, is unequivocal when asked about the assertions made by Coca-Cola and PepsiCo. "Their claim that they're removing all genetically engineered residues is not scientifically defensible," he says. "I'd be happy to stand up in court and say that."

Does it matter? The rapidly growing biotech industry, led by Monsanto, says that genetically modified food promises

BON APPETIT
How safe is genetically modified food?

Are genetically modified crops more dangerous than those produced through traditional breeding? Scientists warn that the long-term, large-scale tests needed to establish the safety of altered food have yet to be done. Researchers have identified several potential risks:

Health risks

■ *Toxicity.* Though no scientifically valid study has shown that altered foods are toxic, some researchers believe it's possible that genetic manipulation could enhance natural plant toxins in unexpected ways—by switching on a gene that, in addition to having the desired effect, pumped out more poison, for example. "We'd never know until people started dropping," says Paul Billings, a medical geneticist at the Department of Veterans Affairs in Grand Prairie, Texas.
■ *Allergies:* People who suffer from allergies could be exposed to proteins they react to without knowing it—if a peanut, wheat, or shellfish gene, for example, ended up in corn. A few years ago, researchers showed that a Brazil nut gene spliced into soybeans induced allergies in people sensitive to the nuts. Though the Food and Drug Administration requires companies to report whether altered food contains any known problem proteins, some scientists fear that unknown allergens could slip through the system.
■ *Bad nutrition;* Scientists also say foreign genes might alter the nutritional value of food in unpredictable ways. A study to be published in the *Journal of Medicinal Food,* for example, found that concentrations of phytoestrogens—compounds thought to protect against heart disease and perhaps cancer—were lower in genetically modified soybeans than in traditional strains.
■ *Antibiotic resistance.* When scientists splice a foreign gene into a plant or microbe, they often link it to another gene, called a marker, that helps determine if the first gene was successfully taken up. Most markers code for resistance to antibiotics. Some researchers warn that these genes might be passed on to disease-causing microbes in the guts of people who eat altered food, contributing to the growing public-health problem of antibiotic resistance.

Environmental risks

■ *Losing a safe natural pesticide.* Among the most popular genetically modified products are crops containing a gene, derived from the soil bacterium *Bacillus thuringiensis,* that produces a protein toxic to insect pests. While these Bt crops have helped farmers cut back on synthetic insecticide use, biologists warn that over exposing bugs to Bt—which for many years has been used in small doses as a safe natural pesticide—will help the insects evolve resistance. If so, both Bt crops and sprays could be rendered useless, depriving organic farmers of the only effective pesticide they have.
■ *Harm to monarchs and other innocents.* In May, Cornell University researchers reported that, in lab studies, monarch butterfly caterpillars that ate milkweed dusted with pollen from Bt corn died or developed abnormally. Ecologists worry that other "non-target species" could be harmed.
■ *Spawning "superweeds."* Biologists fear that genes designed to give crops a competitive advantage—such as insect resistance and herbicide tolerance—may be passed on to wild plants, particularly weeds. Already, scientists have reported that a herbicide-tolerant canola cross-pollinated with a related weed species, producing a herbicide-tolerant descendant. In some cases, such unintended gene transfer has given the weed an edge over competing plant species.

—Laura Tangley

---

a new green revolution. Already, such crops have helped hold down the cost of food production, while also reducing farmers' need for pesticides and herbicides. Modified foods in the works include more nutritious, flavorful, and productive grains, salt- and drought-tolerant crops, and even plants that produce compounds ranging from industrial oils and plastics to drugs and vaccines.

But a growing chorus of critics warns of unintended consequences, ranging from threats to human health and environmental destruction to severe economic dislocations for the world's farmers. In May, Cornell University researchers reported that monarch butterfly caterpillars in the laboratory—fed pollen from a widely used form of genetically modified corn—died or developed abnormally. Though this may happen rarely in nature, the study reinforced the belief held by many scientists that the effects of GMOs on human health and the environment have not been sufficiently studied (*see* box, "How safe is genetically modified food?"). The study has already had a profound political impact overseas, strengthening the hand of environmental groups and foreign governments that want bans on genetically modified food imports.

The stakes for both food producers and consumers are high. During his recent confirmation hearings, Deputy Treasury Secretary-designate Stuart Eizenstat stated that "almost 100 percent of our agricultural exports in the next five years will be genetically modified or combined with bulk commodities that are genetically modified." The European Union's resistance to such crops, he added, "is the single greatest trade threat that we face." Last year, U.S. agriculture exports reached about $50 billion, or more than 7 percent of all American goods bought abroad.

President Clinton formally raised the issue in June with other world leaders at a summit in Cologne, Germany. France, which is Europe's biggest agricultural producer, advocated a new worldwide council to investigate the safety of genetically modified organisms. U.S. negotiators argued that such a move is not needed, suggesting instead that the Europeans form their own food safety and regulatory regime. A compromise was reached by tossing the issue to the Organization for Economic Cooperation and Development.

But the international politicking and intrigue continue. Led by France, the European Union imposed a de facto moratorium in late June on the import of all genetically modified materials not previously approved. Since then, U.S. Agriculture Secretary Dan Glickman has spearheaded the administration's attempts to alternately bully and flatter the Europeans into eating what Washington wants to put on their plates. The bullying comes in the form of continuing threats to take the issue to the World Trade Organization, where the United States has had good luck recently in overturning European trade barriers against bananas and hormone-fed beef. The flattery is no less overt. After flying to Paris to consult with the French, Glickman alluded to Louis Pasteur having been the first great scientist to do significant work on food safety, in hopes of engaging the pride of the country's scientific establishment. It didn't work. Last week, in another effort to mollify the Europeans, Glickman said the United States will for the first time conduct its own long-term studies on the safety of genetically modified organisms.

That move is bound to startle Americans who have been, often unwittingly, eating the stuff for years. Though Americans place more faith than do Europeans in food regulators, there is widespread fear within the food industry that Americans, too, may become phobic about GMOs, especially now that the administration seems to be validating at least some concerns raised by critics of bioengineered food. The Food and Drug Administration requires no special testing of genetically modified foodstuffs, and there are no labeling requirements, either.

Fearing the backlash. The politics of this issue are complex and potentially explosive. Start with the American farmer. Nebraskan Roger Wehrbein is typical in his ambivalence. The entire soybean crop on his family's farm is engineered to resist a powerful weedkiller. A third of the corn crop is either resistant to the weedkiller or designed to repel pests. He'll save $2 to $3 an acre in reduced weedkiller costs and have fewer weeds in the harvested crop. But when he considers biotech's impact on farming, Wehrbein is more hesitant. Are the agribusiness giants that control genetically modified crops going to leave the small farmers and independent seed companies in the dust? "I don't want to say this is necessarily bad," he says, "but it must be done carefully, and we need public debate."

Many farmers believe that genetically altered beans and corn won't hurt humans, but they understand that in the end, regardless of what science may say, consumer taste rules. "We need to make sure we don't introduce new varieties into the marketplace before they receive necessary clearance," says Kirk Leeds, executive director of the Iowa Soybean Association. "In many cases technology is introduced before consumers are ready to accept it." At a time when U.S. farmers are facing declining commodity prices and falling income, U.S. corn exports to Europe have nearly stopped, ultimately because of consumer resistance to GMOs.

Public enemy No. 1. Farmers have to worry, too, about how American consumers will respond as trade frictions and new scientific findings increasingly put genetically modified organisms in the news. It's a threat that probably can't be contained by mere public relations. The British experience suggests that the more effort big biotech companies like Monsanto put into "educating" consumers about GMOs, the more consumers grow wary and resentful. For example, a series of pro-GMO advertisements Monsanto ran a year ago in Britain were criticized as patronizing, and public resistance to genetically modified food actually increased after the campaign. Notes John Vidal, environmental editor of the British newspaper the *Guardian*: "It has become a Monsanto-hate thing. It isn't anti-American; it is anti-overzealous corporations." Liberal Democrat Member of Parliament Norman Baker earlier this year called Monsanto "public enemy No. 1."

Americans may be culturally more inclined to embrace new technology than are Europeans. But this country also has a strong environmental movement that is already beginning to rally against genetically modified food. In February, plaintiffs including Greenpeace, the Sierra Club, and the International Federation of Organic Agricultural Movements filed suit against the Environmental Protection Agency, arguing that it unlawfully approved genetically modified crops. Mothers for Natural Law, an environmental activist group, has collected nearly a half million signatures on a petition calling for mandatory labeling of genetically engineered food.

In the end, the fight over genetically modified food may be much more than a trade war. It could become a domestic donnybrook as well, rivaling the revolt against that other once bright and promising new industry: nuclear power.

With Thomas K. Grose in London, Mindy Charski, Jack Egan, Penny Loeb, Margaret Loftus, and Laura Tangley

Low-calorie sweeteners

Just 'sweet nothings'

Sweetness without calories. No wonder people like low-calorie sugar substitutes.

Drink them in diet soda pop. Eat them in low-calorie baked goods and frozen desserts. Pour them in coffee and sprinkle them on cereal.

Gluttony without guilt. Or is it?

Sweet nothings

Low-calorie sweeteners are chemicals that mimic the sweetness of sugar. They have no appreciable calories or food value.

The Food and Drug Administration (FDA) has approved four low-calorie sweeteners:

■ *Saccharin (sak-UH-rin)*—The FDA attempted to ban saccharin (Sweet'N Low) in 1977, after laboratory studies suggested it may cause bladder cancer. However, Congress overrode the ban, and the FDA granted interim approval in 1991.

Many studies have found no link between saccharin use and cancer in humans. However, there have been suggestions of increased cancer from saccharin use among some groups, such as males who smoke heavily. Products with saccharin must carry a cancer warning.

■ *Aspartame (AS-pahr-tame)*—This substitute was first approved in 1981 for use as a tabletop sweetener and in powdered mixes. Approval was expanded in 1996 for use in other foods and beverages.

Aspartame (NutraSweet, Equal) is often the subject of stories in the popular press and on the Internet claiming that the product causes a variety of health problems, including (among others) headaches, tumors, seizures, panic attacks, hyperactivity and multiple sclerosis.

However, the Centers for Disease Control (CDC) reviewed 600 health complaints against aspartame and concluded it *does not* cause such health problems. In addition, the FDA and the American Medical Association have concluded that aspartame is safe for the general population, all ages.

Aspartame is not safe, though, for people who have the rare hereditary disease phenylketonuria (fen-ul-ke-to-NU-re-uh), or PKU. Products made with aspartame must carry a PKU warning on the label.

■ *Acesulfame-K (uh-SEE-sull-fame)*—The FDA first approved acesulfame-K (Sunett) in 1988. In 1998, approval was expanded for use in soft drinks. Acesulfame-K is often blended with other sugar substitutes to produce a more sugarlike taste. Ninety studies have concluded acesulfame-K is safe.

Low-calorie sweeteners at a glance

Sweetener	ADI*	ADI equivalent**	OK for cooking?
Saccharin	5 mg	8.5 packets of sweetener	Yes
Aspartame	50 mg	5 cans of diet soda	No
Acesulfame-K	15 mg	25 cans of diet soda	Yes
Sucralose	5 mg	5 cans of diet soda	Yes

*FDA-established Average Daily Intake (ADI) limit per kilogram (2.2 pounds) of body weight. ** Product consumption equivalent for a 150-pound person.

8. Low-Calorie Sweeteners

■ *Sucralose (SOO-krah-lose)*—Sucralose (Splenda) is the only sugar substitute made from sugar. It's the newest substitute, FDA-approved on April 1, 1998. More than 100 studies over 20 years have not linked sucralose to any health problems. No warning labels are required.

Safety—and common sense

The FDA has established an "average daily intake" (ADI) for each sweetener. This is the maximum amount considered safe to consume each day over a lifetime. ADIs are intended to be about 100 times less than the smallest amount that might cause an adverse reaction.

But that doesn't mean you *should* consume that much. Removing sugar from a doughnut or cookie doesn't turn these into low-calorie, low-fat foods. And if you consume a lot of these, you may not be eating enough nutritious foods. It's OK to substitute a diet soda for a regular soda, but not for milk.

Some nutritionists recommend limiting yourself to 2 servings a day of foods containing sugar substitutes. As a general rule, that's the amount you can consume without compromising the quality of your diet.

Weight loss— the bittersweet news

Sugar substitutes may help you lose weight if you use them to reduce the number of calories in your diet.

But studies show most people who use sugar substitutes do not lower the total number of calories they consume each day.

In fact, America's weight problem has gotten worse as consumption of low-calorie sweeteners has increased.

It's crunch time for P&G's olestra

Health concerns persist, and consumers are not wowed by snacks with the synthetic fat

By Pamela Sherrid

Frito-Lay didn't become the world's leading chip company by coddling the competition. So when Procter & Gamble's ballyhooed synthetic fat, olestra, was approved for use in salty snacks in 1996, Frito-Lay negotiated hard to get a head start on rivals. In an exchange for buying tubs of olestra, the company landed an exclusive contract to sell snacks with the new ingredient. The result: For the past 16 months, Frito-Lay's Wow! brand potato and tortilla chips were the only widely available munchies with olestra other than P&G's own Pringles brand.

But the chip maker's deal with P&G is set to expire on May 28—and Frito-Lay couldn't be happier. In fact, the company is eager for competition from other snack-food companies. Lots of it. "We'll benefit if olestra becomes part of the mainstream," says a spokeswoman.

She's right about one thing: Olestra is still a long way from achieving mainstream status. Few consumer products have been so controversial. Because it passes through the human body without being digested, olestra adds no fat or calories to foods cooked with it. But olestra causes gastrointestinal upset in some people, and it interferes with the absorption of vitamins and nutrients from foods eaten about the same time.

As a result, the Food and Drug Administration requires a warning label on snacks that contain the product. Consumer activists, most notably firebrand Michael Jacobson, head of the Center for Science in the Public Interest, continue to crusade against it. Even the cultural zeitgeist now seems to be working against olestra. Tom Pirko, a food-industry consultant, notes that the craze for low-fat and no-fat foods peaked in 1996. "People are tired of deprivation," he says.

It's not that olestra has been a bust. Frito-Lay's Wow! brand racked up over $350 million in sales in its first year, making it the most successful food introduction of the 1990s. But Wow!'s sales peaked last June and have not grown since. Given Frito-Lay's enormous clout—it supplies half the nation's potato chips and 73 percent of the tortilla chips—plus its $35 million ad campaign and the revolutionary nature of the product, many analysts were disappointed. "We all thought it would be much bigger news," says Caroline Levy of Schroders & Co.

With its hefty 40 percent price premium compared with regular chips, Wow! can probably turn into a profitable niche product for Frito-Lay. But the stakes are much higher for Procter & Gamble, which spent 25 years and more than $200 million to bring olestra to market.

P&G hopes to interest another food giant in using the synthetic fat. A box of Nabisco Ritz crackers with olestra was even featured in P&G's 1998 annual report. But after a test market of both Ritz and Wheat Thins, Nabisco has decided to bag a national rollout for now. It's the same story at General Mills, which tested Bugles snacks with olestra. The companies' lack of enthusiasm stems in part from the fact that the olestra product took sales away from their own existing low-fat versions.

Chips are down. Despite P&G's wooing, so far only two regional U.S. snack-food companies, Utz and Herr's, are going ahead with olestra chips. They compete in the mid-Atlantic region, where demand for Frito-Lay's Wow! chips was higher than the national average. "A segment of our market definitely wants the benefits," says Richard King, president of Utz. By contrast, Guy's Snack Foods, a big regional firm based in Liberty, Mo., has decided to give olestra a pass. "We don't want to sell any product with a warning on it," says sales manager Jack Salmon. Another obstacle: Unlike regular cottonseed or peanut frying oil, olestra is solid at room temperature, requiring companies to invest in new equipment.

By default, P&G may wind up becoming its own best customer. In 1996 it bought the Eagle brand name and recently completed a test market of newly formulated Eagle snacks, some made with olestra. Food-industry analysts wonder whether Procter & Gamble has the stomach for a bruising head-to-head battle with Frito-Lay, which has in the past spoiled the snack-food ambitions of giants like Anheuser-Busch (which sold Eagle to P&G), Keebler, and Borden. But P&G has staying power. It stuck with languishing Pringles for 20 years before the brand finally took off in the early '90s. Eventually, P&G hopes to get FDA approval to use olestra in many other foods besides salty snacks, everything from ice cream to french fries. But first it will have to counteract apocalyptic oratory from nutrition activists, who say that the nutrient-depleting characteristic of olestra could contribute to serious health problems if people consume small amounts of it throughout the day. If such concerns persist, P&G officials may be the ones suffering from indigestion.

Supermarket Psych-Out

REMEMBER THE AD for Sheba cat food, the one in which the woman with the luxurious voice feeds her luxuriously furry feline from a tin that has large black lettering and a picture of a black cat? Well, it's no accident that the tin has all that black on it.

There was a time when black had a "no-frills association," explains Mona Doyle, president of The Consumer Network, a Philadelphia firm that conducts research on consumer perceptions. "It would have looked doleful" to people shopping for food products," she says. But today, she points out, black has become "a symbol of quality—a status connotation, elegant." In other words, it's associated in people's minds with high-class, expensive goods (a relevant point, since Sheba costs more than twice as much as several other brands).

Color is "a very powerful tool," notes Eric Johnson, head of Research Studies for the Chicago-based Institute for Color Research, which collects scientific information about the human response to color. A customer spends only the briefest amount of time at the supermarket deciding which products and which brands to buy, and the colors food manufacturers use to package their products are chosen with a great deal of care to sway you in what are sometimes split-second decisions.

But color is not all that's used to influence you at what marketers call the "point of purchase." The shape of a food package is meant to entice, too, as are (of course) various price promotions. Here's a look at color, shape, and a couple of other tricks of the trade that companies use to send silent messages to you when you're making choices about which products to buy.

The color of your purchases

There has been "a longstanding understanding in industry that if you want to sell a product, package it in red and white," says The Consumer Network's Ms. Doyle. Think of Campbell's soup, Carnation Instant Breakfast, and Marlboro cigarettes, to name just a few red-and-white-packaged items. But the color field has been thrown open, so to speak. Take a look.

Red Red stimulates feelings of arousal and appetite. Indeed, the Institute for Color Research's Mr. Johnson explains that when the eye sees red, the pituitary gland sends out signals that make the heart beat faster, the blood pressure increase, and the muscles tense—all physiologic changes that can lead to the consummation of a purchase. (No wonder so many foods have red on their packaging.)

Red is also considered a "warm and inviting color," says Paul Brefka, a Boston-area product designer. You'll often see at least some red on boxes of pasta, he says. It evokes shared, hearty Italian meals.

Green "Thirty years ago, green was barf color," Ms. Doyle remarks. But then it "became associated with the environment, and that meant pro-health. It has morphed 180 degrees." Just how much green's reputation has come around has been underscored in a study conducted by Brian Wansink, PhD. The director of the University of Illinois Food & Brand Lab, which looks at how consumers make purchasing decisions at the point of sale, Dr. Wansink did a covert color switch on a popular sweet treat. He put O'Henry candy bars, normally found in yellow wrappers, into green ones. When the bars were seen in green, consumers said they had fewer calories, more protein, and fewer calories from fat than when they were in their usual packaging.

Green's effect is probably why Hershey's reduced-fat Sweet Escapes candy bars have green on their wrappers, just as Healthy Choice frozen dinners are packaged in largely-green boxes. Decaffeinated coffee tends to come wrapped in green, too, while regular coffee often comes in "robust" red.

White By itself, white suggests reduced calories. Sales of sugar-free Canada Dry Ginger Ale increased when its labels incorporated more white, Dr. Wansink says. Silver also means fewer calories. A bottle of Diet Coke is mostly silver; a bottle of regular Coke, mostly red.

Yellow Yellow is the fastest color that the brain processes, Mr. Johnson explains. Thus, he says, it's an "attention getter." There's also "a mythic thing about yellow being a happy color," he notes. For those reasons, it's not surprising that yellow is a very common color in supermarkets, appearing on everything from boxes of Cheerios to Domino Sugar to Triscuit wafers to Hellmann's mayonnaise.

Orange In sociologic studies, Mr. Johnson says, orange indicates affordability. It suggests, "I'm easy, I'm cheap," perhaps because it's not considered a classy color. But its suggestion of accessibility and affordability make it a good color for such "Every-

1 ❖ TRENDS TODAY AND TOMORROW

man" products as Arm & Hammer Baking Soda, Burger King meals, and Stouffer's frozen entrees.

Brown Rich browns indicate "roasted" or "baked" says Mr. Johnson, which is why you'll often see brown as a background color on things like bags and boxes of gravy and cake mixes. Brown also suggests rich flavor—a reason it often appears on cans of coffee.

Blue You won't find a preponderance of foods packaged in blue. People generally want the colors on their boxes, bottles, and cans to reflect what's inside. Mr. Johnson puts it this way: "Human beings require congruency of color in order to buy the goods. People will not buy baked beans in a purple can. Beans are not purple."

Interestingly, that is not so for children, who think incongruously colored foods and food packages are "fun." That's why there has been, for instance, blue Kool-Aid, blue popcorn, and blue candies.

The shape of things to come... into your home

Most instant coffee comes in cylindrical jars—but not Taster's Choice. It's packaged in a deep square jar. The reason: Nestle, Taster's Choice's maker, felt it would provide more of an image of a "hefty" taste if presented that way—a sort of antidote to people's assumption that freeze-dried coffee crystals can't pack a hearty flavor.

Nestle, of course, is not the only company that pays careful attention to the shape of its packaging. "Shape is probably the hottest tactic in differentiating brands," says Jim Peters, editor-in-chief of *BrandPackaging* magazine. Ms. Doyle agrees that package shape has become an extremely important marketing tool.

Just think about the "sensuous, literally provocative shapes of today's packages," she says, giving ice cream containers as an example. They used to be "brick-like," she says—utilitarian. Now, they're "more hand-friendly, sensuous," she notes—round, oval, trapezoidal. It's thought that because ice cream is an indulgence product, she explains, it "should have an indulgent look and feel."

Even dishwashing detergent containers are "tactile, designed for the hand" today, she says. They all have "silhouette shapes—it's easy to look at them as a female form. They have a waist line. They're easy to hold." Which goes to show, she says, that "we're no longer Puritan in many ways."

Bigger seen as better

Consumers often go for the larger size of a product at the supermarket. One reason, of course, is that bigger is generally seen as cheaper on a per-ounce basis. In addition, a larger container is thought to last longer, saving the shopper from having to schlep back to the supermarket as quickly to restock. Neither is necessarily the case.

On a recent trip to the grocery store, we found that a 40-ounce jar of Heinz Tomato Ketchup, at $2.49, cost 6.2 cents an ounce, whereas the smaller, 28-ounce bottle, at $1.49, was only 5.3 cents an ounce. It was a similar story with some cereals. A 24-ounce box of Kellogg's Corn Flakes cost 12.5 cents an ounce, but the littler, 18-ounce box came to just 11.9 cents an ounce.

That happens about 10 percent of the time, Dr. Wansink says. The way around it is simple. Simply check "unit prices" listed on supermarket shelves, which list the price by the pound next to the price for a particular-size container. That way, you can be certain that the size you take is the best buy that day. (Prices and deals change frequently from shopping trip to shopping trip.)

As for the bigger-package-lasts-longer tack, the reason it might not work is that people tend to take bigger portions from bigger containers. Dr. Wansink made the discovery when he asked 98 women in New Hampshire and Vermont to take enough spaghetti from a box to make dinner for two. When they took spaghetti from a 1-pound box, they averaged 234 strands each. When they took it from a larger, 2-pound box

---

Some Grocery Aisle Counter-Tricks of Your Own

To keep from buying too many supermarket products that you didn't plan to buy...

1. Make a grocery list before leaving the house.
2. Write down how many of each item you need so you won't be swayed by signs and placards to buy more than you really want.
3. Don't automatically reach for the largest size; it's not always the cheapest on an ounce-for-ounce basis. Check units prices (price per pound) on shelves to make sure the size you purchase is the best buy.

---

on a separate occasion, they averaged 302 strands each—a 29 percent increase (and a 105-calorie difference per serving).

The same thing happened with cooking oil. The women poured 3.5 ounces into a pan when they poured it from a 16-ounce bottle; 4.3 ounces from a 32-ounce bottle (a difference of 192 calories).

All packaged foods list serving sizes on the Nutrition Facts panel. But, says Dr. Wansink, "few people appear to read them."

"Limit: 2 per customer" and other messages by the numbers

Sometimes it's not the package itself that does the enticing but the sign above it. A limit on how many boxes or bottles the shopper is allowed to take can be particularly effective, as Dr. Wansink demonstrated when he experimented with signs for displays of canned soup in a Sioux City, Iowa, grocery store. When consumers saw soup for 79 cents a can with no limit on how many they could purchase, they typically bought three to four cans. But when the display was changed to limit the purchase to 12 cans, they purchased as many as seven cans each, increasing sales by 112 percent.

Ironically, when supermarkets set a limit like that, they often are not trying to get consumers to buy more of a particular product; they simply are trying to make sure people don't buy too much of it. Such products are frequently loss leaders—items that are marked down so much the store loses money on them in an effort to lead people in so they will end up doing the rest of their shopping there.

"Limit" signs are not the only kind to get people to buy more of a product. Even a sign that says "4 cans for $4" as opposed to "1 can for $1" makes people buy more, Dr. Wansink explains, because it "anchors" people to a higher number. When he manipulated supermarket signs to give prices for multiple units of an item instead of the price for a single package, sales increased 32 percent in 12 out of 13 categories, including cookies, frozen dinners, and soft drinks.

Straightforward suggestions to buy a certain amount, as in "Buy 18 Snickers Bars for Your Freezer," also make people buy more than twice as much as when a sign simply says, "Buy Snickers Bars for Your Freezer." When Dr. Wansink put up a sign for Snickers Bars in a Philadelphia convenience store that did not include any suggestions on how many bars people should buy, they tended to buy one each. But when the sign suggested to people that they buy 18, they bought an average of three.

"People say, 'I'm not going to buy 18!'" Dr. Wansink explains. But they're still influenced to buy more than they would otherwise. Even signs stamped on cartons that say things like "Shipped to stores in boxes of 28 units" make people buy more, Dr. Wansink says.

Fortunately, he points out, the numbers game is very easy to get around. All you have to do is write quantities next to the items on your grocery list. That anchors you to a number of your own choosing before you even walk inside the store.

Unit 2

Unit Selections

11. **Fats: The Good, the Bad, the Trans,** George Blackburn
12. **Should You Be Eating *More* Fat and *Fewer* Carbohydrates?** *Tufts University Health & Nutrition Letter*
13. **Sugar: What's the Harm?** *Consumer Reports on Health*
14. **Vitamin C: Foods Yes, Pills No** *Consumer Reports on Health*
15. **The Best D-Fense** *University of California, Berkeley Wellness Letter*
16. **Can Vitamin E Prevent Heart Disease?** Beth Fontenot
17. **A Disease of Too Much Iron,** Vincent J. Felitti
18. **National Academy of Sciences Introduces New Calcium Recommendations,** Luann Soliah
19. **Fiber: Strands of Protection** *Consumer Reports on Health*
20. **Food for Thought about Dietary Supplements,** Paul R. Thomas

Key Points to Consider

❖ Check out several labels from foods containing fats and oils that you eat frequently. Can you tell how much trans fat each contains? Determine the percentage of your average daily calories that is contributed by total fat and saturated fat. What do your calculations tell you about potential health risks?

❖ Are some nutrients more important than others in maintaining health? Support your answer.

❖ What claims are made for vitamins that you know to be false? Choose one that you aren't sure about and find the answer.

❖ Should fiber be designated a nutrient? Why or why not?

❖ How should one decide whether or not to take supplements? Are the issues involving supplements of a single vitamin or mineral any different than for multivitamins?

Links

www.dushkin.com/online/

10. **Dole 5 A Day: Nutrition, Fruits & Vegetables**
    http://www.dole5aday.com
11. **Food and Nutrition Information Center**
    http://www.nal.usda.gov/fnic/
12. **Nutrient Data Laboratory**
    http://www.nal.usda.gov/fnic/foodcomp/
13. **U.S. National Library of Medicine**
    http://www.nlm.nih.gov

These sites are annotated on pages 4 and 5.

Nutrients

> One cannot think well, love well, sleep well, if one has not dined well.
>
> — Virginia Woolf

Some basic aspects of nutrition have remained relatively unchanged for many years. The list of nutrients is one of these. Even the specific vitamins and minerals have undergone little revision. Nutrients that provide energy are still identified as carbohydrates, fats, and proteins. Fiber is not a nutrient because it is not essential to life, but it is included in this unit because it clearly performs crucial roles in preventing disease and in maintaining normal physiological functions.

Significant concepts about each nutrient, however, have changed, often dramatically. With today's available technology, the turnover in data from nutrition studies is so rapid that information may become obsolete even before it is printed and certainly before it is accepted or acted upon. Nor does the availability of voluminous data mean that theories are proven. Studies and experiments must be replicated, subjected to peer review, refined, and tried again. Conflicts in data, a common occurrence, must be resolved before any actionable conclusions can be reached. And, while epidemiological evidence indicates a relationship, this does not prove cause and effect. Years may pass and numerous other studies be concluded before any firm recommendations for either normal or therapeutic diets can be supported. Outside the scientific community this is frequently misunderstood, and sometimes every media report is taken as a new breakthrough.

Compounding the problem of formulating dietary recommendations is the fact that differences among human beings are truly remarkable; an average human being simply does not exist. Physiological variations preclude accurate predictions of exact nutrient amounts that cause the negative effects of either deficiency or excess. It is the task of the National Academy of Sciences to establish quantity recommendations that more than cover most people's actual requirements but are not high enough to cause harm. Until now, the result has been the periodically revised Recommended Dietary Allowance (RDAs). The more recent DRIs (Daily Recommended Intakes) represent a newer philosophy based on knowledge that nutrients function, not only in the prevention of deficiency symptoms, but preventively to minimize chronic diseases.

The articles in this unit were selected to reflect up-to-date thinking about nutrients that are currently newsworthy or about which we frequently have questions and/or misconceptions. The first article on fat is a good example. A significant health concern today is the consumption of trans-fatty acids, some of which are natural but most of which are formed in the process of hydrogenation. Current knowledge supports the concept that trans fats are as likely to promote disease as is saturated fat. Total fat remains a health issue, too. The average consumer gets between 33 and 34 percent of total calories from fat, somewhat above the current but controversial guideline of no more than 30 percent of calories. The body requires fat for health, yet many consumers try to avoid all or most fat. Americans remain very conscious of fat in food and eagerly look for new products claiming to be low- or no-fat items. The food industry is eager to oblige by offering hundreds of new products yearly. Typical consumers are unaware that lower fat items often have equal or more calories, and they remain paradoxically fanatical about super-premium ice creams and other fat-rich desserts.

Also in this unit you will find two articles on carbohydrates and one on fiber. If high carbohydrate intakes produce lower blood levels of HDL cholesterol in a quarter of our population, as one article reports, then more dietary fat and fewer carbohydrates may be appropriate for those who are vulnerable. In another article, new information suggests that consuming quantities of foods with a high glycemic index may, in fact, trigger the onset of diabetes in people who are insulin resistant. Everyone, however, appears to benefit from a diet high in fiber. But, even here, change is evident, for the newer studies support fiber's protective effect for the heart but find no advantage in preventing colon cancer. Most Americans would benefit from additional fiber to their diets by eating more fruits and vegetables, legumes, and whole grains.

Vitamins remain a topic of significant public interest, and several articles provide interesting insights. For many reasons, supplement sources of vitamins cannot replace a good diet. Vitamins in foods often are absorbed better, interfere with other nutrients less, and seldom reach toxic levels. Foods also contain fiber and other chemicals that are useful in fighting disease. "Food for Thought about Dietary Supplements" by Paul Thomas is crucial because it addresses the fallacious philosophical mindset that, while some amounts of vitamins are good for us, even more will provide benefit. This is not always the case. No doubt vitamins seemed to present "miraculous cures" when they were first discovered as the key to diseases such as pellagra, scurvy, and beri-beri. However, vitamins are not magic bullets but workhorses that go about their everyday jobs of making the body operate smoothly. In large doses they will have pharmacological effects, which may be beneficial but could be harmful as well.

As with vitamins, there is still more to learn about the functions of minerals. Most of us are concerned about obtaining enough dietary iron, but those with hereditary iron overload worry about absorbing too much. For people with this defective gene, it is important to diagnose the problem early.

Calcium recommendations have increased in hopes of preventing the costly and debilitating effects of osteoporosis, from which 28 million men and women in America now suffer. A national survey discovered that fewer than 50 percent of adults consume amounts adequate for maintaining bone health.

Consumers remain concerned about the healthful quality of their food, and scientists continue to work on ways to make it easier for consumers to get high-nutrient foods. One way is to develop "superveggies" such as varieties of onions, peppers, corn, and broccoli that are brimming with disease-fighting compounds. Another way is to fortify foods by adding nutrients that are not there naturally or exist only in smaller amounts. Calcium, for example, has been added to many products, from orange juice to the new Soft Calcium Chews introduced by Mead Johnson Nutritionals which allow chocoholics to get their calcium at the same time that they satisfy their cravings. A recent study seems to show the value of fortification. Indications are that folate deficiency has dropped from 22 percent of the population to under 2 percent as a result of mandatory fortification of enriched grain products with folic acid.

Fats: The Good, the Bad, the Trans

THE STORY

Fats are a dietary paradox. We need them for the essential fatty acids that keep cells healthy, and to help regulate important metabolic processes and transport certain vitamins throughout our bodies. But, for healthy hearts and arteries, we're encouraged to restrict fat to no more than 30 percent of our total daily calorie intake—or about 65 grams a day in a 2,000-calorie diet.

Scientists classify the fatty acids that make up the fat in food as saturated, monounsaturated or polyunsaturated, depending on the degree to which the molecules are saturated with hydrogen atoms (see box "Fat Facts"). While most of the fat we eat contains all three types, one usually predominates. Because saturated fat—the primary fat in red meat and many dairy products—raises blood levels of total and LDL (bad) cholesterol, we're advised to consume no more than 10 percent of total calories as saturated fat. At the other extreme, monounsaturated fats—found abundantly in canola and olive oil—are considered good fats because they lower LDL cholesterol without decreasing HDL (good) cholesterol. Polyunsaturated fats lower both LDL and HDL, but they are also a source of omega-3 fatty acids, which have purported heart-protective properties such as preventing blood clots.

Then there's a fourth category—trans fatty acids (TFAs)—commonly found in cooking oil, margarine, shortening and processed foods made with these ingredients. TFAs arise when hydrogen atoms are added to oils containing mono- or polyunsaturated fats. This so-called hydrogenation process converts liquid oils into a more solid form. Makers of packaged foods and fast-food restaurants use hydrogenated oils extensively because they enhance taste and texture and are more stable during frying and other high-temperature food processing. But a new study suggests that food high in trans fats is just as likely to raise LDL cholesterol as food high in saturated fat—a finding that corroborates results from several other recent studies on TFAs.

To further clarify the effect of TFAs on cholesterol, 36 adults with higher-than-normal blood-cholesterol levels went on five consecutive diets for 35 days each that differed only in trans-fat content. As a benchmark, participants also ate a sixth diet consisting of butter-rich foods (high in saturated fat but low in trans fat) for 35 days. Near the end of each 35-day diet, the Tufts University researchers measured the participants' blood-cholesterol levels.

In all the diets, the fat calories equaled the recommended 30 percent of total daily caloric consumption. Of the five TFA diets, the two diets with the lowest TFA content used liquid oil and semiliquid margarine and had less than 0.5 g of TFAs per 100 g of fat. The diet with the most TFAs included stick margarine and contained 20 g of trans fat. The TFA content of the two remaining diets—made from soft margarine and shortening—fell in the middle of that range. Except for water and noncaloric beverages, participants did not eat or drink anything but the food provided, and no one knew who was getting which diet.

When all the results were compared, the average total and LDL cholesterol levels were highest after people consumed the butter, stick-margarine and shortening diets. The liquid-oil, semiliquid-margarine and soft-margarine diets yielded the lowest average total and LDL levels. When compared with the butter diet, LDL levels from the soft-margarine diet averaged 9 percent lower, those from the semiliquid-margarine diet were 11 percent lower and those from the liquid-oil diet were 12 percent lower.

These findings, in the June 24 *New England Journal of Medicine,* seem straightforward, but how should you apply them to daily food choices?
—*The Editors*

THE PHYSICIAN'S PERSPECTIVE

George Blackburn, M.D.
Associate Editor

This study represents really great science, and for people with cholesterol concerns, it corroborates what other similar studies have found: Foods high in trans fat are just as potentially harmful as foods high in saturated fat. The results are especially believable because researchers carefully controlled the people's diets. This approach is far more reliable than the use of food questionnaires, a more common method of studying the effects of nutrients on health. In questionnaire-based studies, people try to remember what they ate and scientists estimate nutrient intake from those recollections.

But despite the tight dietary controls of this study, we can't generalize the findings to all people, because the participants already had higher-than-normal levels of total and LDL cholesterol. People with normal or low cholesterol levels might not respond the same way. Also, the study involved relatively few people and tracked their cholesterol for a short time. Thus, we don't know if the lower cholesterol levels associated with the low trans-fat diets will last

11. Fats: The Good, the Bad, the Trans

Fat Facts

Type of Fatty Acid	Primary Sources	State at Room Temperature	Effect on Cholesterol
MONOUNSATURATED	Canola* and olive oils; foods made from and prepared in them	Liquid	Lowers LDL; no effect on HDL
POLYUNSATURATED**	Soybean, safflower, corn, and cottonseed oils; foods made from and prepared in them	Liquid	Lowers both LDL and HDL
SATURATED	Animal fat from red meat, whole milk, and butter	Solid	Raises LDL and total cholesterol
TRANS	Partially hydrogenated vegetable oil used in cooking oil, margarine, shortening, and baked and fried foods	Semi-Solid	Raises LDL and total cholesterol

○ = Carbon atom
● = Hydrogen atom

*Many nutritionists consider canola oil the healthiest vegetable oil because it's low in saturated fat, high in monounsaturated fat, and has a moderate level of omega-3 polyunsaturated fat.
**Contain the omega-3 and omega-6 essential fatty acids that the human body can't make on its own.

Chart by Mary Tanner

and eventually translate into healthier hearts. A much larger study of more than 80,000 women two years ago found that those who ate less saturated fat and TFAs and more mono- and polyunsaturated fats substantially reduced their risk of heart disease, but that was a questionnaire-based study.

Even if we assume that trans fats are as unhealthy as saturated fats for most of us, it's not easy to determine how much trans fat we're eating. Food labels don't list trans-fat content. So the best you can do is make ballpark estimates by looking at the ingredient list. Any food that lists partially hydrogenated vegetable oil as one of the first three ingredients is likely to contain a significant amount of trans fat. Unfortunately, "partially" does not tell us how hydrogenated the oil is—and the more hydrogenated the oil, the more TFAs it contains.

Realize, too, that the majority of the TFAs consumed in the U.S. come from baked goods and food purchased in restaurants, the latter of which usually has no labeling whatsoever. So, when dining out, there's no way to assess whether the french fries you are considering with lunch are a less harmful indulgence than an apple-pie dessert.

In the near future, monitoring TFAs in food may become easier. The federal government is currently engaged in an every-five-year review of dietary guidelines and might issue recommendations for trans-fat intake. Of course, new guidelines would be of limited value without more informative labels, and thus the Food and Drug Administration has announced that it will eventually require trans-fat content on food labels.

For now, though, my advice is to place the findings from this new study in the context of generally healthy eating. First, concentrate on making the most of your daily calories that *don't* come from fat by eating a variety of whole foods, including at least five servings of fruit and vegetables a day. **When it comes to fat, stick to the 30 percent/10 percent rule for total and saturated fat, respectively, by cutting back on red meat and dairy products such as butter and whole milk. To control your trans-fat consumption, go easy on food made with hydrogenated vegetable oils and eliminate fried foods altogether. Also, choose soft or semiliquid margarine that lists liquid vegetable oil as the first ingredient and use non-hydrogenated oils for cooking.** With creative use of herbs and spices, it's entirely possible to enjoy satisfying meals that provide the healthy fats while limiting the unhealthy ones.

FOR MORE INFORMATION:

▼*International Food Information Council, 202-296-6547, ificinfo.health.org*

Should You Be Eating *More* Fat and *Fewer* Carbohydrates?

If you have a condition called syndrome X, too many carbohydrates could prove bad for your heart

You've cut out some of the saturated fat found in foods like burgers, whole milk, and cakes and cookies and now fill up on more high-carbohydrate fare like bread and pasta. But rather than going for an extra helping of spaghetti, would you be doing your heart better by having a little extra fatty salad dressing instead? Or a handful of fatty nuts instead of a bagel? As bizarre as it may sound, it goes right to the heart of a fierce debate raging between nutrition and heart disease experts entrenched in opposing camps.

On one hand are those who argue that while the mono- and polyunsaturated fats in foods like salad dressing and nuts don't raise "bad" LDL-cholesterol in the blood the way that saturated fats do, people should still be limiting them. The reason, they say, is that unsaturated fats, just like saturated ones, supply more than twice as many calories as carbohydrates. And that, in turn, contributes to overweight, which in itself raises blood cholesterol and increases the risk for heart disease.

But **those who argue in favor of poly- and monounsaturated fats over starchy foods and other high-carbohydrate choices say that in an estimated 25 percent of the population, piling on carbohydrates lowers "good" HDL-cholesterol.** It also raises triglycerides (fats in the blood that are now thought to raise heart disease risk on their own); renders LDL-cholesterol even more harmful by making the LDL particles smaller and heavier (and therefore more likely to harm arteries); increases the risk for high blood pressure; and makes the blood more likely to form obstructive clots.

The cluster of problems is known as syndrome X, a term coined in 1988 by Stanford University researcher Gerald Reaven, MD. It occurs in people who are hyperinsulinemic, that is, who secrete too much of the hormone insulin. Carbohydrate-rich foods cause the highest spikes in their insulin levels. That's because after carbohydrates are eaten and broken down into blood sugar, or glucose, insulin is needed to get the glucose out of the bloodstream and into all the body's tissues, where it's used as fuel.

In the 75 percent of the population who aren't hyperinsulinemic, eating a lot of carbohydrate isn't a problem. Their bodies' tissues are insulin-sensitive, meaning they "allow" blood sugar to enter even with the secretion of relatively small amounts of insulin. But in those afflicted with hyperinsulinemia, the pancreas must secrete large amounts of insulin to move sugar out of the blood. The more insulin secreted, the worse the untoward effects. (In some people, hyperinsulinemia is a precursor to diabetes.)

Consider a study on a small group of postmenopausal women with an average age of 66 who appeared to be hyperinsulinemic. For three weeks, Dr. Reaven and colleagues put them on an eating plan that contained 60 percent of calories as carbohydrate and 25 percent as fat. For another three weeks, they ate a diet containing only 40 percent of calories as carbohydrate and 45 percent as fat (protein remained constant at 15 percent of total calories). Both diets had the same number of calories.

For the higher-fat diet, the researchers trimmed the women's carbohydrates and upped their fat consumption by serving them, for instance, peanut butter at breakfast rather than bread. The women also received a little more margarine and salad dressing and a little less potato at dinner.

The result: on the higher-fat regimen, they ended up with an average triglyceride level of just 114 milligrams per deciliter of blood. (Research suggests that the closer to 100 the triglyceride level, the better for the heart. Levels below 100 are ideal.) But they had a significantly higher level of 174 on the diet that was higher in carbohydrates. The higher-fat diet also allowed the women to maintain better "good" HDL-cholesterol levels. But presumably because neither diet had much in the way of saturated fat, "bad" LDL-cholesterol levels did not differ from one eating plan to the other.

12. Should You Be Eating *More* Fat and *Fewer* Carbohydrates?

Before you start eating more fat...

Not all researchers are convinced that higher-fat regimens should be recommended for the public at large. They argue that **while people who are *fed* a high-fat diet don't have to worry about overdoing it on calories, men and women *on their own* can easily go calorically overboard** on a high-fat diet—and become overweight—because of the fact that fat has nine calories per gram and carbohydrate, only four. And overweight people, in addition to having higher levels of LDL-cholesterol than others, are much more prone to being afflicted with syndrome X. In fact, the condition usually doesn't manifest itself in someone unless he or she is overweight. Excess weight indirectly leads to the release of more insulin.

Consider that the women in the study, while not obese, were decidedly overweight. The average weight of a woman who was, say, five feet, four inches tall was 157 pounds. Desirable weight for a woman that height is fewer than 145 pounds.

Ernst Schaefer, MD, a heart disease researcher who heads the Lipid Metabolism Laboratory at Tufts, is one of those who firmly believes that advising people to eschew carbohydrates for fat would end up doing more harm than good. He points to research which shows that when people migrate from countries where the diet is low in fat to the U.S., where the diet tends to be relatively fatty, weight—and heart disease deaths—rise substantially.

Because of evidence like that, Dr. Schaefer believes that Americans should try to lower their *total* fat intake, not just their intake of saturated fat. He acknowledges that lower-fat diets automatically raise the proportion of carbohydrates someone consumes, which could be a problem for people with syndrome X. But, he says, the weight kept off—or taken off—with reduced-fat diets will attenuate the effects of syndrome X much better than eating a high-fat, lower-carbohydrate diet without any attendant weight loss.

As proof, he points out that the traditional Japanese diet is extremely high in carbohydrates, with rice being a staple—yet people who follow it are protected from heart disease, largely because they remain quite thin. In addition, when University of California researcher Dean Ornish, MD, put people on extremely low-fat, low-calorie, high-carbohydrate diets in which fully 70 to 75 percent of calories came from carbohydrate-rich foods, there was actually a reversal in the progression of their heart disease—no doubt due in part to the fact that they lost an average of 22 pounds in a year's time.

Those on the other side of the fence agree with Dr. Schaefer that losing, or keeping off, excess weight mitigates the effects of syndrome X much more powerfully than eating a diet relatively high in mono- and poly-unsaturated fats and relatively low in carbohydrates. But, they argue, it is far from proven that eating low-fat foods automatically helps Americans keep trimmer. For instance, **Walter Willett, MD, head of nutrition at the Harvard University School of Public Health, points to the fact that there has been a proliferation of reduced-fat cakes, cookies, ice cream, luncheon meats, salad dressings, and other foods without a national slimming down.** In fact, Americans are only getting heavier.

The reason, at least to some degree, is that Americans have come to equate low-fat with low-calorie, but many of these products have as many—or more—calories than their full-fat counterparts. Worse still, Dr. Willett notes, in many items like reduced-fat cakes and cookies, the calorie count remains high because when fat is taken out, carbohydrates such as sugar and other sweeteners replace it, which only intensifies insulin secretion in people with syndrome X and thereby worsens their condition.

It is not even clear that people who follow a diet with foods *naturally* low in fat, such as fruits, vegetables, and grains, will lose substantial amounts of weight over the long term. Perhaps people just lose weight at first and then the weight loss tapers off. Long-term data do not exist to settle the issue.

All of which begs the question of just what a person is supposed to do. Fortunately, there is actually much more overlap between the two camps than disagreement. But how to proceed depends largely on your own particular situation.

A personalized approach to keeping your heart healthy

Before you make a decision on whether to follow a low-fat diet with lots of carbohydrates or a diet higher in poly- and monounsaturated fats with fewer carbohydrates, **you need to get some results from your physical at the doctor's office.** Your blood pressure will be measured, and the doctor will also withdraw a little of your blood after an overnight fast. From that blood sample a lab can determine your level of LDL-cholesterol, HDL-cholesterol, triglycerides, blood sugar, and insulin. If your blood pressure is fine and your blood levels of these substances are within normal levels, chances are you don't need to worry much about the proportion of fats or carbohydrates you eat.

Here are the normal levels:

- Blood pressure: less than 140/90
- LDL-cholesterol: less than 160 (less than 130 if you already have two other risk factors for heart disease, such as being a male over age 45, a woman over 55, or overweight)
- HDL-cholesterol: at least 35, preferably 60 or higher
- triglycerides: less than 200, preferably less than 100
- blood sugar: less than 110

The more "out of range" you are on LDL-cholesterol (which is not related to syndrome X), the more important it is to cut back on foods high in saturated fat, which include not just burgers and full-fat dairy products like cheese and premium ice cream but also steaks, roasts, doughnuts, cookies, other pastries, and eggs. The doughnuts and other sweets not only have saturated fat, they also often contain substances called trans fatty acids, which are likely to raise LDL-cholesterol just as much as saturated fat does. And the more LDL-cholesterol in your arteries, the more likely they are to become clogged.

People with high LDL-cholesterol should also lose excess weight, if necessary. Extra pounds raise the concentration of LDL particles.

The more "out of range" you are on all the other parameters, the more likely you are to have syndrome X. Syndrome X is not an all-or-nothing condition; it varies by degree, so some people who have it are "off" on certain measurements but not others.

Lifestyle changes specific to syndrome X:

■ If you are overweight, try to lose some excess poundage. Granted, this is easy to say and hard to do, but Stanford's Dr. Reaven estimates that fully 25 percent of the detrimental effects of syndrome X arising from hyperinsulinemia are attributable to overweight. The good news: losing even just 10 to 15 percent of body weight is enough for some people to significantly blunt syndrome X's effects. It makes their tissues more insulin sensitive, thereby requiring less insulin to be secreted. That means that a five-foot, four-inch woman with syndrome X who weighs 157 pounds can substantially improve her health parameters by getting down to 140 pounds; she doesn't need to achieve, say, 120 pounds for highly beneficial results.

Note: Research suggests, but doesn't prove, that it's easier for most people to lose weight on a diet that's high in carbohydrates and relatively low in fat. As long as significant weight loss occurs, a high-carbohydrate diet should not cause further harm to people with syndrome X. But people with syndrome X might not want to go on a very high-carbohydrate, very low-fat diet that has only about 15 percent of calories as fat. Since carbohydrates do cause higher-than-normal spikes in their insulin levels, they should consider a more moderately reduced-fat diet that has at least 20 percent of calories as fat, if not more. Either way, losing weight is more a matter of reducing *calories* by keeping portion sizes moderate rather than simply choosing anything that has a "low-fat" burst on the label.

■ If you're sedentary, engage in some vigorous physical activity, perhaps for 30 minutes a day, three to five times a week. A sedentary lifestyle, just like excess weight, Dr. Reaven says, is responsible for about 25 percent of the effects of syndrome X.

■ If you're already a healthy weight and moderately active and your blood tests still indicate that you have syndrome X, eat a little less in the way of carbohydrates and a little more poly- and monounsaturated fats. Admittedly, that could be hard to do without weight gain. Just a handful of nuts could contain a couple of hundred calories. A little extra oil in your stir-fry or margarine on your toast could add 100 calories or more here and there, too. Thus, **as you remove carbohydrates from the diet, be sparing with the amount of fats you add back in.**

And try to remove carbohydrates that are high in sugar and relatively low in nutrients, such as cakes, cookies, and the like (including the reduced-fat varieties). *Don't* remove high-carbohydrate vegetables and fruits. "You should have most of your calories from carbohydrates, no matter what kind of diet" you're on, Harvard's Dr. Willett says. And he and others agree that your high-carbohydrate choices should be items that are naturally low in fact, including beans, vegetables, and fruits.

As far as grains, whole grains are better than refined grains like those in pasta, white bread, and white rice, Drs. Schaefer and Willett say. The fiber they contain may help to slow the rush of sugar into the blood during digestion—and consequently blunt the flow of insulin.

Sugar: What's the harm?

Critics swarm to the sweetener like flies to a sugar bowl. We'll sift through the charges.

In 1986, the Food and Drug Administration said that sugar consumption in the U.S. had probably peaked: Sugar makers supposedly couldn't boost production, and consumers—who were getting an average of 11 percent of their daily calories from added sugar—supposedly couldn't gobble up any more.

But the average sugar intake has soared to about 18 percent of calories since then. The 20 teaspoons of sugar that the typical American now consumes each day—primarily from commercially prepared food, snacks, and drinks—is approximately twice the upper limit recommended in the USDA's familiar food pyramid. (Artificial sweeteners are also being consumed in record amounts—see "Sweet Substitutes".)

At the time, the government had declared that sugar posed no health risks other than tooth decay. Concerned about the jump in sugar intake, a growing number of researchers—as well as a few self-styled diet gurus—have taken a new look at sugar's safety. Here's the latest on the sweet stuff.

Insulin resistance: The newest concern

The most serious—and the most controversial—charges against sugar stem from three recent Harvard studies, involving a total of more than 100,000 people, which have resurrected the notion that sugar increases the risk of developing diabetes and possibly of having a heart attack. The three studies assessed consumption of foods that have a high "glycemic index," a measure of how fast the body converts the carbohydrates (sugars and starches) in those foods into sugar in the blood. (High-glycemic foods include most sugary items as well as refined-grain products, such as white bread, regular pasta, and white rice. In contrast, whole grains and most fruits and vegetables have a low glycemic index.) Two of those studies linked consuming a diet rich in high-glycemic foods with a roughly 40 percent rise in the risk of diabetes; the third study, not yet published, linked that diet with an increased heart-attack risk in women.

The Harvard researchers suspect that those effects may be limited to the 10 to 25 percent of people who are already at risk for developing diabetes due to a condition called insulin resistance; those people need unusually large amounts of the hormone insulin to handle the sugar entering the bloodstream. When those insulin-resistant individuals consume large amounts of foods with a high glycemic index, according to one theory, the pancreas has to work even harder than usual to produce enough insulin to control the repeated sharp rises in the blood-sugar level. That may eventually exhaust the pancreas, leading to a chronically elevated blood-sugar level—in other words, diabetes.

In addition, insulin-resistant individuals tend to have both a high level of triglycerides (a potentially artery-clogging type of fat in the blood) and a low level of HDL cholesterol, the "good," artery-clearing kind. Some evidence suggests that meals with a high glycemic index are particularly bad for triglyceride and HDL levels, and may thus increase the risk of heart attack in those people.

Many researchers remain skeptical about that theory, due to the difficulty of untangling the effects of high-glycemic foods from the many other factors that contribute to diabetes and coronary disease. And since all carbohydrates are eventually converted to sugar in the blood and tend to worsen both HDL and triglyceride levels, the skeptics still think the total amount of carbohydrates consumed by people with diabetes or insulin resistance is far more important than whether those carbohydrates tend to have a high or low glycemic index.

But virtually all researchers agree on one thing: Sugar provides only empty calories with no other nutritional value and can thus crowd important nutrients out of the diet. So one simple, healthful way for diabetic or insulin-resistant individuals to limit their total carbohydrate consumption is to cut back on sugar. If that doesn't help, refined-grain products should be the next items to go. (In addition, those individuals should avoid heavy consumption of alcoholic beverages, which also tend to worsen triglyceride and HDL levels.) The *possibility* that high-glycemic foods may increase the risk of diabetes in insulin-resistant people should provide further incentive for those people to limit their intake of high-glycemic foods, particularly sugar.

But most people don't know they may be insulin resistant unless they have a strong family history of diabetes, they develop unfavorable triglyceride and HDL levels, or they develop diabetes itself. So the advice to eat a relatively low-glycemic, low-fat diet, including lots of produce and whole grains, seems sensible for everyone—particularly since that's the cornerstone of a healthy diet anyway.

Weight gain: Sugar plays the heavy

The best-selling diet book "Sugar Busters!" argues that the jump in insulin sparked by consuming sugar and other foods with a high glycemic index causes calories to be stored in the body as fat rather than burned as energy. But that claim makes little biological sense. And several trials have shown that weight changes due to diet depend entirely on how many total calories are consumed, not where those calories come from—even in people who are insulin-resistant.

However, sugar may indeed contribute to America's swelling weight problem in another way. Some researchers believe that calories from fat are more fattening than calories that come from other foods. That's partly because some evidence has suggested that the body may store those fat calories more readily than it stores calories from protein or carbohydrates. But the bulk of the evidence still indicates that the total calorie intake, not the calories' source, is what really counts.

And consuming lots of sugar certainly will supply lots of calories. For example, drinking three 12-ounce cans of regular soda rather than water would provide an extra 480 calories. The average person who did that every day, without eating less or exercising more, would gain roughly a pound a week.

In addition, sugar and fat often go together in many foods. Such items—cakes, cookies, ice cream, candy bars, and the like—tend to be crawling with calories. Diet studies suggest that overindulgence in such treats may indeed

Is 'natural' better than white?

Many people believe that white table sugar is somehow worse for you than "natural" sweeteners like brown sugar, corn syrup, fruit sugar, honey, or maple syrup. But apart from their taste and physical form, all those sweeteners, including table sugar, are virtually indistinguishable.

Table sugar, or sucrose, is actually a compound of two simpler sugars, glucose and fructose. All other sweeteners contain either sucrose, fructose, glucose, or some combination of those sugars.

All sweeteners—except blackstrap molasses, which contains calcium, iron, and other nutrients—essentially supply nothing but nutritionally empty calories. (Concentrated fruit juices do contain some vitamins and minerals, but the tiny amount used in juice-sweetened cookies and other products has no significant nutritional value.)

Further, honey and syrups are more concentrated than granulated sugar, so they pack more calories per teaspoon. Syrups are also stickier than granulated sugars and thus potentially worse for the teeth.

Pure fructose does have a somewhat lower glycemic index than sucrose or glucose, meaning it raises the blood-sugar level more gradually (see story). But that difference is modest and has little practical significance. More important, foods are rarely sweetened with pure fructose. The most common sources of that sugar—concentrated fruit juice, honey, and high-fructose corn syrup—typically contain nearly the same proportions of glucose and fructose as sucrose does.

be a major cause of obesity in American women.

But choosing sweets that were manufactured to have little or no fat won't necessarily help either—and might actually set you back. No-fat and low-fat items often contain so much extra sugar that they end up packing nearly the same number of calories as the original. Again, the healthiest way to cut calories is to follow a diet high in produce and whole grains and low in sweets and fat.

Cavities: Another charge with teeth

There's no controversy here: Consuming sugar definitely can promote tooth decay. While fluoride, plastic sealants for children's teeth, and improved oral hygiene have all sharply cut the incidence of cavities, it's still important to protect your teeth by watching what you eat—and when you eat it.

The bacteria that are found in plaque, the sticky film that tends to accumulate on the teeth, can convert all types of carbohydrates—which include starches as well as sugars—into tooth-dissolving acid. Since the plaque bacteria break down sugar faster than they break down starch, sweets do pose a special risk of promoting cavities. Nevertheless, starch can be equally harmful if it lingers on the teeth long enough to get broken down by the plaque bacteria. In fact, starch tends to stick to the teeth longer than even the sugar in sticky treats like caramel. So the worst enamel eaters are probably sweet baked goods like cookies and cakes, which tend to linger longer on the teeth *and* contain both sugar and starch.

To minimize the cavity risk, it's wise to consume carbohydrates mainly with meals. That way, the accompanying foods will stimulate the secretion of saliva, which helps neutralize the plaque acids and wash away or dissolve food particles and sugar. (Chewing sugarless gum after eating can serve the same purpose.) For between-meal snacks, choose fruit or raw vegetables.

Sweet substitutes

The quest for good-tasting, noncaloric substitutes for sugar sweeteners has stimulated sales of a potent sweetener derived from a South American shrub called stevia. The Food and Drug Administration says stevia can't be sold as a food or used to manufacture food, since its safety is unknown. But a legal loophole lets companies market stevia as a "dietary supplement," provided they don't directly encourage its uses as a food. At least one company, Now Foods, sells stevia powder in what look like standard sugar packets—a practice that may be stretching the FDA rule.

Of course, would-be dieters can choose from an array of artificial sweeteners that do have the FDA's blessing. Those products can help control your caloric intake, provided they don't serve as an excuse to indulge in other high-calorie treats. And unlike sugar, the substitutes generally don't affect the blood-sugar level—a big plus for people with diabetes—and don't promote cavities; in fact, some substitutes may actually retard cavities. Here's a rundown on the currently available alternatives:

■ **Sucralose** *(Splenda)*. The newest artificial sweetener on the market, sucralose is the only one that's made from sugar. It's chemically altered so it slips undigested through the intestinal tract, but apparently it still tastes like sugar and poses no known health risks. Sucralose is now making its debut in beverages such as *Diet RC Cola* and *Diet Very-Fine* juice drinks. Tabletop packets should follow soon, and sucralose could eventually show up in everything from baked goods to chewing gum.

■ **Saccharin** *(Sweet 'N Low)*. In 1977, the Food and Drug Administration proposed banning saccharin because animal studies suggested a cancer risk. Pressured by the artificial-sweetener industry, Congress indefinitely suspended the proposed ban and mandated a warning label instead. In 1991, the FDA quietly withdrew its proposed ban; the warning label remains.

■ **Aspartame** *(Equal, NutraSweet)*. This sugar substitute appears to be safe except in people who have the inherited disorder known as phenylketonuria (PKU), which affects roughly 1 in 15,000 Americans. (Afflicted individuals must limit their intake of the amino acid phenylalanine, a component of aspartame.) But don't cook with aspartame, since heat tends to destroy the sweetness of the product sold in stores.

■ **Acesulfame potassium** *(Sunette)*. Also known as ace-K, it's used almost exclusively in soft drinks (notably *Pepsi One*). Like sucralose, it poses no known health hazards.

■ **Sorbitol and xylitol.** These sugar alcohols are not really artificial sweeteners, but they're often used as sucrose substitutes, in part because they contain far fewer calories and have hardly any effect on the blood-sugar level. Sugar alcohols are used particularly often in products such as sugarless gum, mints, and toothpaste, since they don't promote tooth decay. In fact, some evidence suggests that xylitol may actually help prevent cavities—though the minimum amount needed to fight decay is not known.

Most raw fruits contain relatively little sugar and aren't very sticky. The exceptions are bananas, which are loaded with sugar, and dried fruits, which are sugary *and* sticky.

Low blood sugar: Not to worry

Some people believe that increased consumption of sugar can trigger symptoms of hypoglycemia, or low blood sugar, such as sweating, trembling, rapid heartbeat, and hunger. It's true that the extra insulin secreted to handle an influx of sugar can push some individuals' blood-sugar level below normal. But such modest drops in blood sugar will spark symptoms only in certain prediabetic individuals who have a condition called reactive hypoglycemia. In everyone else, the symptoms have some other cause, such as panic attacks or an overactive thyroid gland. People who suspect hypoglycemia should ask their physician to determine whether their symptoms do, in fact, coincide with a blood-sugar slump.

Hyperactivity: Sugar absolved

The number of children with attention deficit disorder, or hyperactivity, seems to have soared in recent years. And the simultaneous rise in kids' sugar consumption seems to support the common belief that sugar makes kids "bounce off the walls." But the apparent epidemic of overactivity almost surely stems solely from increased diagnosis, due to heightened awareness of the problem and relaxed diagnostic criteria. And the already strong evidence absolving sugar has gotten even stronger.

In the most recent study, researchers from Vanderbilt University pooled the results of 16 clinical trials where kids ate meals prepared either with lots of sugar or with artificial sweeteners. The researchers found no evidence of hyperactivity—in behavior or mental sharpness—after the high-sugar meals. In the trials that included parents' evaluations of their kids, even they couldn't tell the difference.

If anything, sugar may have the opposite effect. In one study, kids fed a high-sugar diet actually learned slightly faster and showed slightly less physical speed and agility than other kids. The authors concluded that sugar tends to *relax* children slightly. At least half a dozen other trials have suggested that meals high in carbohydrates, including sugar, have that mellowing effect, perhaps because they boost levels of serotonin, a brain chemical that regulates mood.

Quick energy: Usually not

Many people assume that a shot of sugar right before or during a workout will provide a burst of energy by boosting their blood-sugar level. But the body gets its energy mainly from a stored form of glucose in the muscles and liver—not from sugar circulating in the blood—during the first hour or two of vigorous exercise. Consuming carbohydrates—not necessarily sugar—a few hours before a workout should provide all the stored glucose that most exercisers need. Only people doing prolonged, extremely vigorous exercise, like a marathon or a soccer game, may benefit from an immediate sugar fix.

Summing up

Contrary to popular belief, sugar does not make kids hyperactive, seldom causes problems with low blood-sugar, and won't provide quick energy for the average exerciser. But other claims about the sweetener may have more substance:

Sugar provides nothing but empty calories and tends to crowd other nutrients out of the diet. It promotes tooth decay and can contribute to weight gain. Whether sugar and other high-glycemic foods increase the risk of developing diabetes or having a heart attack in the insulin-resistant minority is not clear. But even the possibility adds another reason for everyone to eat less sugar and more fruits, vegetables, and whole grains.

Vitamin C: Foods yes, pills no

Megadose supplements may be worse than worthless. But a high-C diet is a different story.

In his popular web site, best-selling author and alternative-health guru Andrew Weil, M.D., recommends taking a daily minimum of 2,000 milligrams of vitamin C—33 times higher than the government's recommended intake—to fight cancer and bolster immunity. Weil is only the latest in a long succession of vitamin-C enthusiasts, including the late Nobel laureate Linus Pauling, who've pushed megadoses of the vitamin.

There's little evidence to support that recommendation. In fact, a pivotal study from the National Institutes of Health has shown that high doses of vitamin C are generally useless, since the body absorbs only a limited amount. Other research suggests that excessive vitamin C may be harmful.

But the same NIH study that debunked megadoses of the vitamin demonstrated that smaller doses, readily obtainable from a healthy diet, can make a big difference in how much vitamin C reaches the blood and other tissues. The NIH findings may help explain the results of large studies on vitamin C and disease risk: While high-dose pills appear to offer little protection, a *diet* rich in the vitamin may indeed help ward off a number of deadly or disabling illnesses—including coronary heart disease and cancer. This report will help you draw the line between enough and too much vitamin C.

The absorbing facts

The NIH study graphically demonstrated just how tightly the body limits the amount of vitamin C it retains. The researchers recruited seven young men to live in a hospital for four to six months, where they were fed a controlled diet that supplied all necessary nutrients except vitamin C. After the diet had depleted their bodies of the vitamin, the volunteers took progressively larger daily doses of supplementary vitamin C, increasing from 30 to 2,500 milligrams (mg).

Blood levels of vitamin C rose quickly at first, from 30 percent saturation at 60 mg—the currently recommended intake—to 72 percent saturation at 100 mg—the amount in an 8-ounce glass of orange juice—to 86 percent saturation at 200 mg. Higher doses yielded only marginal increases—to 91 percent saturation at 400 mg and total saturation at 1,000 mg. Those increases probably offer little or no significant benefit, particularly since some of the body's tissues are already saturated at doses lower than 200 mg.

Based on those findings, the researchers urged the National Academy of Sciences to raise the recommended daily intake of vitamin C from 60 to 200 mg. While that's more than most people consume, you can readily get that much from a healthy diet.

Studies suggest modest amounts of vitamin C may help prevent cancer.

Food, pills, and disease

The NIH study strongly suggests that the body can't utilize more than a moderate amount of vitamin C. Studies of the vitamin's effect on disease risk support that conclusion, by showing protection mainly at the amounts supplied by diet rather than by big supplements.

■ **Coronary disease.** Vitamin C is an antioxidant. So it theoretically should help prevent the oxidation, or chemical damage, that causes the "bad" LDL cholesterol to stick to the artery walls. Observational studies suggest that the vitamin may further protect the heart by boosting blood levels of the "good" HDL cholesterol. Several clinical trials, which pitted vitamin-C pills against a placebo, have seemingly failed to confirm that benefit. But when Tufts University researchers reanalyzed the results of one trial, they found that the vitamin did boost HDL in the many volunteers whose blood was less than 70 percent saturated with vitamin C.

Observational studies of vitamin C and actual coronary disease, rather than just cholesterol levels, suggest a similar effect. Two Harvard studies of health professionals, who typically consumed lots of the vitamin in their diet, failed to find any benefit. But research in other populations with a lower average intake has generally been positive. In a study of some 2,400 Finnish women, for example, those who consumed the most vitamin C—at least 90 mg a day—had only half the coronary mortality of those who consumed 60 mg or less. Another study, of nearly 7,000 Americans, found that those with a low or low-normal blood level of the vitamin had one-third more cardiovascular deaths than those whose blood was nearly saturated.

■ **Cancer.** In theory, vitamin C may help protect against cancer by inhibiting oxidation, which can damage the DNA and turn normal cells cancerous. Observational research suggests that the vitamin may indeed provide protection—and that modest doses will generally do the trick. According to one recent review, 36 of 48 observational studies have shown that people who get the most vitamin C in their diet are less susceptible to cancer—particularly of the gastrointestinal and respiratory tracts—than those who consume the least. But only 8 of 24 studies have suggested that taking supplements may reduce the risk. One possible explanation: Those who didn't take supplements were already getting enough of the vitamin, on average, to help ward off the disease.

Vitamin C's ability to fight oxidation may be particularly useful in the stomach, where the ulcer bacterium *Heliobacter pylori* produces oxidizing molecules known as free radicals. In addition, vitamin C helps neutralize potentially cancer-causing nitrates in the diet. Those actions of vitamin C may help explain why 14 of 16 observational studies have linked a high dietary intake of the vitamin with a lowered risk of stomach cancer.

■ **Other diseases.** In theory, oxidation can damage both the retina and the lens of the eye, causing macular degeneration and cataracts, respectively. To ward off such damage, the lens normally contains high concentrations of antioxidants, including vitamin C; the retina also contains some of the vitamin. Observational research on whether vitamin C helps prevent either disease has yielded mixed results. But most of the positive studies involved amounts of the vitamin obtainable from diet alone.

VITAMIN C IN FRUITS AND VEGETABLES [1]	
Food	Vitamin C (mg)
FRUITS	
Strawberries (7 medium)	127
Orange, California navel (1)	80
Cantaloupe (¼)	58
Kiwi (1)	57
Black currants (¼ cup)	51
Grapefruit, pink or red (½)	47
Papaya (¼)	47
Watermelon (1 slice)	46
Mango (½)	29
Star fruit (carambola) (1)	27
VEGETABLES [2]	
Bell peppers, sweet red, raw (½ cup)	95
Chili peppers, red, raw (¼ cup)	91
Broccoli (½ cup)	62
Brussels sprouts (½ cup)	48
Bell peppers, sweet green, raw (½ cup)	45
Cauliflower (½ cup)	28
Sweet potato, baked (1 medium)	28
Kale (½ cup)	27
Potato, baked (1 large)	26
Avocado, Florida, raw (1)	24
Tomato, raw (1 medium)	24
Spaghetti sauce, marinara (½ cup)	21
JUICES (6 fl oz)	
Orange	93
Grapefruit	70
Tomato	34
Pineapple	20

[1] Table lists fruits and vegetables containing at least 20 mg of vitamin C.
[2] Cooked, unless otherwise specified.

The evidence for vitamin C's protective benefits is even weaker for arthritis, asthma, and cognitive impairment than for eye disease. But again, the few supporting studies involved food, not supplements.

It's possible, of course, that at least some of vitamin C's apparent benefits stem from other components of the vitamin-rich foods. For example, fruits and vegetables, the best sources of the vitamin, are loaded with other potentially disease-fighting compounds (see our June report). But whether the likely benefit stems from vitamin C, other substances, or both, the bottom line is the same: It helps to eat plenty of foods rich in the vitamin.

High-dose harm

Large doses of supplementary vitamin C may have unpleasant or harmful effects, in part because the excess amount pours into the kidneys and intestines for elimination. For example, high doses can cause flatulence and diarrhea. More important, doses over 1,000 mg increase the urinary concentration of uric acid and oxalate, the building blocks of kidney stones. So high-dose supplements theoretically could increase the risk of stones in susceptible individuals.

Some evidence has raised the possibility that high doses of vitamin C might sometimes help cause rather than prevent disease. In the most alarming study, published last year in the journal Nature, researchers reported that vitamin C changed from an antioxidant to a *pro*-oxidant—and started damaging cells—at doses as low as 500 mg a day. Other scientists subsequently spotted major flaws in that study, and most other research has discounted the vitamin's pro-oxidant potential in ordinary circumstances.

However, test-tube studies suggest that vitamin C may still promote oxidation when it's exposed to high levels of iron. In a recent clinical trial, volunteers who started with a high blood level of vitamin C and then took iron supplements and vitamin-C pills developed white-blood-cell damage, apparently due to oxidation. Other research has shown that the vitamin can become a pro-oxidant in people who have a genetic disorder that causes excessive iron buildup.

Summing up

The National Academy of Sciences has pegged the recommended daily intake of vitamin C at 60 mg, mainly because that's more than enough to prevent scurvy, the vitamin-C-deficiency disease. But it's not enough to maintain even a moderate blood level of the vitamin—or to reduce the risk of other, more common diseases.

Eating the widely recommended five to nine daily servings of fruits and vegetables will supply about 200 to 350 mg of the vitamin. That should almost completely saturate the blood—and may help ward off coronary disease, cancer, cataracts, and possibly arthritis, asthma, cognitive impairment, and macular degeneration. It will also supply a host of other potentially disease-fighting compounds. For a list of fruits and vegetables that are high in vitamin C, see the table at right.

Taking higher doses of vitamin C has no known benefit—including any effect on the common cold (see box below). And it may cause intestinal side effects, kidney stones, and possibly a harmful interaction with high levels of iron.

C is not for colds

Just about every victim of the common cold has heard this confident advice from some well-meaning friend: "Take loads of vitamin C." If you point out that it hasn't helped you in the past, you're likely to hear some variation on this stock response: "You took only 1,000 milligrams? Linus Pauling recommended 20,000."

There's a more likely reason why the pills haven't helped: They simply don't work.

C for protection?

Since Pauling first lionized megadoses of vitamin C in the late 1960s, researchers have conducted more than 20 clinical trials of the pills' supposed cold-shielding powers. Not one of those trials found that supplements reduced the chance of catching cold.

By searching for flaws in those studies, Finnish researcher Harri Hemila, Ph.D., has almost single-handedly kept the controversy alive. Even Hemila now acknowledges that the evidence fails to show that vitamin C can prevent colds in the average person. He does claim, based on analyses of a few studies, that the vitamin may help people who have a low level to start with. If Pauling's approach does work, Hemila concludes, it's probably "not due to the high dosage per se, but rather to the correction of a marginal deficiency."

While the evidence for even that point is weak, at least it's somewhat consistent with other research on vitamin C. That evidence shows that the body can't absorb high doses of the vitamin. And it suggests that while modest amounts of vitamin C—particularly from food—may help ward off several diseases, higher amounts offer no additional protection (see story).

C for cure?

A few studies have suggested that vitamin C may slightly reduce the severity of cold symptoms. But most of the research shows no such benefit. The evidence that vitamin C affects the *duration* of colds—a far more objective, reliable measurement than symptoms—is even weaker. When researchers analyzed the combined results of the eight best trials, they concluded that vitamin C does not speed recovery from colds. Those findings, combined with the similarly negative evidence on prevention, suggest that popping vitamin-C pills to cure a cold is a waste of time and money.

In theory, it's still possible that modest doses of vitamin C might help people who have a borderline deficiency of the vitamin. But while there is a smidgen of evidence to support that notion for prevention, there's no such evidence for treatment.

The best D-fense

Does vitamin D, or the lack of it, have anything to do with breast cancer? With prostate cancer? An interesting new theory says it may. Mortality rates for both cancers are lower in regions where sunlight is most plentiful. Since sunlight is responsible for producing vitamin D in the human body, researchers have wondered if this could be the connection. Some test-tube studies have shown that vitamin D inhibits the growth of cancer cells, including those in the breast and prostate.

Last year a research team at the Northern California Cancer Center analyzed statistics from a survey of a large group of American women and found that women with higher sun exposure and those with a high dietary intake of vitamin D had a lower risk of breast cancer. This was backed up by a study from the University of North Carolina at Chapel Hill.

Any news that might help unravel cancer mysteries is welcome, but this is very preliminary research. Some evidence also points to a link between vitamin D and reduced risk of colon cancer. But all this does not mean you should move south or start sunbathing.

What is this thing called vitamin D?

Unique among the vitamins, vitamin D is a hormone, and like other hormones it is manufactured in the body. It helps the body utilize calcium and phosphorus and builds bones and teeth. Like many other nutrients, it probably has a beneficial effect on the immune system. You don't actually need to consume vitamin D, provided you get a minimal amount of sunlight, which causes your skin cells to manufacture the vitamin.

Some groups of Americans, especially those over 60, tend to be deficient in vitamin D. Thus, last year the Food and Nutrition Board of the National Academy of Sciences revised its vitamin D recommendations upwards for older people: while those under 50 need only 200 IU (international units) daily, those 50 to 70 should get 400 IU, and those over 70 need 600 IU.

If you get even 10 or 15 minutes of sunlight on your arms and face two or three times a week, you will probably manufacture enough vitamin D to meet your needs. And because it is a fat-soluble vitamin, you can store enough to supply you in the days, or even months, when you don't get any sun exposure.

Nevertheless, it's a good idea to drink milk—for many reasons, among them that milk is fortified with vitamin D. Each cup contains 100 IU. Other foods containing vitamin D are fatty fish such as salmon and sardines, egg yolks, and fortified breakfast cereals. (Yogurt is *not* made from fortified milk.) Too much vitamin D can be toxic, but it's nearly impossible to get too much from food, and it is impossible to get too much from sun exposure.

Is geography a problem? Skin type?

Your ability to make vitamin D from sunlight varies according to your location and the time of year. According to Dr. Michael Holick, an expert in vitamin D at Boston University Medical Center, those who live at a latitude of 42° (a line that runs through Boston, Detroit, Chicago, the middle of Iowa, and southern Oregon) can manufacture sufficient vitamin D from a minimal amount of sun exposure between April through October. That is generally sufficient, because you will store enough vitamin D for the winter. People farther south—in Washington, D.C., for example—can manufacture the vitamin from March through November. The darker Canadian winter may have six months or more when the sun isn't sufficient to manufacture D. But most Canadians (and those living in the northern U.S.) will be all right, particularly if they get some dietary vitamin D.

If you have dark skin, especially if you are African-American, you may need longer exposure to sunlight—perhaps up to twice as much as a light-skinned person—since skin pigmentation screens sunlight and reduces vitamin D production.

Is your age a problem?

As you grow older, your ability to manufacture vitamin D in the sunlight declines, and just increasing your exposure time won't do the trick. By the time you are 70, your vitamin D production is only 30% of what it was when you were 25. That's why you need to increase your dietary intake. Anyone over 60 who doesn't get adequate amounts of vitamin D from foods and also lacks sun exposure will need supplements. Those at highest risk are the homebound or institutionalized, as well as those living in the northern third of this country and in Canada. Vegans and others who don't drink milk may also need to take a supplement.

Supplements are tricky, however, because even small overdoses of D can be toxic, leading to kidney stones, kidney failure, muscle and bone weakness, and other problems. Danger starts at 2,000 IU a day. *Nearly all documented cases of vitamin D toxicity were caused by supplements.* A daily multivitamin with 400 IU of vitamin D is usually the best solution. But it makes sense to discuss your risk of vitamin D deficiency with a health professional.

Sunscreen note

Sunscreen can reduce or even shut down the synthesis of vitamin D. This is a problem chiefly for older people, who are often more conscientious about using sunscreen than the young, but who also produce less D. Try to get 15 minutes exposure without sunscreen in the early morning or late afternoon, when the sun is less damaging. Then apply sunscreen if you plan to stay out longer, particularly if you are fair-skinned.

Final word: *You should consider taking 400 IU of vitamin D daily if you fall into one of the following categories:*

- *Housebound, get little sun.*
- *Vegan (consume no animal products, and thus no milk, eggs, or fish).*
- *Over 60, seldom get sun,* and *drink little or no milk.*
- *over 70.*

Best source: a multivitamin.

Can Vitamin E Prevent Heart Disease?

To E or not to E?

by Beth Fontenot, MS, RD

Some of the most interesting nutrition research in recent years has produced preliminary evidence that large doses of vitamin E may reduce the occurrence of heart attacks. As a result, vitamin E has received a great deal of media attention, prompting consumers to spend $300 million a year on vitamin E supplements. A few health and nutrition experts are ready to jump on the bandwagon and recommend supplementation, but others are asking whether the evidence really warrants such a move.

Judging by sales, vitamin E is one of the most sought-after dietary supplements among Americans. The nutrient is popular, it seems, even among professionals.

And no wonder. The claims for the nutrient's benefits are prevalent and appealing. "Health-food" literature and the media would have us believe that taking vitamin E will prevent arthritis, cataracts, stroke, diabetes, cancer, and heart disease. In addition, it's supposed to boost the immune system, ease symptoms of premenstrual syndrome, delay symptoms of Alzheimer's disease, and protect the body from aging.

Vitamin E Basics

Vitamin E was discovered in the 1920s when rats fed a basic diet became unable to reproduce viable offspring but were cured when given tocopherol, a substance that had been isolated from vegetable oils. In fact, the term "tocopherol" comes from greek words meaning "to bear offspring." Vitamin E became the name given to a group of eight fat-soluble compounds—four tocopherols (designated alpha, beta, gamma, and delta) and four tocotrienols (designated with the same Greek letters). It was not until 1966 that vitamin E was considered essential for humans.

All of these compounds have different degrees of biological activity. The most active form of the vitamin is the "d" isomer of alpha-tocopherol, which is found in many supplements. Recent research has indicated that other forms, such as gamma-tocopherol, may also be important to the body. Though gamma-tocopherol has only one-tenth the biological activity of alpha-tocopherol, it is more widely distributed in foods. It's found in foods such as sunflower seeds, almonds, and wheat germ.

Vitamin E requires the presence of fats and bile in the gut to be absorbed. The degree to which vitamin E is absorbed by the body is dependent on the total absorption of dietary fat. Absorption can be as high as 70%. However, when taken in doses well above the Recommended Dietary Allowance (RDA), the absorption rate of vitamin E drops to less than 10%. Vitamin E travels through the body by way of chylomicrons and other lipoproteins, and it is distributed to almost all tissues in the body. It is most concentrated in tissues containing an abundance of fatty acids, such as cell membranes.

The primary function of vitamin E appears to be to act as an antioxidant. When incorporated into the lipid portion of cell membranes and carrier molecules, it protects these structures from toxic compounds, heavy metals, drugs, radiation, and free radicals. It also appears to protect cholesterol from oxidative damage.

The recommended intake for vitamin E is expressed in alpha-tocopherol equivalents (alpha-TE). One alpha-TE is equal to 1 mg of alpha-tocopherol. Vitamin supplement labels usually express vitamin E content in IUs (international units). One IU is equal to 1 mg of synthetic vitamin E or about 0.74 mg of natural alpha-tocopherol. The current RDA for vitamin E is 10 mg for men (15 IU) and 8 mg (12 IU) for women. The RDA can be met with a tablespoon of corn oil.

Since many people medicate themselves with large amounts of vitamin E, it is fortunate that its toxicity is relatively low. However, the known toxicity of the other fat-soluble vitamins suggests that caution should be taken with long-term megadoses of vitamin E. High intakes of vitamin E can interfere with intestinal absorption of vitamins A and K. And at dosages exceeding 1,000 mg per day, vitamin E has been shown to enhance the effects of Coumadin therapy and to be antagonistic to the blood-clotting action of vitamin K.

Vitamin E and Heart Disease

The oxidation of lipoproteins appears to play an important role in the development of atherosclerosis, the disease process that leads to heart attacks as well as strokes. Considerable evidence exists that antioxidant vitamins from both the diet and from supplements may prevent lipoprotein oxidation and its biological effects in the body. The strongest evidence seems to be for vitamin E.

Support for the role of antioxidant vitamins in heart disease prevention has come from observational studies, particularly two cohort studies that were published in 1993. In the first study, the Nurses' Health Study, the researchers concluded that among over 85,000 middle-aged women in the study, there was a 40% reduced risk of coronary artery disease for those who took vitamin E supplements compared to those who did not (*N Engl J Med* 1993;328: 1444–9). The second study, the Health Professionals Follow-up Study, involved over 39,000 males and provided evidence of a significant association between a high intake of vitamin E from supplements and a lower risk of heart disease (*N Engl J Med* 1993;328:1450–1456).

Though these observational studies have pointed to the *possibility* of beneficial effects of vitamin E, they cannot establish cause and effect. And there has been very little direct evidence of benefit from randomized trials, which can establish a causal connection. Recently published results from the Alpha-Tocopherol, Beta-Carotene Cancer Prevention (ATBC) Study did not support the results of the observational studies. This randomized trial tested the effects of daily doses of 50 IU of vitamin E, 20 mg of beta carotene, both, or placebo on over 29,000 male smokers for five to eight years. The researchers found that with vitamin E supplementation, there was an increase in the risk of hemorrhagic stroke. And with beta-carotene supplements, there was an increase in mortality from lung cancer and ischemic heart disease. This trial raised the possibility that antioxidant supplements may have harmful as well as beneficial effects (*N Engl J Med* 1994:330:1029–1035).

Two more recently published observational studies produced conflicting results. In a seven-year study of over 34,000 postmenopausal women, researchers found that the intake of vitamin E from food was inversely associated with the risk of death from heart disease and concluded that postmenopausal women could lower their risk of heart disease without using supplements (*N Engl J Med* 1996;334:1156–1162). However, in the Rotterdam Study, researchers did not find an association between dietary vitamin E and heart disease in an elderly population (*Am J Clin Nutr* 1999;69: 261–266).

Last March at the Conference on Cardiovascular Disease Epidemiology and Prevention, Dr. Lori Mosca of the University of Michigan presented a study suggesting that vitamin E supplements provide little benefit to health and may cause harm in women after menopause. The study found that women who obtained vitamin E from their diet experienced significant reductions in LDL oxidation while the women who obtained vitamin E from supplements experienced increased LDL oxidation. Dr. Mosca believes that it may be the gamma-tocopherol in food that is protective instead of alpha-tocopherol found in supplements.

The results of secondary prevention trials (and those with known heart disease) have been more supportive of potential benefits of antioxidant vitamins. The Cambridge Heart Antioxidant Study (CHAOS) examined the effects of 400 to 800 IU of alpha-tocopherol on subsequent cardiovascular events. The risk of heart attack and other cardiovascular events was reduced in the group receiving vitamin E supplements (*Lancet* 1996;346:781–786). A secondary analysis of the ATBC study also found that the risk of a second heart attack was reduced in those taking vitamin E supplements (*Lancet* 1997;349:1714:1720).

AHA Position

According to a recent Science Advisory from the American Heart Association (AHA), there are not enough data on the long-term safety and efficacy of vitamin E supplementation to justify any population-wide recommendations for supplementation for the primary prevention of heart disease. The advisory also states that the role of vitamin E in secondary prevention is encouraging and leaves open the possibility of future recommendations regarding vitamin E supplementation in those with heart disease if further studies confirm the findings (*Circulation* 1999;99:591–595).

It is still unknown whether there are serious negative effects associated with taking vitamin E supplements. It is also unknown whether some other unidentified component in foods may actually be responsible for a reduced risk of heart disease. The Food and Drug Administration (FDA) is examining the scientific data to determine whether there is adequate evidence to support a health claim for antioxidants and disease prevention. A decision is expected next year.

Over time, a clearer picture should emerge, but for now, the AHA advises that based on current knowledge about vitamin E (and other antioxidant vitamins), "the most prudent and scientifically supportable recommendation for the general population is to consume a balanced diet with emphasis on antioxidant-rich fruits and vegetables and whole grains."

Beth Fontenot is a freelance nutrition writer and the Nutrition Coordinator on the faculty of the Louisiana State University Medical Center-Shreveport Family Practice Residency Program at Lake Charles Memorial Hospital in Lake Charles, LA.

A Disease of Too Much Iron

THE STORY

When it comes to vitamins and minerals, most of us probably worry more about getting too little than too much. But for some people with a little-known—but surprisingly common—genetic disorder called hereditary hemochromatosis, the problem is too much of a good thing.

In hereditary hemochromatosis, also known as iron overload, a genetic abnormality causes the body to absorb greater than normal amounts of iron from food. Over several decades, the accumulated iron exceeds the body's normal iron storage capacity, and the excess gets deposited in various tissues. Whereas a healthy person may store 1 gram or less of iron, people with hemochromatosis may accumulate as much as 15 to 30 grams (0.5 to 1 ounce). In the most severe cases, the amount of iron in the body is reportedly enough to set off airport metal detectors. Ultimately, this buildup can damage organs and cause chronic fatigue, arthritis-like joint pain, diabetes or other symptoms. Because so many of these symptoms can easily be confused with other medical conditions, hemochromatosis often goes undiagnosed.

Recent evidence indicates that the problem is much more common than was once believed, affecting anywhere from 1 in 200 to 1 in 500 Americans, according to Adele Franks, MD, of the Centers for Disease Control and Prevention (CDC), who wrote the introduction to a special supplement on hemochromatosis in the Dec. 1 *Annals of Internal Medicine*. Those most at risk are people of Mediterranean, Northern-Eastern European and Hispanic descent. People of Irish descent are three times more likely to carry the defective gene than other Europeans. The disorder is recessive, meaning that it takes two copies of the abnormal gene, one from each parent, to cause disease symptoms. People with a single defective gene are carriers but don't show any signs of illness themselves. About one in eight Americans is a carrier.

Typically, the disorder becomes apparent in middle age, when, for example, an arthritic patient requires a joint replacement, or when the skin becomes characteristically discolored (called bronze diabetes for the skin's tanned look). Men are more likely to be affected than women because women, until menopause, lose blood—and excess iron—through menstruation and childbirth.

Early detection can stave off the organ damage that, left untreated, may eventually lead to heart or liver failure. The CDC is considering blood screening for everyone, but for now there is no consensus on when or how this would be done. Meanwhile, should you talk to your doctor about getting tested?—*The Editors*

THE PHYSICIAN'S PERSPECTIVE

Vincent J. Felitti, M.D.
Not many problems in medicine are totally preventable, but the damage due to hemochromatosis is one. When diagnosed early, a simple and inexpensive treatment program can prevent significant, debilitating and potentially fatal illness. But getting that early diagnosis is problematic.

Most physicians were trained to believe that hemochromatosis was dismissibly rare. Only in the last 15 years or so have we learned that it is much more common than previously thought. Two years ago, researchers discovered the defective gene that causes 95 percent of hemochromatosis. Studies conducted since support an estimated incidence of 1 in 250 people in the United States. But because current practice has not caught up with the recent findings, hemochromatosis is still often overlooked.

One of the difficulties with hemochromatosis is that its major symptoms are often seen as independent conditions by different physicians, with no one recognizing the grouping of problems as evidence of an underlying iron overload. Moreover, by the time these symptoms are apparent, the disease is usually advanced, and the opportunity to prevent or reverse organ damage has often been lost. Some problems, such as arthritis, generally do not get better with treatment, while others, such as impotence or depression, usually go away once treatment begins. Others still, such as diabetes, are sometimes reversible if treatment is started early.

These difficulties are why screening is so critical. **The only way to catch the disorder before damage occurs is for everyone to get a once-in-a-lifetime test to determine if body iron levels are elevated.** At the

HEMOCHROMATOSIS SIGNS AND SYMPTOMS

◆ Profound fatigue
◆ Joint pain or arthritis
◆ Elevated blood sugar or diabetes
◆ Abdominal pain
◆ Fatigue
◆ Irregular heartbeat
◆ Chronic intermittent diarrhea
◆ Changes in skin color
◆ Loss of libido or impotence
◆ Lack of menstruation or early menopause
◆ Enlarged spleen or liver
◆ Congestive heart failure
◆ Cirrhosis   ◆ Hypothyroidism
◆ Depression   ◆ Loss of body hair

large HMO where I work, we're screening 50,000 people per year.

Testing for the condition is simple, but it's important to use the right test. There is a genetic test, but it currently identifies only 85 percent of people affected. This is likely because another, still-undiscovered gene is involved. The most reliable analysis is a blood test known as serum iron saturation or transferrin saturation, available at any standard medical lab. If the test is elevated, then hemochromatosis is suspected and a second test, after fasting, will be done to confirm the results. Another common blood test, ferritin, typically used to evaluate anemia, can be misleading, since ferritin levels are generally normal early in the course of hemochromatosis. Surprisingly, people with hemochromatosis can also be anemic, since the high iron levels have a toxic effect that suppresses the bone marrow's production of red cells. Testing can be done at any time after age one.

Treatment is also relatively simple. Iron is an unusual material in that once it gets into the body, it stays there forever. The only easy way to remove it is by removing blood. Patients typically have a pint of blood removed (just like donating blood) each week until iron levels return to normal. This "de-ironing" may take from several months to a couple of years. Then patients must return for treatment several times a year for the rest of their lives to maintain normal iron levels.

People with hemochromatosis should avoid multivitamins containing iron, as well as vitamin C, which can increase the body's absorption of iron from food. And because excess iron damages the liver and makes it more vulnerable to disease, patients should limit alcohol to reduce the risk of cirrhosis.

An important step for anyone who tests positive for hemochromatosis should be to encourage family members to get tested. Unlike so many genetic diseases for which we now have tests but no treatment, hemochromatosis is a problem we can do something about.

Vincent J. Felitti, MD, is director of the Department of Preventive Medicine at Kaiser Permanente in San Diego, CA.

FOR MORE INFORMATION

The Iron Disorders Institute, (864) 241-0111; www.irondisorders.org

NATIONAL ACADEMY OF SCIENCES INTRODUCES NEW CALCIUM RECOMMENDATIONS

LUANN SOLIAH, PhD, R.D., CFCS,
Associate Professor and Dietetics Director, Department of Family and Consumer Sciences, Baylor University

ABSTRACT

Osteoporosis is a serious, chronic condition of porous (easily fractured) bones. It develops silently and slowly over time and is directly related to decreased calcium storage in the bones. New calcium recommendations have been published by the National Academy of Sciences. The new guidelines recommend increased calcium intake to prevent bone deterioration. This article reviews these new guidelines, food sources of calcium, and common calcium supplements. Attaining the increased calcium recommendations is possible, but it does require balanced, healthful food choices.

Osteoporosis is a preventable disease of porous, easily fractured bones. It afflicts more than 28 million Americans—most of them women (Wilde, Economos, & Palombo, 1997). Women are most at risk because bone decreases rapidly after menopause. Prevalence of osteoporosis increases with age; however, prevention strategies can begin at any time in one's life. For adults, proper nutrition, balanced meals, and generous calcium intakes are reasonable preventive recommendations. Specifically, the role of calcium nutrition in bone health is well established (National Institutes of Health [NIH], 1994). High calcium intakes have been shown to reduce the loss of bone in postmenopausal women (Dawson-Hughes et al., 1991) and decrease fractures in persons who had fractures previously (Chapuy et al., 1992).

NEW CALCIUM RECOMMENDATIONS

Scientists agree that bone strength later in life depends on how well the bones are developed during youth and that adequate calcium nutrition during the growing years is essential to achieving optimal peak bone mass (National Academy of Sciences [NAS], 1997; NIH, 1994). On the basis of this agreement, the National Academy of Sciences has released a new report that revises calcium requirements for Americans. For the first time since 1989, the federal government has increased its recommendations for calcium intake (NAS, 1997).

The Food and Nutrition Board at the National Academy of Sciences reviewed, adjusted, and increased the recommendations for calcium because of new research findings. The new recommendations are called Dietary Reference Intakes (DRI), and they expand the scope and application of the former Recommended Dietary Allowances (RDAs; National Research Council [NCR], 1989; see also NAS, 1997). The new DRIs provide two sets of measures for each nutrient: Adequate Intakes (similar to RDAs) and Tolerable Upper Intake Levels (maximum nutrient intake guidelines; NAS, 1997; "Higher Levels of Calcium," 1997). The concept of the DRIs extends the RDA goal of avoiding nutrient deficiency. DRIs quantify the relationship between a nutrient and the risk for disease (e.g., calcium intake and osteoporosis prevention). Thus, the new DRIs are designed to reflect the latest research about nutrient requirements based on optimizing health among all life-stage groups (NAS, 1997; "Higher Levels of Calcium," 1997).

Table 1 illustrates the new (1997) Adequate Intake (AI) calcium recommendations for each life-stage group. AIs are the observed or experimentally set intake by a defined population or subgroup that appears to sustain a defined nutritional status, such as growth rate, normal circulating nutrient values, or other functional indicators of health (NAS, 1997).

The new DRIs (AI) state that adults between the ages of 19 and 50 years should consume 1,000 mg of calcium

> **For the first time since 1989, the federal government has increased its recommendations for calcium intake.**

18. National Academy of Science Introduces New Calcium Recommendations

per day, and all adults older than 50 years should consume 1,200 mg of calcium per day (NAS, 1997). Some authorities suggest even higher levels of calcium (1,500 mg/day) for postmenopausal women who are not receiving estrogen replacement therapy (Gums, 1996; NIH, 1994; Whitney & Rolfes, 1996). These recommendations are considerably higher than the former 1989 RDAs of 800 mg per day for most adults (NRC, 1989). The calcium recommendations were increased because adults lose bone mass as they age and are, therefore, at increased risk for osteoporosis. The government scientists were responding to the mass of accumulated evidence that the need for calcium is high throughout life (Matkovic & Heaney, 1992; NAS, 1997; NIH, 1994). Research evidence from several controlled, randomized trials verified that the 1989 RDA (10th edition) for calcium was too low and understated the true need for maximum bone accretion (Johnston et al., 1992; Lloyd, Andon, & Rollings, 1993; Recker, Davies, & Hinders, 1992).

There is general agreement that consuming the recommended amount of calcium will help protect bones and teeth over a lifetime. Unfortunately, a relatively small percentage of women (20%–50%) consistently meet their daily calcium requirement (Crane, Hubbard, & Lewis, 1998; Eck, Relyea, & Klesges, 1997; Galvacs, 1997). The challenge is even greater for female adolescents. The new guidelines recommend that adolescents between the ages of 9 and 18 years should receive 1,300 mg of calcium per day (see Table 1). Data from the Continuing Survey of Food Intakes by Individuals (CSFII) indicate that the proportion of female adolescents who regularly consumed the recommended amount of calcium-rich foods was only about 10% (United States Department of Agriculture [USDA], 1988; see also Crane et al., 1998).

In contrast, young boys and men generally obtain more calcium from their diets because they eat more food (Crane et al., 1998; NRC, 1989; Whitney & Rolfes, 1996). They also have a higher reported intake of mean dairy products (beginning at age 2) compared to girls and women of the same age (USDA, 1988).

SOURCES OF CALCIUM

Bone requires several nutrients to develop normally and to maintain itself after growth ceases. The most important nutrients for proper bone development are protein, calcium, phosphorus, vitamin D, vitamin C, vitamin K, and a few trace minerals (Heaney, 1996). The nutrients most likely to be deficient in western nations are calcium and vitamin D (Heaney, 1996; Ryan, Eleazer, & Egbert, 1995). For this reason, food sources of calcium and vitamin D are important to include in the daily diet.

Dairy foods are excellent sources of both calcium and vitamin D. Milk is fortified with vitamin D and is thus the best guarantee that people will meet their daily requirement (Ryan et al., 1995). In addition, with proper exposure to sunlight, ample vitamin D can be synthesized within the body (Ryan et al., 1995).

Milk, cheese, and yogurt are the primary food sources of calcium (NRC, 1989). In addition, these foods provide multiple nutrients (vitamin D, phosphorus, lactose, and calcium), rather than a single nutrient. The presence of vitamin D and lactose increases the absorption of calcium (Heaney, 1996). Also, calcium appears to be used better if accompanied by a reasonable amount of phosphorus (Spencer, Kramer, & Osis, 1988).

Milk contains about 300 mg of calcium per cup. To consistently meet the 1,200 mg calcium guidelines (for adults 51 years of age and older), a person would have to consume approximately four dairy products or the equivalent each day. Examples of calcium-rich foods are shown in Table 2.

Unfortunately, many adults do not like dairy products or cannot comfortably drink milk. Twenty-five percent of U.S. adults are lactose intolerant (Suarez, Savaiano, & Levitt, 1995). Lactose-intolerant adults need information on lower lactose-content dairy foods (e.g., yogurt and cheese), and they need encouragement to drink small amounts of milk (e.g., 4-oz portions) several times each day. They also need education on calcium-fortified foods such as specially formulated fruit juices. High-calcium dairy products (milk and yogurt with added calcium) and calcium-fortified breads are sold at some supermarkets. Calcium-fortified breakfast cereals provide additional calcium. Powdered nonfat milk can be added to soups and casseroles to augment calcium intake.

A variety of other foods also supply calcium (see Table 2). Leafy green vegetables, legumes, sardines, and some homemade breads provide additional calcium. Dark green, leafy vegetables contain a reasonable amount of calcium, but absorption and binding problems occur, so there is little, if any, calcium

Table 1. **Dietary Reference Intakes for Calcium**

LIFE STAGE GROUP	CALCIUM MG/DAY ADEQUATE INTAKE
Infants	
0–6 months	210
6–12 months	270
Children	
1–3 years	500
4–8 years	800
Males/Females	
9–18 years	1,300
19–50 years	1,000
>51 years	1,200

[a] Adequate Intake is the observed or experimentally set intake by a defined population or subgroup that appears to sustain a defined nutritional status, such as growth rate, normal circulating nutrient values, or other functional indicators of health.

Source: National Academy of Sciences–Institute of Medicine (1997). *Dietary Reference Intakes.* Washington, DC: National Academy Press.

2 ❖ NUTRIENTS

Table 2. Food Sources for Calcium [a]

Food	Portion size	Calcium(mg)
Dairy		
Skim milk	1 cup	301
2% milk	1 cup	298
Whole milk	1 cup	290
Swiss cheese	1 oz	272
Yogurt	1/2 cup	207
Cheddar cheese	1 oz	204
Processed cheese	1 oz	174
Vanilla pudding	1/2 cup	139
Ice cream	1/2 cup	86
Cottage cheese	1/2 cup	63
Vegetables		
Broccoli	1/2 cup	36
Spinach	1/2 cup	27
Okra	1/2 cup	27
Green beans	1/2 cup	17
Protein Foods		
Sardines with bones	3 oz	433
Salmon with bones	3 oz	242
Tofu (soybean curd)	1/2 cup	130
Almonds	1/3 cup	129
Breads		
Waffle	7" waffle	191
Biscuits (two)	3" biscuits	134
Pancakes (two)	4" pancakes	68

[a] ESHA Research and West Publishing Company (Nutripro Plus) ® (1993). (Macintosh Version 3.0). Salem, OR.

available for the body's uptake (Weaver & Plawecki, 1994). Specifically, oxalates greatly reduce the absorbability of calcium from vegetarian sources (Weaver, Heaney, Proulx, Hinders, & Packard, 1993). Another dilemma to consider is the enormous quantity of green vegetables (15 cups) that would have to be consumed each day to reach the 1,000 to 1,200 mg recommendation.

Consumers need to read food labels to identify the calcium content of canned, frozen, and packaged foods. If possible, one calcium-rich food needs to be consumed at each meal. A balanced diet that includes all food groups is the best assurance of nutrient adequacy.

CALCIUM SUPPLEMENTS

When calcium requirements cannot be consistently met by eating calcium-rich food, a calcium supplement is recommended. During the menopausal years, calcium supplements of 1,000 mg per day may slow, but cannot fully prevent, the inevitable bone loss of aging (Reid, Ames, Evans, Gamble, & Sharpe, 1993). Nevertheless, supplements are frequently used as a part of therapy for osteoporosis prevention as well as osteoporosis treatment.

A number of types and brand names of calcium supplements are available (see Table 3). The "ideal" calcium supplement would have the following characteristics: reasonable size for comfortable swallowing, no unpleasant side effects, quick dissolving action, highly absorbable, affordable, and the appropriate calcium dosage could be easily achieved. In general, these characteristics are difficult to accomplish.

One of the most important factors to consider is how well the body absorbs and uses calcium from various supplements. The elemental calcium content (absorbable quantity) varies from product to product and directly influences the amount required to achieve the recommended guidelines. For example, calcium carbonate has a 40% absorption rate, thus a 1,200-mg dose provides 480 mg calcium (Gums, 1996). In contrast, calcium gluconate only has a 9% absorption rate and thus would require a 5,333-mg dose to provide an equal quantity of calcium (Gums, 1996).

Basically, three major types of calcium supplements are sold (Whitney & Rolfes, 1996). First, there are purified calcium compounds, such as calcium carbonate, citrate, gluconate, lactate, or phosphate. Second, there are mixtures of calcium with other substances, such as calcium with magnesium, aluminum salts, or vitamin D. Finally, there are powdered calcium products such as bone meal, oyster shell, and dolomite. Dolomite is a "natural" calcium compound (from limestone and marble), but it may be contaminated with hazardous toxic minerals such as cadmium, mercury, or lead (Whitney & Rolfes, 1996).

Only proven bioavailable supplements (e.g., chewable or tablets that meet U.S. Pharmacopeia standards for disintegration) are recommended (Packard & Heaney, 1997). A quick and easy household test for dissolving action is to add one calcium tablet to 6 ounces of vinegar. A high-quality product will dissolve within 30 minutes (Whitney & Rolfes, 1996).

Calcium carbonate is one of the most frequently used supplements, but it may not dissolve in the stomach as easily as some of the other calcium compounds, because it requires gastric acid for optimal absorption. In general, calcium carbonate is absorbed best when it is taken with meals and distributed in small doses throughout the day (Packard & Heaney, 1997).

Calcium citrate is an alternative to calcium carbonate and it offers some unique advantages. Calcium citrate does not require gastric acid for absorption, thus it may be taken with or without meals and it does not interfere with the absorption of other nutrients (McKane et al., 1996). In addition, calcium citrate is available in several forms (effervescent liquitabs, caplets, and tablets).

Calcium lactate and calcium gluconate are much less concentrated than either calcium carbonate or calcium citrate, thus much larger doses have to be taken to receive an equivalent amount (see Table 3). The absorption of calcium from antacids (e.g., Tums or Rolaids) or from powdered materials such as oyster shells is poor.

As previously stated, calcium supplements will not cure osteoporosis, but they may decrease the risk. Along with this advantage, taking calcium supplements may present some disadvantages. For example, some calcium compounds may impair iron, magnesium, and zinc absorption (McKane et al., 1996). Some individuals may be at increased risk for urinary tract stones or kidney damage (Gums, 1996). Other considerations include nutrient-drug interactions. An example of a calcium-drug interaction is calcium and tetracycline. The two together may form an insoluble complex that impairs both mineral and drug absorption. To avoid these problems, consumers should disclose and discuss all the medicine and supplements they take with their health care professionals.

As awareness of osteoporosis increases, more people are seeking advice about calcium supplementation. Consumers need to read the labels of the supplements to determine how many tablets they will have to take each day to receive the appropriate amount. The product's cost can be reduced by choosing generic supplements rather than name brand products. Some of the common side effects of calcium supplements include bloating, gas production, constipation, and reduction in stomach acid. Consumers should be prepared to go through a stage of "trial and error" until they find a product that is the most comfortable choice for them.

CONTEMPORARY APPLICATIONS

Experts agree that it is highly desirable to eat a nutritious diet containing rich sources of calcium. Young adults who achieve a higher bone density are less likely to experience health problems as they grow older. In contrast, low calcium uptake by the bones during the growing years makes a person vulnerable to osteoporosis.

Health policy makers for the government have assessed the situation and concluded that Americans need more calcium in their daily diets to delay bone loss and prevent osteoporosis. Food is always the preferred method for providing calcium. Creative menu planning requires effort; but if at least one calcium-rich food or beverage is provided at each meal on a consistent basis, most of the calcium recommendation can be obtained. For those who cannot drink milk or do not like dairy products, several calcium-fortified foods are available, and they should be included in the diet as often as possible. Furthermore, calcium supplements can increase total calcium provision and help achieve at least part of the new NAS recommendations.

For older adults, proper nutrition, regular physical activity, and health education can decrease the risk of osteoporosis and related bone injuries. Family and consumer science professionals employed in home health care agencies, county extension offices, rehabilitation centers, and area agencies for senior citizens should provide information on healthful food choices and calcium supplements for individuals with

Table 3. **Common Calcium Supplements**

Product	Source of calcium and mg of elemental calcium/tablet	Number of tablets/day to provide about 900–1,000 mg calcium
Caltrate 600®	carbonate (600 mg)	1.5
Caltrate 600 + Vitamin D®	carbonate (600 mg)	1.5
Os-Cal 500®	carbonate from oyster shell (500 mg)	2
Os-Cal 500 + Vitamin D®	carbonate from oyster shell (500 mg)	2
Posture® (600 mg)	phosphate (600 mg)	1.5
Posture-Vitamin D®	phosphate (600 mg)	1.5
Citracal®	citrate (200 mg)	5
Citracal® + Vitamin D	citrate (315 mg)	3
Citracal Liquitab®	citrate (500 mg)	2
Tums® 500 mg	carbonate from limestone (500 mg)	2
Tums E-X® 300 mg	carbonate from limestone (300 mg)	3.5
Tums Ultra®	carbonate from limestone (400 mg)	2.5
Calcet® + Vitamin D	carbonate, lactate, gluconate (300 mg)	3.5
Fosfree®	carbonate, gluconate, lactate (175 mg)	6

calcium-related concerns. Community outreach programs on osteoporosis should be developed for middle-aged and senior citizens because they have the potential to reach the largest number of people within a community.

All consumers should be made aware that bone building is not a static process. Osteoporosis is a gradual thinning or weakening of the bones that develops over several decades. The value of consistently healthy lifestyle choices is important to reinforce for good consumer compliance and healthy outcomes. Therefore, even though bone loss is an inevitable consequence of older age, broken bones and osteoporosis can be prevented.

References

Chapuy, M., Arlot, M., Duboeuf, F., Brun, J., Crouzet, B., Arnaud, S., Delmas, P., & Meunier, P. (1992). Vitamin D3 and calcium to prevent hip fractures in elderly women. *New England Journal of Medicine, 327,* 1637–1642.

Crane, N. T., Hubbard, V. S., & Lewis, C. J. (1998). National nutrition objectives and the Dietary Guidelines for Americans. *Nutrition Today 33*(2), 49–58.

Dawson-Hughes, B., Dallal, G., Krall, E., Harris, S., Sokoll, L., & Falconer, G. (1991). Effect of vitamin D supplementation on wintertime and overall bone loss in healthy postmenopausal women. *Annals of Internal Medicine, 115,* 505–512.

Eck, L. H., Relyea, G., & Klesges, L. M. (1997). Awareness of nutrient intake adequacy in adult women. *Journal of The American Dietetic Association Abstracts, 97*(9), A–20.

ESHA Research and West Publishing Company [Nutripro Plus] ® (1993). (Macintosh Version 3.0). Salem, OR.

Galvacs, K. G. (1997). Dietary calcium intake and the prevalence of calcium supplement use among well-educated women. *Journal of The American Dietetic Association Abstracts, 97*(9), A–17.

Gums, J. G. (1996). New methods of diagnosis and treatment of osteoporosis. *U.S. Pharmacist, 21*(9), 85–93.

Heaney, R. P. (1996). Bone mass, nutrition, and other lifestyle factors. *Nutrition Reviews, 54*(4), S3–S10.

Higher levels of calcium recommended in the new Dietary Reference Intakes. (1997). *Nutrition Week, 27*(31), 1, 6.

Johnston, C. C., Miller, J. A., Slemenda, C. W., Reister, T. K., Hui, S., Christian, J. C., & Peacock, M. (1992). Calcium supplementation and increases in bone mineral density in children. *New England Journal of Medicine, 327,* 82–87.

Lloyd, T., Andon, M. B., & Rollings, N. (1993). Calcium supplementation and bone mineral density in adolescent girls. *JAMA, 270,* 841–844.

Matkovic, V., & Heaney, R. P. (1992). Calcium balance during human growth: Evidence for threshold behavior. *American Journal of Clinical Nutrition, 55,* 992–996.

McKane, W. R., Khosla, S., Egan, K. S., Robins, S. P., Burritt, M. F., & Riggs, B. L. (1996). Role of calcium in modulating age-related increases in parathyroid function and bone resorption. *Journal of Clinical Endocrinology Metabolism, 81,* 1699–1703.

National Academy of Sciences-Institute of Medicine. (1997). *Dietary Reference Intakes.* Washington, DC: National Academy Press.

National Institutes of Health Consensus Development Conference. (1994). Optimal Calcium Intake. *JAMA, 272,* 1942–1948.

National Research Council-Food and Nutrition Board. (1989). *Recommended Dietary Allowances* (10th ed.). Washington, DC: National Academy Press.

Packard, P. T., & Heaney, R. P. (1997). Medical nutrition therapy for patients with osteoporosis. *Journal of The American Dietetic Association, 97*(4), 414–417.

Recker, R. R., Davies, K. M., & Hinders S. M. (1992). Bone gain in young adult women. *JAMA, 268,* 2403–2408.

Reid, I. R., Ames, R. W., Evans, M. C., Gamble, G. D., & Sharpe, S. (1993). Effect of calcium supplementation on bone loss in postmenopausal women. *New England Journal of Medicine, 328,* 460–464.

Ryan, C., Eleazer, P., & Egbert, J. (1995). Vitamin D in the elderly. *Nutrition Today, 30,* 228–233.

Spencer, H., Kramer, L., & Osis, D. (1988). Do protein and phosphorus cause calcium loss? *Journal of Nutrition, 118,* 657–660.

Suarez, F. L. Savaiano, D. A., & Levitt, M. D. (1995). A comparison of symptoms after the consumption of milk or lactose-hydrolyzed milk by people with self-reported severe lactose intolerance. *New England Journal of Medicine, 333,* 1–4.

United States Department of Agriculture. (1988). *Food Consumption Nationwide Survey* (Continuing Survey of Food Intakes by Individuals [CSFII]; USDA NFCS, CFS2, Rep. No. 86–93).

Weaver, C. M., Heaney, R. P., Proulx, W. R., Hinders, S. M., & Packard, P. T. (1993). Absorbability of calcium from common beans. *Journal of Food Science, 58,* 1401–1403.

Weaver, C. M., & Plawecki, K. L. (1994). Dietary calcium: Adequacy of a vegetarian diet. *American Journal of Clinical Nutrition, 59,* 1238S–1241S.

Whitney, E. N., & Rolfes, S. R. (1996). *Understanding nutrition* (7th ed.). Minneapolis, MN: West Publishing Company.

Wilde, A., Economos, C., & Palombo, R. (1997). Focus group research in the development of an osteoporosis educational program targeting seniors. *Journal of The American Dietetic Association Abstracts, 97*(9), A–86.

Fiber: Strands of protection

Conflicting news on fiber weaves a tangled web. We'll untangle it.

A decade ago, reports that fiber lowers cholesterol levels led many Americans to forsake a cherished sensual pleasure in their morning routine: They switched from danishes to oat-bran muffins. Since then, fiber's image has repeatedly seesawed as studies first refuted, then confirmed, its effects on cholesterol. The most recent news on fiber seems only to make the seesaw rock harder.

In January, a large Harvard study announced that, contrary to previous reports, fiber doesn't protect against colon cancer. Five months later, the same researchers reported that fiber did protect against coronary heart disease—but not primarily by lowering blood-cholesterol levels. That undoubtedly comes as a surprise to fans of *Cheerios* and *Quaker Oats*, whose cereal boxes say that fiber cuts the risk of coronary disease because it lowers cholesterol.

Fortunately, some reasonably clear threads run through the seemingly snarled research.

Fiber for the heart

The Harvard study, involving some 69,000 female nurses, is the largest and latest of several studies suggesting that fiber may protect the heart. The researchers found that after ten years, the women who ate the most fiber had a 23 percent lower heart-attack rate than those who ate the least. A previous Harvard study, this one involving men, linked a high-fiber diet with a 36 percent reduction in heart attacks. In both cases, the researchers controlled for fat consumption, addressing concerns that the apparent benefit of fiber might actually have stemmed from the lower amount of fat in a high-fiber diet.

Several smaller studies have reported similar findings. And more-recent results from that same Harvard study in men suggested that a fiber-rich diet may slightly reduce the risk of stroke as well.

Extrapolating from other data, the researchers calculated that only about one-fifth of the apparent coronary benefit comes from fiber's much-touted ability to lower the cholesterol level. Indeed, it's true that reduced cholesterol is only one of many likely reasons why fiber helps the heart. But it's the best-documented effect. And despite its modest impact, it's still probably more important than any of the others, which have even smaller individual effects.

The cholesterol benefit comes from soluble fiber, the kind that dissolves in hot water and abounds in beans, oats, most fruits and whole grains, and some vegetables. Such fiber may work by inactivating digestive acids that are made from cholesterol, forcing the liver to pull cholesterol out of the blood to make more acids. Moreover, the fermentation of soluble fiber during digestion creates chemicals that may slow the liver's production of cholesterol itself.

In a separate recent Harvard study, researchers analyzed 67 clinical trials on soluble fiber and cholesterol. They found that consuming 5 extra grams of soluble fiber a day—an amount that most Americans could easily add to their diet and that many *should* add just to reach the recommended minimum—typically lowers the total-cholesterol level by about 8 points. For someone with average cholesterol, an 8-point drop should generally lower the risk of heart attack by about 12 percent. The actual percentage may be greater

Reprinted with permission from the August 1999 issue of *Consumer Reports on Health,* pp. 1, 3-5, for educational purposes only. © 1999 by Consumers Union of U.S., Inc., Yonkers, NY 10703-1057, a nonprofit organization. The information and images you receive online regarding Consumer Reports material are protected by the copyright laws. We prohibit any commercial use of our material, including copying, redistributing, or retransmitting. To subscribe, call 800-234-1645 or visit us at www.ConsumerReport.org.

than that, since nearly all of the total-cholesterol reduction comes from the harmful LDL cholesterol, not the good HDL. And some evidence suggests that soluble fiber lowers cholesterol levels more than average in the people who need it most—those with elevated cholesterol levels.

More than cholesterol

Here are the other possible reasons why fiber seems to provide cardiovascular protection:

- **Lower insulin levels.** Fiber, particularly soluble fiber, slows the body's conversion of carbohydrates into sugar in the blood. But refined gains such as white rice, white bread, and regular pasta, which are high in carbohydrates, have had most of their fiber removed. Digestion of those foods may send so much sugar into the blood that the body churns out extra insulin to handle the extra sugar. At least in the 10 to 25 percent of people who are "insulin resistant"—and thus require even more of that hormone to do the job—the extra insulin may contribute to coronary risk in several ways: It can raise blood pressure and the level of triglycerides (a fat in the blood that, like cholesterol, can help clog the arteries); reduce the level of good HDL cholesterol; and increase the risk of diabetes, which multiplies the heart-attack risk.

- **Reduced blood pressure.** Researchers from Tulane University recently analyzed 20 clinical trials that compared high-fiber diets with low-fiber fare. The researchers concluded that an extra 14 grams of total fiber per day—again, an increase that most people could readily achieve—lowered both systolic and diastolic blood pressure (the upper and lower numbers, respectively) by about 2 points, and slightly more than that in hypertensive individuals. Such a decline typically lowers heart-attack risk by about 5 percent, stroke risk by 8 percent. While fiber's effect on insulin may explain some of that benefit, other mechanisms as yet unknown probably contribute as well.

- **Weight loss.** Extra weight puts a direct burden on the heart; it also hurts the heart indirectly, by promoting the development of several coronary risk factors, including high cholesterol levels, physical inactivity, and diabetes. Soluble fiber mixes with liquids in the stomach to form a gelatinous mass, reducing appetite by making a meal feel larger and linger there longer. Several clinical trials comparing similar weight-loss regimens have shown that the addition of fiber helps people lose an average of 4 extra pounds over a two-to-three-month period; people who get the additional fiber by switching from a typical American diet to one rich in fruits, vegetables, grains, and beans theoretically should shed more weight than that, since those foods are typically low in calories.

- **Reduced risk of blood clots.** Laboratory evidence suggests that chemicals formed by the fermentation of soluble fiber in the gut may indirectly inhibit the formation of blood clots, which can trigger a heart attack or stroke. A few small studies suggest that people who eat lots of fiber may indeed have lower levels of those clot-promoting compounds.

> "Doe we not see the poore man that eateth browne bread [hath] fuller, stronger, fayrer complectioned and longer living than the other that fare daintelie every day."
> —Dr. P. Stubs, 1585

Colon and breast cancer

The recent Harvard study of colon cancer, part of the same ongoing nurses' study, failed to find any evidence that fiber reduces that cancer risk. That's a major setback for fiber—but not a fatal one.

Researchers have identified two ways that fiber, particularly the insoluble kind—abundant in whole grains, beans, most vegetables, and some fruits—theoretically might cut the colon-cancer risk. The most likely possibility is that insoluble fiber speeds potentially cancer-causing wastes through the colon and enlarges the stools, thus diluting their concentration. In addition, the colonic fermentation of insoluble fiber in whole grains appears to create cancer-fighting chemicals (just as soluble-fiber fermentation creates clot-blocking and cholesterol-lowering compounds). But even the women who ate the most fiber overall in the nurses' study got little of it from whole grains—which might explain the failure to find any effect on colon-cancer risk.

How to figure your fiber intake

Public-health organizations typically recommend that normal, healthy adults get between 20 and 35 grams of fiber each day. That's a big jump for most people: American adults consume roughly 16 grams of fiber daily, on average.

To get a sense of how much fiber you consume in a day, complete the simple worksheet below. For each food category, multiply the number of servings you had yesterday by the value listed. Then add up your score to get the total amount of fiber you ate.

Of course, that score provides just a rough idea of the amount of fiber in your diet. And it doesn't distinguish soluble from insoluble fiber. (Roughly one-third of your fiber should be soluble—anywhere from 7 to 12 grams per day.) To estimate your fiber

Food	Servings	Grams
Vegetables (Serving size: 1 cup raw leafy greens; ½ cup other vegetables.)	× 2 =	
Fruits (Serving size: 1 whole fruit; ½ grapefruit; ½ cup berries or cubed fruit; ¼ cup dried fruit.)	× 2.5 =	
Beans, lentils, split peas (Serving size: ½ cup, cooked.)	× 7 =	
Nuts, seeds (Serving size: ¼ cup; 2 tbsp peanut butter.)	× 2.5 =	
Whole grains (Serving size: 1 slice whole-wheat bread; ½ cup whole-wheat pasta, brown rice, or other whole grain; ½ bran or whole-grain muffin.)	× 2.5 =	
Refined Grains (Serving size: Same as above. Includes white or wheat bread, white or spinach pasta, white rice or other processed grains, and refined-flour bagels or muffins.)	× 1 =	
Breakfast cereals (Serving size: Check package or table at right for serving size and amount of fiber per serving.)	× fiber per serving =	
	TOTAL GRAMS OF FIBER =	

Moreover, despite the size of that study, its conclusions were based on only 671 cases of colon cancer. An analysis of 13 previous observational studies, which compared a total of some 5,300 colon-cancer patients with some 10,500 other people, suggested that a high-fiber diet may cut the risk nearly in half.

Those 13 studies were all retrospective, a somewhat weaker design than the prospective approach in the Harvard study. But five other observational studies *were* prospective—and three of them did find an apparent benefit. The most recent of those studies, published this spring in the International Journal of Cancer, was considerably smaller than the Harvard study but nine years longer; that's potentially important, because colon cancer develops over a long period of time. The new study involving men from seven different countries, suggested that a 10-gram increase in fiber intake may reduce colon-cancer deaths by one-third, even after adjustment for fat intake, exercise, and other colon-cancer risk factors.

Of course, even prospective observational studies can only suggest a causal connection; proving the link requires clinical trials, where researchers assign volunteers to consume either fiber or a placebo. While there have been no such trials on fiber and colon cancer, several small trials have found that insoluble fiber from wheat bran inhibits the formation of colon polyps, which sometimes turn cancerous. Findings from two larger and longer clinical trials involving polyps—one using a wheat-bran supplement, the other a high-produce diet—are expected early next year.

As for breast cancer, the evidence on fiber is similarly hopeful but inconclusive. Clinical trials have generally shown that insoluble fiber lowers the level of estrogen, which fuels the growth of breast-cancer cells. The first major observational study on fiber and breast cancer found no signs of any protective benefit. But the next one did—and that study, involving some 60,000 Canadian women, controlled for several potentially confounding factors that were not addressed in the earlier study. Several smaller observational studies of fiber intake have also pointed to possible protection against the disease.

Other gut benefits

Researchers used to think that fiber caused diverticulosis, in which small pouches form in the wall of the colon, usually its lower part. Those pouches, or diverticula, can become infected, bleed, and even rupture. But researchers now know that fiber can actually help prevent diverticulosis by warding off the constipation and resulting increase in colonic pressure that contribute to pouch formation.

In addition, the Harvard study in men found that those who ate the most fiber, particularly from fruits and vegetables, had only about half the ulcer risk of those who ate the least. And an Italian study published this year linked a high fiber intake with a 30 percent drop in the likelihood of gallstones.

Food over fiber

The link between fiber and reduced coronary risk is strong and getting stronger. But the link for fiber-rich *foods*—fruits, vegetables, and whole grains—is stronger still. And while the evidence that those foods help ward off stroke, colon cancer, and breast cancer is not conclusive, it's more solid than the evidence for fiber itself. For that reason, it's usually better to rely on foods than on fiber supplements such as *Fiberall, Metamucil,* and *Mylanta Natural Fiber.*

Foods contain numerous other substances that may help fend off one or more of those diseases. They also tend to be low in calories and fat, particularly saturated fat, the artery-clogging kind. And they may protect against numerous other diseases as well, including other kinds of cancer.

So despite the often inconclusive evidence on fiber itself, the practical message is clear: Eat a wide variety of fiber-rich whole foods. Those foods should provide you with 20 to 35 grams of fiber each day, depending on how many calories you consume. The average woman, who consumes about 1,600 calories a day, should get at least the lower number; the average man, who consumes about 2,500 calories, should aim for at least 30 grams. To get a rough idea of how much fiber you consume, complete the worksheet on preceding page. (For a more precise tally, consult the table on this page and read the labels on packaged foods.)

FIBER CONTENT OF SELECTED FOODS

Food	Serving size	Total fiber (g)	Soluble fiber (g)	Insoluble fiber (g)
BREAKFAST CEREALS [2]				
All-Bran Bran Buds	⅓ cup	13.0	4.0	9.0
All-Bran Extra Fiber	½ cup	13.0	1.0	12.0
Fiber One	½ cup	13.0	1.0	12.0
Quaker Oat Bran	½ cup	6.0	3.0	3.0
Raisin Bran	½ cup	4.0	0.5	3.5
Cheerios	1 cup	3.0	1.0	2.0
Grape Nuts	¼ cup	2.5	0.5	2.0
Shredded Wheat	1¼ large	2.9	0.2	2.7
Oatmeal	½ cup	2.0	1.2	0.8
Corn Flakes	1 cup	1.0	0.0	1.0
LEGUMES (cooked)				
Lentils	½ cup	9.2	1.5	7.7
Red kidney beans	½ cup	8.2	3.4	4.9
Split peas	½ cup	8.1	2.5	5.6
Pinto beans	½ cup	7.4	2.7	4.6
Great Northern beans	½ cup	6.2	1.1	5.1
Navy beans	½ cup	5.8	1.7	4.1
Lima beans	½ cup	4.9	1.2	3.8
BREADS/GRAIN/PASTA				
Barley	½ cup	6.8	1.4	5.4
Whole-wheat spaghetti	½ cup	3.2	0.4	2.7
Whole-wheat bread	1 slice	2.2	0.5	1.7
Oat-bran muffin	½	2.1	0.7	1.5
Rye bread	1 slice	1.9	0.8	1.0
Brown rice	½ cup	1.8	0.2	1.6
Wheat bread	1 slice	1.6	0.2	1.4
Bagel	½ medium	1.3	0.5	0.8
Spaghetti	½ cup	1.1	0.5	0.6
White bread	1 slice	0.6	0.3	0.3
White rice	½ cup	0.6	0.1	0.4
NUTS AND SEEDS				
Almonds	¼ cup	3.9	0.4	3.5
Sunflower seeds	¼ cup	2.2	0.7	1.5
Peanut butter, smooth	2 tbsp	2.1	0.6	1.5
Filberts	¼ cup	2.1	0.7	1.4
Walnuts	¼ cup	1.4	0.5	0.9
FRUITS (fresh)				
Apple, with skin	1 large	4.2	1.6	2.6
Pear, with skin	1 medium	4.0	0.8	3.2
Blackberries	½ cup	3.8	0.9	2.9
Florida orange	1	3.6	2.1	1.5
Prunes, dried	4	3.1	1.3	1.8
Banana	1	2.8	0.9	1.9
Kiwi fruit	1	2.6	0.9	1.7
Peach/nectarine, with skin	1	2.1	0.8	1.3
Grapefruit, pink or red	½ large	1.8	1.3	0.5
Strawberries	½ cup	1.7	0.6	1.1
VEGETABLES (cooked)				
Artichoke hearts	½ cup	4.8	0.6	4.2
Corn	½ cup	4.7	0.2	4.4
Green peas	½ cup	4.4	0.6	3.8
Avocado	½ cup	3.8	1.5	2.2
Brussels sprouts	½ cup	3.6	1.7	1.9
Sweet potato, without skin	1 medium	3.4	1.7	1.7
Potato, without skin	1 large	2.8	0.7	2.1
Broccoli	½ cup	2.3	1.0	1.3
Carrot slices	½ cup	2.3	1.0	1.3
Spinach	½ cup	2.1	0.6	1.4
Green beans	½ cup	2.0	0.8	1.2
Cauliflower	½ cup	1.5	0.2	1.3
VEGETABLES (raw)				
Tomato	1 medium	1.3	0.3	1.0
Celery	½ cup	0.9	0.2	0.7
Pepper, green	½ cup	0.9	0.3	0.6
Romaine lettuce	1 cup	0.7	0.3	0.4

[1] The recommended daily intake for fiber is 20 to 35 grams.

[2] All cold cereals based on a serving size of approximately 1 ounce; volume varies due to differing densities. Servings of hot cereals (*Quaker Oat Bran* and oatmeal) weigh more than 1 ounce.

Sources: ESHA Research, Salem, Ore., and manufacturers' data.

Fiber power

To reach the recommended minimum intake, most American men need to add at least 12 grams of total fiber to their daily diet; most women need to add at least 6 grams. But don't go overboard: Getting a lot more than the recommended maximum of 35 grams a day can interfere with the body's absorption of nutrients such as calcium, iron, and zinc; huge amounts can even cause intestinal blockage. And don't rush: Boosting fiber intake too fast can cause flatulence, bloating, cramps, and diarrhea.

You're much less likely to encounter any of those problems—and you'll get innumerable other benefits as well—if you eat fiber-rich whole foods instead of relying on fiber supplements or high-fiber cereals. (Such supplements may be useful only for people who are constipated or who have trouble eating the grains, beans, and produce that supply fiber naturally.) Eating at least five servings per day of fruits, vegetables, or beans and at least six servings of whole grains—the government-recommended amounts—generally ensures an ample intake of fiber.

Here are several ways to boost your fiber intake:

■ Choose breads made from whole-wheat flour. Most breads called "wheat" or "multigrain" are made primarily from refined flour, with a smattering of whole-grain flour plus some molasses or caramel coloring to give the bread that brown, "natural" look. To make sure you get whole-wheat products, look on the label for any of these reassurances: the words "whole wheat" or "100 percent whole grain"; whole-wheat flour listed as the first ingredient; or at least 2 grams of fiber in each slice of bread.

■ Bake with whole-grain instead of refined flour.

■ Choose brown rice over white rice, and whole-wheat pasta over regular or even spinach pasta.

■ Substitute whole, unpeeled fruits for fruit juices. Eat them as an appetizer, dessert, or snack. If you treat yourself to ice cream or cake, top it with fruit.

■ Add fruit, brown rice, or whole-grain cereals to yogurt.

■ Add beans, barley, or other whole grains to soup. Snack on cooked, cooled beans seasoned with garlic powder, chili powder, or Cajun spice. Or make them into a bean dip for raw vegetables.

■ Prepare cold salads that combine cooked whole grains, pasta, or beans with chopped raw vegetables. (Don't spend on lettuce-based salads for fiber.)

■ Make meatless entrees by cooking grains in seasoned stock and tossing them with vegetables or beans.

Summing up

Despite the sometimes conflicting research, fiber is almost surely good for the heart in many small ways that add up to a significant benefit. In particular, fiber helps reduce cholesterol, blood pressure, and body weight; it may also help the heart by warding off blood clots and reducing insulin levels. Most of those benefits have been linked specifically to soluble fiber.

The gastrointestinal tract may benefit from fiber, too, especially the insoluble kind. At the very least, fiber helps prevent constipation and diverticulosis, and it may reduce the risk of ulcers and gallstones. More important, some evidence suggests that fiber may help fend off colon cancer—and possibly breast cancer, too. But for nearly all those benefits, the evidence for high-fiber *foods* is stronger than for fiber itself.

The best sources: beans, high in both types of fiber; whole grains and most vegetables, especially rich in insoluble fiber; and oats and most fruits, especially high in soluble fiber (see table). But if you eat at least five daily servings of produce or beans and six servings of whole grains, you should automatically get enough fiber without worrying about the specific type.

Food for Thought about Dietary Supplements

The surge of public interest in nutrition supplements has been fired by the recently enacted federal regulations governing health claims, which permits the health food industry to make claims about the function of nutrients not permitted for food products. This article provides healthy skepticism about the common rationales for the use of supplements.

PAUL R. THOMAS, ED.D. R.D.

Paul Thomas, currently a Fellow at the Georgetown Center for Food and Nutrition Policy, Georgetown University, previously served as a staff scientist for the Food and Nutrition Board, Institute of Medicine, National Academy of Sciences. He is a registered dietitian who received an Ed.D. degree in nutrition education from Columbia University. He is an author and editor of several books on contemporary nutrition issues. Correspondence can be directed to him at the Georgetown Center for Food and Nutrition Policy, 3240 Prospect Street, N.W., Washington, DC 20007.

The dietary supplements industry is very healthy. Sales of vitamins, minerals, and other food concentrates are roughly $4 billion per year. Although at least one quarter of American adults swallow these pills, powders, and potions daily,[1] probably the majority of us take them at least occasionally. What are we getting in return?

I've asked myself this question since the 1960s when, as a teenager, I began taking dozens of supplements after reading about their magical powers in *Prevention* and *Let's Live* magazines, and books by

> **The Food and Nutrition Board recommends that those who choose supplements limit the dose to levels of the RDA or less.**

Adelle Davis. Surely they would help cure my adolescent acne; I just needed to find the right combination. But my pizza face only improved when I took tetracycline and topical retinoic acid (the drug, not the vitamin) prescribed by a dermatologist. Growing out of adolescence also helped.

My education about dietary supplements became more comprehensive when I discovered the medical library during my college education as a biology ("pre-med") major. I learned that the hype surrounding them in the popular press was rarely supported by studies in the journals. Dietary supplements have benefited me in that they developed my interest in nutrition to the point where I chose to make a career in this discipline. But over time, and despite the growing popularity of supplements even among nutrition professionals, I have gone from being an enthusiastic vitamin promoter to a skeptic.

Most of us would agree that it's best to meet our nutritional needs with food, which means that everyone should eat a healthy, balanced diet. I believe that, short of that, dietary supplements are at best a poor and inadequate substitute. Supplements are appropriate for some people for specific purposes. But should they be taken every day, by everybody? I don't think so, and I make my case with the following eight points.

POINT 1: NO EXPERT BODY OF NUTRITION EXPERTS RECOMMENDS THE ROUTINE USE OF SUPPLEMENTS

A small number of nutritionists support regular supplement use. But no scientific body of nutrition experts recommends that everyone take supplements on a routine basis as dietary insurance or for optimal health. Expert bodies are by nature conservative and unlikely to recommend a practice until the evidence is convincing and perhaps even overwhelming. That's the point, since dietary guidance for most people should be based on strong evidence.

In 1989, the Food and Nutrition Board of the National Academy of Sciences issued a comprehensive review of the relationships between diet and health.[2] The report stated that dietary supplements should be avoided at levels above the Recommended Dietary Allowances (RDAs). Finally, however, a group of nutrition experts was not warning people to stay away from supplements with pronouncements of dire risks from their use. The recommendation was not to stay away from supplements, but to take them in no more than RDA amounts. The Food and Nutrition Board acknowledged that the long-term potential risks and benefits of supplements had not been adequately studied and called for more research.

> *Some proponents feel that supplements are "magic bullets" for cancer, heart disease, and other maladies.*

The latest pronouncements on supplements are found in the new (4th) edition of *Dietary Guidelines for Americans*, which was released in January.[3] The report states that "diets that meet RDAs are almost certain to ensure intake of enough essential nutrients by most healthy people," and that people with average requirements are likely to have adequate diets even if they don't meet RDAs.

About supplements, the report states: "Daily vitamin and mineral supplements at or below the Recommended Dietary Allowances are considered safe, but are usually not needed by people who eat the variety of foods depicted in the Food Guide Pyramid." It acknowledged, however, that some people might benefit from supplements. These include older people and others with little exposure to sunlight who may need extra vitamin D. Women of childbearing age might reduce the risk of neural-tube defects in their infants with folate-rich foods or folic acid supplements. Pregnant women usually benefit from iron supplements. And vegans, who avoid animal products, might need some nutrients in pill form. The report urges the public not to rely on supplements.

Surveys show that most supplementers take a one-a-day multiple-vitamin-mineral product. But some take large doses of single nutrients or nutrient combinations as self-prescribed medication for disease or to try to reach a more optimal state of health, the latter fueled most recently by the enthusiasm for antioxidants. The practices of these aggressive supplementers merit some concern.

POINT 2: NUTRITION IS ONLY ONE FACTOR THAT INFLUENCES HEALTH, WELL-BEING, AND RESISTANCE TO DISEASE

The major chronic diseases that prematurely maim and kill most Americans have multiple causes. However, just as the advent of antibiotics and vaccines led many to think that the cure of diseases awaited specific "magic bullets," some proponents of supplements seem to think that these products are nutritional magic bullets for cancer, heart disease, and other maladies.

Health reporter Jane Brody calls us "a nation hungry for simple nutritional solutions to complex health problems."[4] Edward Golub, in his recent book, *The Limits of Medicine*, warns us against "thinking in penicillin mode."[5] It can be easy to do in

20. Food for Thought about Dietary Supplements

> *Supplements are not the answer to health and disease for the vast majority of people.*

nutrition because the first identified nutrient-related diseases (*eg*, scurvy and beriberi) were caused by dietary deficiencies. Anyone who doesn't get enough of the proper nutrient will eventually succumb to the relevant deficiency disease. No matter how much you exercise, who your parents are, or whether or not you smoke, you will become scorbutic without sufficient vitamin C.

Unfortunately, there is no such simple cause-effect relationship for diseases such as cardiovascular disease, cancer, stroke, and diabetes. Large doses of vitamin E, for example, may or may not influence the risk of developing heart disease. For some people, it may potentially be important. For most, however, it is at best one factor, and probably not a major one.

A primary contributor to chronic disease risk is our genetic heritage. Nutritionist Elizabeth Hiser writes, "Genes have a powerful influence over body size and disease risk, and though diet helps temper unwanted tendencies, *who* you are is often more important than *what* you eat. ... Because of genetics, diet helps some people a lot, some people a little, and a very few people not at all."[6] Genetic endowment accounts in large measure for why some people get heart disease when young, for example, no matter how well they care for themselves, and why others live long lives even when they violate many of the commandments of healthy living.

Chronic disease risk is also affected by whether or not we exercise, refrain from smoking, avoid drinking to excess, limit exposure to unproductive stressors, and have sufficient rest, relaxation, and fun—and, of course, eating a diet that meets dietary guidelines and the

RDAs. In our enthusiasm for supplements, however, we run the risk of reducing the importance of these factors.

One example of "thinking in penicillin mode" is linking calcium with the treatment, and especially prevention, of osteoporosis. However, bone health is influenced by many factors, including smoking, alcohol consumption, exercise, and intake of nutrients such as phosphorus, protein, and boron that affect calcium absorption, utilization, and excretion. In fact, osteoporosis is uncommon in several countries with relatively low calcium intakes.

> *Even, when and if, phytochemicals are reliably found in supplements, it will never be appropriate to take them in that form rather than from foods that contain them.*

Social commentator H. L. Mencken said, "For every complicated problem there is a simple solution—and it is wrong."[7] Supplements are not the answer to health and disease for the vast majority of people. Who our parents are, how we live our lives, and the food we put into our mouths several times a day affect our health more profoundly.

POINT 3: FOOD IS MORE THAN THE SUM OF ITS NUTRIENTS

Nutritionists used to think that macro- and micronutrients made a food nutritious and good for health. Other food constituents, such as fiber, were seen as nonessential, and therefore unimportant, since death is not directly associated with fiber deficiency. However, we have learned that, while fiber is not essential in the traditional sense, its presence in the diet makes it much easier to defecate and influences blood cholesterol levels and risk of diseases such as diverticulosis and certain cancers.

Many compounds in food that are not classical nutrients can apparently influence health and risk of disease. Several hundred studies show that heavy fruit and vegetable eaters have approximately half the risk of cancer compared with those who don't eat these foods, but the results are not consistently related to one or several nutrients. New biologically active constituents found mostly in plant foods—phytochemicals (or "phytomins" as *Prevention* magazine calls them)—are being discovered regularly. They include flavonoids, monoterpenes, phenolics, indoles, allylic sulfides, and isothiocyanates. Phytochemicals became a "hot item" in 1994 when they were the subject of a cover story in Newsweek that April.[8] The title: "Better than Vitamins: The Search for the Magic Pill." (There's that word too often linked with supplements: magic! So is "miracle.")

Whole natural foods, to quote *Newsweek*, "harbor a whole ratatouille of compounds that have never seen the inside of a vitamin bottle for the simple reason that scientists have not, until very recently, even known they existed, let alone brewed them into pills." Even when phytochemicals can reliably be found in supplements, it will never be appropriate to swallow pills (or consume specially fortified processed foods) instead of eating recommended amounts of the foods that contain them, such as vegetables, fruits, whole grains, and legumes. To do so would be to inappropriately rely on preliminary science, when the future will bring the discovery of new phytochemicals that have always been available from today's natural foods. Determining whether and how isolated food constituents with biological activity may improve health, treat disease, or extend life is a daunting task that will occupy researchers for decades or longer.

Scientists continue to learn more about the complexity of foods and the myriad of biologically active constituents they contain that can influence health and disease risk. How ironic, then, that the calls this research generates for renewed efforts to persuade people to eat healthier diets—the tried and true—often seems to be drowned out by the acclaim for dietary supplements.

POINT 4: DEVELOPING RDAs AND OPTIMAL NUTRIENT RECOMMENDATIONS IS VERY DIFFICULT

As a staff scientist with the Food and Nutrition Board, I worked with the subcommittee that developed the most recent (10th) edition of the RDAs. I was surprised to learn that the research base for the RDAs is quite limited. There are not as many studies as one would like to determine minimum and average nutrient requirements for each age-sex group, estimate the population variability in need, and to feel more comfortable about the judgments made to derive nutrient allowances. Setting RDAs is tough work!

> *Developing recommendations for optimal nutrient intakes will be many times more complex than developing RDAs.*

Now there is substantial discussion about so-called optimal intakes of nutrients, levels of intake that might allow people to be healthy and fit for a longer time. Some nutrition scientists believe optimal nutrient intakes will typically exceed RDA levels and may require supplements in some cases to achieve. Still, no one doubts that developing optimal nutrient intakes will be orders of magnitude more complex than developing RDAs.

The optimal intake of any nutrient will probably vary substantially among individuals and even throughout the person's life from infancy to old age. It will probably also depend on the parameter of interest. For example, an optimal intake of a nutrient to reduce the risk of heart disease might not be optimal to decrease cancer risk and might actually increase it. Defining, understanding, and assessing optimal nutrition is becoming one of the most exciting challenges for investigators in the nutrition and food sciences.

Clinical studies help identify cause-and-effect relationships, whereas epidemiologic studies can only identify whether variables are related.

POINT 5: TAKING SUPPLEMENTS OF SINGLE NUTRIENTS IN LARGE DOSES MAY HAVE DETRIMENTAL EFFECTS ON NUTRITIONAL STATUS AND HEALTH

On April 14, 1994, the *New England Journal of Medicine* published the infamous Finnish study.[9] In this clinical trial, 29,000 male smokers in Finland were randomly divided into four groups, receiving either a placebo, 20 mg beta-carotene (approximately four to five times the amount in five servings of fruits and vegetables), 50 IU of vitamin E (about three to four times average dietary intakes, but still a small dose as a supplement), or both the beta-carotene and vitamin E. After 5 to 8 years, the beta-carotene takers had an 18% *higher* incidence of lung cancer, with hints that this carotenoid might also have raised their risk of heart disease. Vitamin E seemed to reduce the risk of prostate cancer but increased the risk of hemorrhagic stroke.

This study is noteworthy, both because of its surprising findings and the fact that it is one of the few large clinical trials on supplements and disease risk. The majority of studies investigating this relationship are epidemiologic in nature. Clinical trials in which subjects are randomly assigned to treatment or control groups help to identify cause-and-effect relationships. Epidemiologic studies, in contrast, can only identify whether the variables under study are related in some way.

The Finnish study showed that antioxidant nutrients might harm rather than help male smokers, so it has been scrutinized intensely. Blumberg, for example, noted that those with the highest plasma concentrations of vitamin E and beta-carotene at the start of the study had the lowest risk of developing lung cancer[10]; therefore, these nutrients may have provided some protection to some smokers. But for those who would suggest that the subjects should not have expected any benefits from supplements, given their deadly habit, two points should be made. First, several epidemiologic studies show that fruit and vegetable consumption reduces the risk of lung cancer in smokers— again, foods (containing beta-carotene and many other carotenoids and phytochemicals), not supplements. Second, dietary supplements are often promoted to smokers and those who are not eating or taking care of themselves as well as they should with claims that the products protect health.

A major concern with supplements is potential toxicity.

The Center for Science in the Public Interest, a consumer advocacy group that had recommended antioxidants to its readers, changed its position after the Finnish study.[11] "Shelve the beta-carotene," it said, or take no more than about 3 mg per day, the amount found in many multivitamins. It also advised people to "reconsider taking vitamin E." *New York Times* medical writer Nicholas Wade, commenting on the Finnish study, said: "The vitamin supplement industry... would like everyone to believe the issue of benefits is settled.... For all who assumed the answer was already known, the Finnish trial offers two lessons. One is that science can't be rushed. The

Large doses of one nutrient can adversely affect nutritional status in relation to another nutrient.

other is not to put all your bets on those convenient little bottles: back to broccoli and bicycles."[12]

Time shows the wisdom of Wade's advice. Two large clinical trials were completed in January of this year that further debunk beta-carotene as a magic bullet. After 12 years of taking either 50 mg beta-carotene or a placebo every other day, 22,071 physicians learned that the phytochemical provided no protection against cancer or heart disease. In the second trial, 18,314 men and women at risk for lung cancer due to smoking or exposure to asbestos were given supplements of beta-carotene (30 mg/day), vitamin A (25,000 IU/day), or a placebo. Those receiving the supplements had a *higher* rate of death from lung cancer and heart disease; although the results were not statistically significant, the study was halted. Dr. Richard Klausner, the director of the National Cancer Institute, which financed both trials, concluded, "With clearly no benefit and even a hint of possible harm, I can see no reason that an individual should take beta-carotene."

A major concern with supplements is potential toxicity. Fat-soluble vitamins like A and D, which are stored in the body, are obviously harmful in excess, but so are some water-soluble nutrients. Large doses of vitamin B6, for example, can produce neuropathy in the arms and legs, leading to partial paralysis. Some people taking tryptophan have developed and died from eosinophilia-myalgia syndrome, a connective tissues disease characterized by high levels of eosinophils, severe muscle pain, and skin and neuromuscular problems. (It is not yet certain whether the syndrome was caused by the tryptophan itself, by a contaminant produced in the manufacturing process, or by the two in combination.) High-dose niacin supplements, especially in the time-released form, have caused liver damage. Large amounts of beta-carotene can be dangerous to alcoholics with liver disorders. And antioxidant nutrients can act as prooxidants under certain conditions, generating cell-damaging free radicals.[13]

Another concern with supplements is the possibility of adverse nutrient interactions. Calcium, for example, affects the absorption of iron and vice versa. Various amino acids compete with each other for absorption from the small intestine and to cross the blood-brain barrier. Large doses of one nutrient or phytochemical can adversely affect nutritional status in relation to another. In one study, for example, very large doses of beta-carotene, 100 mg/day given for 6 days, decreased the concentration of another important carotenoid, lycopene, in the low-density lipoproteins by 12 to 25%.[14] Beta carotene is not the only carotenoid of benefit to health, or perhaps even the most important one. I am reminded of Walter Mertz, the renowned nutrition and trace mineral expert, who was asked if he took beta-carotene as a supplement. He replied he would be "afraid" to take it, not knowing how extra beta-carotene would affect the balance of all the other carotenoids in his body that he obtained from food.

Little information is available to demonstrate that the long-term and possibly lifetime intake of large doses of nutrients is completely safe. Studies on the consequences of large nutrient intakes in humans rarely have a large sample size and go beyond several months. If high levels of iron in the body, for example, really increase the risk of heart disease, as at least one study suggests,[15] the chances are remote that a physician will think that a patient who died of a heart attack possibly did so because of supplemental iron. In other words, nutrient toxicity may be a cause of more illness and death than suspected, because the problems will not be linked (or even thought to have a possible link) to use of supplements.

POINT 6: DIETARY SUPPLEMENTS VARY SUBSTANTIALLY IN QUALITY

Few federal manufacturing and formulation standards exist for supplements, in part because they fall into a regulatory gray area between food and drugs.[16] A decade ago, investigators discovered that many calcium supplements did not disintegrate or dissolve in the digestive tract; the calcium was simply excreted. These results prompted the development of disintegration and dissolution standards for some types of supplements by the US Pharmacopoeia, the scientific organization that establishes drug standards....

Garlic supplements provide an example of not necessarily getting what you think you paid for. They have become popular because several studies suggest that garlic may help to lower blood cholesterol and reduce the risk of cancers of the breast, colon, and other organs. Attention has focused on two compounds that may be responsible for these effects: allicin and s-allyl cysteine. The Center for Science in the Public Interest analyzed garlic powder and various garlic pills and found major differences by brand in their content of these two compounds.[17] Plain garlic powder was best and least expensive, whereas the most popular brand of garlic supplement contained no allicin (Table 1). Similarly, Consumers Union recently found that ginseng products varied greatly in their content of ginsenosides, the root's supposed active ingredients.[18]

It is difficult to find a comprehensive, one-a-day type of supplement that supplies nutrients at RDA levels. Most products are not well balanced. They contain, for example, many times the recommended amount of inexpensive B vitamins like thiamin and riboflavin but only small amounts of calcium and magnesium, because recommended amounts of these minerals can add substantially to the size of the pill. Some supplements contain superfluous ingredients such as bee pollen, hesperidin complex, and PABA, which do little more than boost the price (see Refs. 19 and 20 for good advice on choosing a supplement).

POINT 7: SUPPLEMENTS ARE PROMOTED BY COMMERCIAL AND OTHER FORCES ON THE BASIS OF INCOMPLETE OR PRELIMINARY SCIENCE

I stated earlier that the bulk of evidence linking supplements to reduced risks of heart disease, cancer, and other diseases is epidemiologic in nature, or based on *in vitro*, mechanistic, or biochemical studies. They show correlations and indicate the possibility of protective effects, but do not prove cause and effect. So we do not know whether most of these suggestive data are of practical importance to people over the long run as they eat good or bad diets, smoke or refrain from smoking, live in polluted or clean environments, and are either exercisers or couch potatoes.

The scientific community tends to blame journalists for distorted reporting about nutrition. True, there are both good and mediocre reporters on the subject. And too often the

Table 1
Comparison of Garlic Supplements

Name of Supplement	Cost per Tablet* (cents)	Allicin (µg)†	SAC (µg)‡
McCormick Garlic Powder§	6	5,600	590
KAL Beyond Garlic	18	4,800	270
Garlique	33	3,840	130
Garlicin	18	2,165	145
Nature's Way	8	1,530	140
Kwai	11	815	60
Quintessence	9	535	185
Natural Brand (GNC)	10	300	45
P. Leiner (private label)‖	5	115	45
Kyolic¶	11	0	255

© 1995, CSPI. Adapted from *Nutricion Action Healthletter* (1875 Connecticut Ave., N.W., Suite 300, Washington DC 20009-5728. $24.00 for 10 issues).
* Based on list price when available or average price paid.
† One large clove of fresh garlic supplies about 5,000 µg allicin.
‡ S-allyl cysteine.
§ One-third teaspoon.
‖ Product usually carries the name of the drugstore or other chain where it is sold.
¶ The best-selling garlic supplement.

reporting is bad, incomplete, prepared from press releases, or focused on one study without placing it in perspective—a poor foundation for people to make intelligent decisions.

A recent study illustrates this point, Houn and colleagues examined popular press coverage of research on the association between alcohol consumption and breast cancer.[21] Of the 58 published journal papers on this topic over 7 years, only 11 were cited by the press. Three studies published in the *New England Journal of Medicine* and the *Journal of the Medical Association* were featured in more than three quarters of the news stories. And almost two thirds of the stories gave recommendations to women on alcohol consumption based on one study. Reporters ignored the published review articles and editorials that would have provided a better basis for advice. This highlighting of a few studies, which seems to occur in many other nutrition areas, tends to confuse people and lead them to think that a new study will undoubtedly contradict the findings of the previous one. It's the new math of media nutrition coverage: 1 + 1 = 0. As syndicated columnist Ellen Goodman puts it, "Fresh research has a sell-by date that is shorter than the one on the cereal box."[22]

Responsibility for distorted reporting of nutrition does not rest with the media alone. Increasingly, it involves nutrition scientists. Although they tend not to make exaggerated claims when reporting their work at scientific meetings, some are more bold when they speak to reporters or the public. Sometimes their institution's press office encourages this boldness. As research funds become harder to secure, scientists and their employers are

> *Responsibility for distorted reporting of nutrition rests as much with some nutritional scientists as with the media; many major journals reach reporters before medical professionals.*

learning that being in the news raises their visibility, which can help to raise money.

Now, major journals like the *New England Journal of Medicine* and *Journal of the American Medical Association* reach reporters before they reach biomedical professionals. And because a growing amount of research is financed by industry, a company might seek publicity about a new finding to enhance the value of its stock or draw attention to itself. A good book on the changing nature of reporting scientific advances is *Selling Science*, by sociologist Dorothy Nelkin.[23]

The dietary supplements industry is busy making bold claims for its products on the labels, in advertising, and in product literature using preliminary science. The 1990 Nutrition Labeling and Education Act, which resulted in the new nutrition labels on packaged foods, allows supplement manufacturers to present the same health claims that are allowed on foods—claims supported by "significant scientific agreement" and preapproved by FDA. Two of the authorized health claims are relevant to supplements: the links between calcium and osteoporosis and between folate and neural tube defects.

However, the Dietary Supplement Health and Education Act passed in 1994 allows the industry to make claims pertaining to the structure and function of a nutrient. For example, a supplement could not claim that it helps cure AIDS, but it might be possible to state that the product "boosts the immune system." The legal basis for a claim is that (1) some substantiation exists, (2) FDA be notified of the claim within 30 days of its presence on the label, and (3) two additional sentences be added to such claims: "This statement has not been evaluated by FDA. This product is not intended to diagnose, treat, cure, or prevent any disease." Along with these so-called "structure-function" claims, a retailer may now provide literature on supplements, although it is supposed to be balanced scientifically and not be misleading. Some members of the dietary supplements industry are fighting even these limitations, arguing that their absolute freedom of speech to provide whatever information they think is appropriate is being threatened.

An advertisement in *Time* magazine last October for Bayer Corporation's One-A-Day Brand Vitamins suggests the growing boldness of claims for even mainstream dietary supplements. The copy states: "It's been all over the news. Findings on folic acid studies were announced recently at a medical conference in Bar Harbor, Maine, suggesting that adequate intake of folic acid may significantly lower elevated homocysteine levels, one of the risk factors for heart attacks and strokes in men. One-A-Day Men's Formula contains 100% of the US RDA of folic acid. Why not start taking your One-A-Day today?"

Public health may benefit from the promotion of supplements by increasing the public's awareness of nutrient, diet, and disease relationships. But I fear the risks outweigh the benefits. The promotional copy typically fails to give information on food-related alternatives to supplements. In addition, the public rarely has the expertise to evaluate the information in the promotion. Furthermore, consumers' expectations of a product's effectiveness may be heightened by the hype and lead to irrational use of the product.

There can be a great difference between *a* truth and *the* truth. A truthful statement may inevitably be misleading. This lesson was made clear in the plethora of ridiculous health claims on foods back in the late 80s and early 90s. Some high-fat products, for example, were truthfully labeled as being cholesterol free, because manufacturers knew many people would think the product was more healthful.

> **Dietary supplements provide a false sense of security.**

> **Concentrating anything in the food chain, be it vitamin C, beta-carotene, salt, or fat, increases the likelihood of mistakes.**

Supplements supplying nutrients at levels beyond what can reasonably by obtained from food should be viewed as nonprescription drugs. High-potency products should not be used without careful thought and perhaps expert help.

POINT 8: FOCUSING ON NUTRIENTS AND SUPPLEMENTS CAN TAKE ATTENTION AND CONVICTION AWAY FROM IMPROVING ONE'S LIFESTYLE

Nationally representative surveys of American adults show that approximately one third are interested in nutrition and think they are on the right track to healthy eating. In contrast, another third couldn't care less about meeting dietary guidelines. Those in the middle third claim they are trying to eat better, but find it difficult.

So, the good news is that two thirds of adult Americans say they care about their nutrition. But the bad news is that perhaps only 5 to 10% of the US population meets dietary recommendations regularly, such as eating five or more servings of fruits and vegetables per day and limiting fat to no more than 30% of calories. Furthermore, obesity is a growing epidemic in this country, now affecting one third of adults and one quarter of children. The irony is that people who eat well are most likely to take supplements, whereas those most likely to benefit from higher nutrient intakes are least likely to take them.

My greatest concern about dietary supplements is the false sense of security it provides some people, those who use supplements to an extent as substitutes for a good diet. It is natural for us to want an easier way or, ideally, some magic bullet, to achieve health short of being vigilant or saintly all the time. We're especially likely to cut corners when we are short of time and feeling stressed, such as by choosing foods on the basis of convenience and ease of preparation and by not exercising. Taking a basic supplement as one small part of a health-promoting lifestyle may be reasonable and perhaps even prudent. But taking supplements is a problem for people, probably the majority, who are not making the lifestyle changes they know they should. A recent advertisement by Hoffman-La Roche, Inc. for vitamin E states... "Many doctors... believe taking supplements or eating fortified foods containing vitamins and minerals is a sound health measure, particularly for people who don't eat a good diet...." Unfortunately, some people use supplements as a deliberate or unconscious excuse for not trying to improve their diets and lifestyles.

A reporter called me some time ago to ask how people could use vitamins to stay healthy. I replied that people should pay more attention to their diets. He told me to be realistic and used himself as an example. He said he leads a very busy life, has little time to shop for food and prepare it, and there are few places near work that serve nutritious lunches. So what supplements would help him cope more productively with his situation? Here is an example where supplements may harm more than help, by being used as a surrogate for tackling the hard things that would really improve his nutritional status, such as preparing lunches the night before, convincing nearby restaurants to offer more nutritious fare, and making sure he eats a very nutritious breakfast and dinner. This reporter was looking for what he acknowledged to be a second-best solution, but taking a supplement will make him even less likely to attempt the best but more difficult solution.

CONCLUDING THOUGHTS

... Those who recommend that healthy people supplement their diets with extra vitamins and minerals often call it a form of dietary insurance, as essential to have as car or home insurance. I disagree. When you purchase insurance, the benefits and costs of the policy are detailed and you choose a specific level of protection. The terms of a dietary insurance policy, though, can never be known, much less specified. Taking supplements without a clear need is more analogous to playing the lottery. You hope to win some money, and ideally the jackpot, by buying lottery tickets. You won't hurt yourself unless you buy more tickets over time than you can afford, but you are not likely to win anything either, especially the big prize.

Even comprehensive dietary supplements are, at best, poor substitutes for nutrient-rich foods. Foods, about which we know little, are more than the sum of their parts, about which we have some knowledge. Furthermore, it's harder to hurt yourself with foods than with supplements. Concentrating anything in the food chain—be it vitamin C, beta-carotene, salt, or fat—increases the likelihood of mistakes. Nutrients and other nonnutrient substances relevant to health are readily available in familiar and attractive packages called fruits, vegetables, legumes, grains, and animal products. And they come in concentrations and in combinations with which humans have had long cultural familiarity.[29] ...

REFERENCES

1. Slesinski MJ, Subar AF, Kahle LL. Trends in use of vitamin and mineral supplements in the United States: The 1987 and 1992 National Health Interview Surveys. *J Am Diet Assoc* 1995; 95: 921–3.
2. National Research Council. *Diet and Health: Implications for Reducing Chronic Disease Risk.* Washington, DC: National Academy Press, 1989.
3. US Department of Agriculture, Department of Health and Human Services. *Nutrition and Your Health: Dietary Guidelines for Americans,* 4th ed. Washington, DC: Government Printing Office, 1995.
4. Brody J. Personal health: Sorting out the benefits of taking extra vitamin E. *New York Times,* July 26, 1995: C8.
5. Golub E. *The Limits of Medicine: How Science Shapes Our Hope for the Cure.* New York: Times Books, 1994.
6. Hiser E. Getting into your genes. *Eating Well* 1995; 6 (1): 48–9.
7. Herbert V, Kasdan TS. Misleading nutrition claims and their gurus. *Nutr Today* 29 (3): 28–35, 1994.
8. Begley S. Beyond vitamins: The search for the magic pill. *Newsweek,* April 25, 1994: 45–9.
9. The Alpha-Tocopherol, Beta-Carotene Cancer Prevention Study Group. The effect of vitamin E and beta carotene on the incidence of lung cancer and other cancers in male smokers. *N Engl J Med* 1994; 330: 1029–35.
10. Blumberg JB. Considerations of the scientific substantiation for antioxidant vitamins and B-carotene in disease prevention. *Am J Clin Nutr* 1995; 62: 1521S–1526S.
11. Liebman B. Antioxidants: Surprise, surprise. *Nutr Action Healthletter* 1994; 21 (5): 4.
12. Wade N. Method and madness: Believing in vitamins. *New York Times Magazine,* May 22, 1994: 20.
13. Herbert V. The antioxidant supplement myth. *Am J Clin Nutr* 1994; 60: 157–8.
14. Graziano JM, Johnson EJ, Russell RM, Manson JE, Stampfer MJ, Ridker PM, Frei B, Hennekens CH, Krinsky NI. Discrimination in absorption or transport of B-carotene isomers after oral supplementation with either all-*trans*- or 9-*cis*-β-carotene. *Am J Clin Nutr* 1995; 61: 1248–52.
15. McCord JM. Free radicals and prooxidants in health and nutrition. *Food Tech* 1994; 48 (5): 106–11.
16. Anon. Buying vitamins: what's worth the price? *Consumer Rep* 1994; 59: 565–9.
17. Schardt, D. Schmidt S. Garlic: Clove at first sight? *Nutr Action Healthletter* 1995; 22(6): 3–5.
18. Anon. Herbal roulette. *Consumer Rep* 1995; 60: 698–705.
19. Anon. A 9-point guide to choosing the right supplement. *Tufts Univ Diet & Nutr Letter* 1993; 11(7): 3–6.
20. Liebman, B, Schardt D. Vitamin smarts. *Nutr Action Healthletter* 1995; 22(9): 1, 6–10.
21. Houn F, Bober MA, Huerta EE, Hursting SD, Lemon S, Weed DL. The association between alcohol and breast cancer: Popular press coverage of research. *Am J Publ Health* 1995; 85: 1082–6.
22. Goodman E. To swallow or not to swallow. *Liberal Opinion Week,* April 24, 1994.
23. Nelkin D. *Selling Science: How the Press Covers Science and Technology,* revised edition. New York: WH Freeman and Company, 1995.
24. Anon. Many shoppers not yet aware of nutrition facts label. *Food Labeling News* 1995; 3(32): 21–3.
25. Gussow JD. *A Word on Behalf of Food.* Presentation at the Alumni Advances Conference of the dietetic internship program at Oregon Health Sciences University, Portland, OR, May 1995.
26. Shepherd SK. Nutrition and the consumer: Meeting the challenge of nutrition education in the 1990s. *Food & Consumer News* 1990;62 (1): 1–3.
27. Goodman E. Food literacy. *Liberal Opinion Week,* December 14, 1992.
28. Stacey M. *Consumer: Why Americans Love, Hate, and Fear Food.* New York: Touchstone Books, 1994.
29. Gussow JD, Thomas PR. *The Nutrition Debate: Sorting Out Some Answers.* Palo Alto, CA: Bull Publishing Co., 1986.

The views expressed in this article are those of the author and do not reflect the position of the Center for Food and Nutrition Policy.

Unit 3

Unit Selections

21. **Disease-Fighting Foods? (Many Are Overhyped. But All Offer Important Lessons about Good Nutrition),** Consumer Reports on Health
22. **"Mediterranean Diet" Reduces Risk of Second Heart Attack** The Cleveland Clinic Heart Advisor
23. **Homocysteine: "The New Cholesterol"?** The Cleveland Clinic Heart Advisor
24. **Soy: Cause for Joy?** Jack Raso and Ruth Kava
25. **False Alarms about Food** Consumer Reports on Health
26. **Questions and Answers about Cancer, Diet and Fats,** International Food Information Council
27. **How to Grow a Healthy Child,** Dairy Council Digest
28. **A Focus on Nutrition for the Elderly: It's Time to Take a Closer Look,** Nutrition Insights
29. **Physical Activity and Nutrition: A Winning Combination for Health,** Dairy Council Digest
30. **Alcohol and Health: Straight Talk on the Medical Headlines,** Charles H. Hennekens

Key Points to Consider

❖ Pretend that you are planning research projects relative to nutrition and your age group. Rank by order of importance your top three priorities and defend them.

❖ What changes should you make in your lifestyle in order to conform to the best current knowledge about your nutrient needs? Choose one change and brainstorm ways to achieve it.

❖ Support the concept that variety is one of the key factors in an appropriate diet. Are there any disadvantages?

❖ Are you and your friends as sedentary in your lifestyles as the average American of the same age? If so, what could you do to change that?

❖ The decision to use or not use alcohol and the decision about how much to use are not always easy ones. List the reasons for your decisions and evaluate them.

DUSHKIN ONLINE Links   www.dushkin.com/online/

14. **American Cancer Society**
    http://www.cancer.org/frames.html
15. **American Heart Association**
    http://www.americanheart.org
16. **The Food Allergy Network**
    http://www.foodallergy.org
17. **Go Ask Alice! from Columbia University Health Services**
    http://www.goaskalice.columbia.edu
18. **Heinz Infant & Toddler Nutrition**
    http://www.heinzbaby.com
19. **LaLeche League International**
    http://www.lalecheleague.org
20. **National Osteoporosis Foundation**
    http://www.nof.org
21. **Nutrition for Kids: 24 Carrot Press**
    http://www.nutritionforkids.com
22. **Vegetarian Resource Group**
    http://www.vrg.org

These sites are annotated on pages 4 and 5.

Through the Life Span: Diet and Disease

> Food improperly taken, not only produces diseases, but affords those that are already engendered both matter and sustenance; so that, let the father of disease be what it may, intemperance is its mother.
>
> —Richard E. Burton

Perhaps you have heard the old adage "You are what you eat." Your parents may have read a book by Adelle Davis in which she claimed that aging will not occur on the days one eats right. We all know that neither of these statements is literally true, but scientists are constantly supporting the concept that what we eat does affect what we are.

It is commonly agreed that a good (balanced) diet throughout life will help us all reach our genetic potentials and avoid premature aging, disease, and untimely death. Studies of other populations often provide clues to diet/disease connections. Researchers must interpret them cautiously, however, as such studies cannot prove all-inclusive cause-and-effect relationships; sometimes the results even appear contradictory.

From time to time, scientific evidence does consolidate into a very clear health message. One case in point is the protective qualities of many chemicals in our foods, especially in fruits and vegetables. The need for antioxidants to scavenge and disarm damaging free radicals seems clear. Some antioxidants are known nutrients such as vitamins E and C; others are also part of the chemical structure of our foods, but until recently we have known little about them. This information represents a significant breakthrough in our understanding of how the body works, but the reader should be cautious about interpreting it to mean that bottles of supplements would be a wise investment. The first article in this unit addresses this topic.

Several articles in this unit were selected because they discuss common chronic diseases of concern to large numbers of people. During our youth we tend to feel invulnerable, but then life moves on, slipping eventfully and uneventfully through a few decades. Soon the fiftieth birthday is celebrated, with the golden years just beyond. Typically, we have gained weight, probably more than currently is considered healthy. And, as we reach our sixties and seventies, more and more of us will be dealing with high blood pressure, coronary disease, cancer, osteoporosis, and other conditions that cause varying degrees of disability. Now major lifestyle changes become inevitable. However, these diseases might have been avoided altogether, or at least delayed, if we had made the appropriate lifestyle choices while we were young.

Heart disease is one of the biggest health concerns in this country and is the topic of several articles. Blood cholesterol, which is partially dependent upon one's consumption of saturated and trans fats, has been considered one of the primary diet-related risk factors. However, high homocysteine levels may be equally serious, and some research suggests that a low folacin intake is responsible. Other news that an egg a day does not increase a risk of heart disease in most people is supported by the findings of two recent studies and by the evidence that eggs contain little harmful fat, as well as less cholesterol than previously thought. Moderate consumption of caffeine (the International Food Information Council suggests a daily limit of 3 cups of coffee or 300 mg. of caffeine) does not appear to be harmful either; nor is red meat harmful if it is lean and limited to moderate portions. For those with high blood cholesterol, the food industry is promoting two margarines containing stanol esters that are touted to effect as much as a 14 percent cholesterol reduction after as little as 8 weeks. And, interestingly, the Bureau of Alcohol, Tobacco, and Firearms has given permission for wine labels to include statements that suggest beneficial effects.

Another article specifically addresses the diet/cancer connection, one that is still somewhat controversial. By some estimates, diet may account for 30 percent of cancers and worldwide dietary patterns generally find higher cancer rates linked to populations that eat lots of red meat and lower rates linked to plant-based diets. It has been estimated, therefore, that eating the recommended 5 or more fruits and vegetables daily would cause a cancer decline in the United States of 20 percent, with even higher reductions for lung, colon, and rectal cancers. But, if this is true, does it represent a clear cause-and-effect? And, if so, is it the high fat content of the meat, the compounds produced during cooking, the lack of protective chemicals such as antioxidants in plant foods, or something else altogether? Once again we find strong support for finding protection in diet rather than in a pill.

Endless subsets of any large population have special needs. In this edition, these groups are represented by children and the elderly. Eating habits are established early that affect development and later health. According to some sources, teenagers achieve 92 percent of their bone mass by the time they are 18, yet only 60 percent of them consume the recommended calcium intake. High-fat foods such as cake and cookies are among children's top sources of protein, fiber, calcium, and iron. And, according to a government study, cold breakfast cereals are the primary sources of vitamins and minerals for American children. With a quarter of our children overweight, it is clear that some changes are appropriate.

The elderly have somewhat better eating habits than their grandchildren. Thirteen percent of us are now over 65 years of age, and an increasing number of us reach 85 years and beyond. With declining energy needs, it is difficult to consume enough nutrient-dense foods. Absorption rates have declined, and risks of many chronic diseases have now been realized. Other factors such as physical limitations and lack of mobility may also interfere with consuming a good diet.

Finally, there are two articles on unrelated topics that affect us. Exercise is not strictly a nutrition topic, but the need for it is so interrelated with the amounts of food we eat and with the same diseases affected by nutrition that it seems irresponsible not to include it. The same applies to the use of alcohol, where some consumers will benefit and some will be harmed.

One should remember that there is still much we do not know about nutrition and that even within age, gender, and ethnic groups, people are physiologically different. Connections between food/nutrition and health can be found in other units in this book. Unit 1 has articles on protective qualities of fruits and vegetables. Articles on vitamins, lipids, and other nutrients are found in unit 2, and unit 6 discusses information leading to harmful dietary practices. The reader might also review articles in previous *Annual Editions: Nutrition* and in periodicals to appreciate the extent of the information—and the confusion—surrounding nutrition.

Article 21

Disease-fighting foods?

Many are overhyped. But all offer important lessons about good nutrition.

Sometimes the news about nutrition sounds too good to be true. Pizza may prevent prostate cancer. Wine protects the heart. Garlic may prevent heart disease *and* cancer. Even when the food doesn't make you drool, you may still be excited to read that ordinary tea or broccoli may work wonders.

But today's wonder foods can easily lose their luster overnight—or regain it just as fast—when a new headline highlights a contradictory finding. One reason for those dizzying swings is that virtually all individual foods have at most only a modest affect on health, since any one item makes up only a small part of

RESEARCH ROUNDUP ON HOT FOODS

Dietary item	Supposed benefit	Evidence on active ingredients	Evidence on the food itself	Recommendations
Broccoli and other cruciferous vegetables	Cancer protection	**Isothiocyanates** (most notably **sulforaphane**) and two antioxidants, **vitamin C** and **beta-carotene** (in dark-green crucifers), help prevent and inhibit cancer growth. **Indoles** help convert estrogen into a harmless hormone.	Numerous observational studies have linked cruciferous vegetables with reduced cancer risk. Broccoli and cauliflower sprouts, which contain far more sulforaphane than mature vegetables, fight cancer in animals.	Eat cruciferous vegetables regularly. Adding broccoli or cauliflower sprouts is theoretically beneficial, though there's no supporting evidence in humans. (Other cruciferous vegetables include brussels sprouts, cabbage, cauliflower, kale, and turnips.)
Tomatoes and tomato products	Cancer protection	The antioxidants **lycopene** and **vitamin C** help prevent and inhibit cancer growth.	Several recent studies have linked high intake of lycopene from tomatoes and tomato products with reduced risk of prostate and other cancers.	The suggestive evidence adds another possible reason—beyond the many nutrients in tomatoes and tomato products—to eat those foods and possibly other items high in lycopene, including apricots, guavas, pink grapefruit, and watermelon.
Oats and oat bran	Heart protection	**Soluble fiber** reduces blood-cholesterol level.	Clinical trials indicate that the amount of bran in 1½ cups of oatmeal, eaten daily, can reduce total-cholesterol level by about 6 points.	Eating enough oatmeal or oat bran to affect your cholesterol levels significantly may be difficult. But consuming lots of soluble fiber, from oats as well as beans, produce, and nuts, is a good idea, especially if your cholesterol level is high.
Garlic and other allium vegetables	Heart protection	**Allicin** inhibits blood clots, reduces cholesterol production in the liver, and helps open arteries.	Studies have linked high intake of garlic and other allium vegetables with reductions in cholesterol and blood pressure. Three recent well-designed, though relatively small, trials of garlic pills have yielded little or no evidence of those effects.	It's probably not worth taking garlic pills. Whether whole garlic and related vegetables help protect against cancer or coronary disease is unclear. (Other allium vegetables include chives, leeks, onions, and scallions.)
	Cancer protection	**Sulfur-allyl cysteine** and other sulfur compounds block formation and effects of cancer-causing chemicals.	One large observational study has linked garlic with reduced colon-cancer risk. Several weaker studies suggest a possible stomach-cancer connection.	
Olive oil	Heart protection	**Monounsaturated fat** lowers "bad" LDL cholesterol. **Oleic acid, polyphenols,** and **vitamin E** inhibit the oxidation that turns LDL cholesterol bad.	Mediterranean people, who consume lots of olive oil, have low rates of coronary disease. But whether that's due to the oil or other health habits is not known.	There's no convincing evidence that any of the nontropical vegetable oils—whether predominantly monounsaturated (like olive oil) or polyunsaturated—is better than the others for the heart. But choose any of those oils over tropical oils or butter, high in saturated fat, or partially hydrogenated oils, high in equally harmful trans fat.
	Breast-cancer protection	**Monounsaturated fat**, unlike polyunsaturated fat, does not promote cancer in animals. **Oleic acid, polyphenols,** and **vitamin E** inhibit the oxidation that can turn normal cells cancerous; polyphenols help neutralize cancer-causing substances in several other ways as well.	A few observational studies have linked olive oil with reduced breast-cancer risk. However, a smaller but far more rigorous study found no connection.	Preferring olive oil to other oils in hopes of reduced breast-cancer risk can't hurt, but the supporting evidence is slim at best.
Nuts	Heart protection	**Monounsaturated fat, polyunsaturated fat,** and **soluble fiber** reduce cholesterol levels. **Arginine** widens arteries and inhibits clotting. **Vitamin E** and **flavonoids** fight the oxidation that turns LDL cholesterol bad.	Four large observational studies, including Nurses' Health Study and Physicians' Health Study, have linked nuts with reduced coronary risk.	Consider adding some nuts to your diet—particularly if they replace fatty meat or full-fat dairy foods as a source of protein.

Reprinted with permission from the March 1999 issue of *Consumer Reports on Health*, pp. 8-9, for educational purposes only. © 1999 by Consumers Union of U.S., Inc. Yonkers, NY 10703-1057, a nonprofit organization. The information and images you receive online regarding Consumer Reports material are protected by the copyright laws. We prohibit any commercial use of our material, including copying, redistributing, or retransmitting. To subscribe, call 800-234-1645 or visit us at www.ConsumerReport.org.

21. Disease-Fighting Foods? Many Are Overhyped

the total diet. So a benefit may be too subtle for some studies to detect. In fact, the apparent benefit may be too small to merit focusing on that one food. And for most foods, studies have only suggested a benefit, they haven't proved it.

But whether or not the evidence warrants paying special attention to a particular food, it usually does point to a larger lesson. For oat bran, for example, that's to eat plenty of other foods high in soluble fiber, since fiber is what lowers cholesterol.

Other reports, about broccoli, olive oil, tomatoes, and perhaps garlic, are significant because they too point to an entire family of less famous foods. Research on nuts highlights the potential coronary benefits not only of soluble fiber but also of unsaturated fats from most any food. While much of the evidence on fish and soy foods is still equivocal, eating them instead of fatty meat clearly is healthful.

The possible benefits of ordinary tea illustrate the most important point of all: There's a cornucopia of obscure, potentially protective compounds in virtually all plant foods. So it's wise to consume a wide variety, since new research may turn today's nutritional lightweight into a heavyweight—or vice versa.

RESEARCH ROUNDUP ON HOT FOODS

Dietary item	Supposed benefit	Evidence on active ingredients [1]	Evidence on the food itself	Recommendations
Fish and fish oil	Heart protection	**Omega-3 fatty acids** reduce triglyceride levels, inhibit blood clots and abnormal heart rhythms, and reduce blood pressure.	Fish oil seems to reduce blood pressure only slightly; evidence linking fish with reduced risk of *developing* coronary disease is inconsistent. However, stronger evidence links fish with reduced risk of cardiac *death*, theoretically caused by blood clots or abnormal heart rhythms. And fish oil may help lower triglycerides.	It's not worth taking fish-oil capsules for the heart (except under doctor's supervision for very high triglycerides). But eating fish once or twice a week, particularly to replace fatty meat, is worthwhile. At the very least, fish is generally low in fat, particularly saturated fat.
	Rheumatoid arthritis relief	**Omega-3 fatty acids** inhibit production of inflammatory chemicals that worsen rheumatoid arthritis.	Clinical trials suggest that fish oil may reduce arthritis symptoms.	Rheumatoid-arthritis patients may want to try fish-oil pills, under doctor's supervision. To benefit from fish itself, you'd probably have to eat a lot every day.
Green or black tea	Cancer prevention	**Flavonoids** and other **polyphenols** are potent antioxidants, and help neutralize cancer-causing substances in several other ways as well.	Tea does help prevent and fight cancer in animals. Observational studies in humans have linked tea with reduced cancer risk, particularly in the digestive tract.	Despite limited evidence in humans, drinking this inexpensive beverage can't hurt and might help (unless you're one of the few people who should avoid caffeine).
	Heart protection	**Flavonoids** and other **polyphenols** inhibit the oxidation that turns LDL cholesterol bad, reduce LDL level, inhibit blood clots, and may raise "good" HDL level.	Limited observational research suggest that tea may reduce LDL level and possibly raise HDL level. Two studies have linked a high intake of flavonoids with a reduced risk of coronary death.	
Soy foods, such as tofu and soy milk	Cancer protection	**Isoflavones** are plant estrogens. The isoflavone **genistein** reduces cells' intake of human estrogen, which fuels breast cancer. Genistein also suppresses enzymes and new blood vessels that stimulate tumor growth.	Chinese and Japanese women, who consume lots of soy foods, have a lower incidence of breast cancer. But there's little other support for soy's anticancer action in humans.	Regard any anticancer effect of soy foods as theoretical.
	Heart protection	**Soy protein** and possibly other substances reduce cholesterol level. **Genistein** inhibits blood clots, blockage in blood vessels, and the oxidation that turns LDL bad.	Clinical trials suggest that a high soy intake may reduce the total-cholesterol level by as much as 6 to 10 percent.	Consuming roughly four servings of soy foods or beverages per day may help improve cholesterol levels—particularly if those servings replace fatty meat.
	Menopausal relief and bone protection	**Soy protein** and **isoflavones** may ease menopausal hot flashes and slow postmenopausal bone loss.	Menopausal flashes are less common in Far East, and two small clinical trials suggest soy may reduce frequency. Some evidence links soy with fewer fractures in postmenopausal women; one small trial suggests a possible increase in bone density.	Trying a high-soy diet for menopausal flashes can't hurt, though there's only limited supporting evidence.
Red wine and other alcoholic beverages	Heart protection	**Alcohol** raises level of "good" HDL cholesterol and inhibits blood-clot formation. **Flavonoids** and **resveratrol** (both in red wine) inhibit the oxidation that turns LDL bad. Flavonoids inhibit clots, too.	Alcohol is by far the most important ingredient in these drinks. The overall evidence on coronary disease suggests no advantage for red wine over white, or for any wine over beer or spirits.	Moderate intake of any alcoholic beverage—no more than two drinks a day for men, one for women—may be good for the heart. But don't *start* drinking unless you've discussed it with your doctor—and avoid alcohol entirely if you're susceptible to addiction or have any medical reason for not drinking.

[1] Includes both preliminary and established findings, almost entirely from laboratory and animal studies.

"MEDITERRANEAN DIET" REDUCES RISK OF SECOND HEART ATTACK

For years now, we've heard that Mediterranean cuisine is not only tasty but good for the heart. The most recent data come within the past few months as researchers in Lyons, France, announced that the so-called Mediterranean diet—based on fish, fruits, vegetables, cereals, beans, grains and olive oil—can reduce the risk of a second heart attack or other cardiac "event" by as much as 50–70%.

Results of the Lyons Diet Heart Study

Cardiac Event	Mediterranean Dieters (219 patients)	Western Dieters (204 patients)
Cardiac deaths	6	19
Nonfatal Heart Attacks	8	25
Unstable angina	6	24
Heart failure	6	11
Stroke	0	4

Source: Mediterranean Diet, Traditional Risk Factors, and the Rate of Cardiovascular Complications After Myocardial Infarction, Circulation, 1999; 99:779-785.

In the study, published in the Feb. 16 issue of the American Heart Association's journal Circulation, half the participants ate a diet low in saturated fat and cholesterol, high in fiber, and rich in omega-3 fatty acids (believed to protect against heart disease). The other half were the "control" group, eating a "prudent" Western-type diet relatively low in fat, cholesterol and saturated fat. Other variables—including blood pressure, cholesterol levels and weight—were largely similar between the two groups. Nearly 20% of each group continued to smoke throughout the study. All had had a previous heart attack.

The research was an extension of the original 27-month Lyons Diet Heart Study, which was halted in 1994 to allow the control group to switch to the Mediterranean diet since its benefits proved overwhelmingly positive. For the continuing study, 219 original participants were located, followed and compared with a new control group of 204 for 19 months.

The study showed that eating a Mediterranean-style diet not only lowered the chances of cardiac death and heart attack but protected against heart-related complications such as unstable angina (severe, uncontrollable chest pain), stroke, heart failure, and blood clots in the lungs or elsewhere (pulmonary or peripheral emboli). A subanalysis of the original study showed that the Mediterranean diet also substantially reduced the risk of certain cancers, especially of the urinary and digestive tracts and the throat.

Fat: the surprise ingredient

Surprisingly, the Mediterranean dieters enjoyed a fair amount of the fat consumption, often thought to be linked to cancer and heart disease.

The type of fat eaten is apparently significant. The Mediterranean dieters consumed 30% of their calories from fat—exactly in accordance with recommendations promoted by the National Cholesterol Education Program (NCEP) and the American Heart Association (AHA) for the general public. But most of the fat was taken in the form of unsaturated oils: either fish, olive, nut (walnut) or seed (flaxseed) oils. Saturated fat—as found in butter, for example—contributed only 8% of this group's calories. Saturated fat is known to raise blood cholesterol level more than anything else.

Those in the control group—whose diet more closely resembled a traditional American diet—got 34% of their calories from fat, nearly 12% of it saturated. The differences may seem slight, but they make a difference; the AHA and NCEP recommend that anyone who has already had a heart attack follow a diet known as the "Step II" diet, in which less than 30% of total calories come from fat and less than 7% from saturated sources. (See "What are the Step I and II diets?)

Participants on the Mediterranean diet also ate more omega-3 fatty acids, including alpha linolenic acid (LNA), eicosapentaenoic acid (EPA) and docosahexenoic acid (DHA). Omega-3 fatty acids have been shown in many studies to protect against coronary artery disease and may also

What are the Step I and II diets?

The American Heart Association and the National Cholesterol Education Program recommend the Step I and step II diets to reduce the risk of coronary heart disease. The Step I guidelines are designed for the general public. Step II is for people who have cholesterol levels in the high-risk range (240 mg/dL and higher) or who have had a heart attack. These changes in diet should be carried out under a physician's guidance, along with regular physical activity and weight reduction as needed.

Complete information on the Step I and Step II dietary guidelines is contained in NCEP's "Step by Step: Eating to Lower Your High Blood Cholesterol." It can be found on the Internet at www.nhlbi.nih.gov/nhlbi/cardio/chol/gp/stepb.htm .
Or call 1-301-592-8573 or fax 1-301-592-8563.

Sources: American Heart Association and National Cholesterol Education Program

---

prevent sudden cardiac death. LNA is found in tofu, nuts, soybeans, flaxseed and canola oil. EPA and DHA are found in seafood, especially cold-water seafood such as codfish and sardines. Along with being an excellent source of omega-3 fatty acids, fish is also a good protein source that is low in saturated fat.

Cholesterol and fiber count, too

More cholesterol was consumed by those on the "Western" diet; approximately 30% more, or 312 mg/day. The Step II diet limits daily cholesterol intake to 200 mg, in line with the Mediterranean group. Dietary fiber intake was about 3 grams higher in the Mediterranean diet. (Fiber intake came from fruits, vegetables and whole-grain products, which also provide large amounts of antioxidant vitamins and important trace elements.) Animals foods were mostly of the fish, yogurt and low-fat feta cheese variety. Meat was eaten only occasionally in the Mediterranean group and rarely as the main ingredient in a meal.

Some professionals call for revised guidelines

The Lyons Diet Heart Study results are so impressive that some prominent researchers are urging that NCEP and AHA reconsider dietary recommendations contained in the Step I diet. Specifically, they suggest that those guidelines for saturated fat intake may be too high, and for omega-3 fatty acids too low.

Researchers are also considering whether taking cholesterol-lowering medication in combination with the Mediterranean-style diet might be even more protective. But until clinical trials are done and results are in, check with your doctor to see if such a diet is suited for you. Considering that most of the Mediterranean dieters were still following the diet years after it began, it doesn't seem to be a hardship either on your taste buds or your willpower.

HOMOCYSTEINE: "THE NEW CHOLESTEROL"?

A substance in the blood called homocysteine has made headlines repeatedly over the past few years as a possible new risk factor for cardiac disease. But is it? And if so, what should you do about it? *Heart Advisor* asked Killian Robinson, M.D., a Cleveland Clinic cardiologist who has published widely on the topic of homocysteine, for the facts.

What is homocysteine?

Homocysteine (pronounced HO-mo-SIS-teen) is an amino acid. Several amino acids, including methionine, are essential in human nutrition. Homocysteine is produced when methionine is metabolized. Homocysteine normally stays in the blood only for a short time and is then cleared from the body by the liver.

What makes levels of homocysteine rise? Men have higher levels of homocysteine than women. Medications such as niacin (which is sometimes used for cholesterol lowering) and antifolate drugs (which are used to fight malignant disease) can cause elevated levels. Aging also causes homocysteine to rise.

High levels of homocysteine also occur in a rare inherited disease, homocystinuria, in which a genetic error makes the liver unable to dispose of homocysteine normally. The artery walls of children with this disorder are abnormally thickened and diseased. Patients with homocystinuria may die from blood clots in the brain, heart and kidneys.

Why is homocysteine suspect?

Despite the appearance of the arteries of young victims of homocystinuria, no one suspected that homocysteine played a role in heart disease until a young medical school graduate, Kilmer S. McCully, M.D., published a research paper in 1969. Based on his observations of homocystinuria, Dr. McCully proposed that homocysteine buildup may in fact also be responsible for atherosclerosis. For the most part, the medical community ignored or scoffed at this theory.

Over the past few years, however, the relationship between atherosclerosis and high levels of homocysteine has become a hot "new" topic. In his book *The Homocysteine Revolution*, Dr. McCully surmises that this may be because, over time, physicians have begun to see that traditional risk factors (such as cholesterol and hypertension) cannot account for a large percentage of heart attacks. In fact, people with no recognized risk factors can have coronary disease.

Researchers from Australia and then Europe published the earliest studies revisiting the homocysteine question. The papers strongly suggested a relationship between homocysteine and cardiovascular disease. In this country, a study by The Cleveland Clinic published 1995 in *Circulation* found that high levels of homocysteine increased the risk of heart disease fivefold. That same year, Tufts University researchers found that subjects who had higher levels of homocysteine were also more likely to have blockage of the carotid (neck) artery, a warning sign of the possibility of a stroke or coronary artery disease. They published their findings in *The New England Journal of Medicine*.

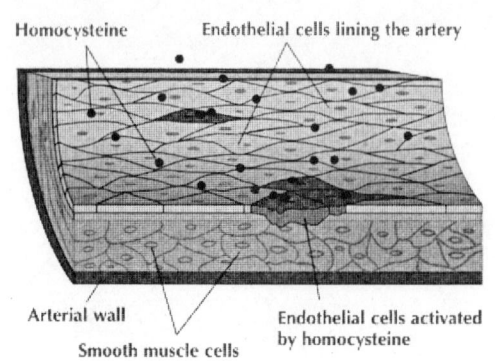

In 1997, the *Journal of the American Medical Association (JAMA)* reported that people with the highest levels of homocysteine in the blood had more than twice the risk of clogged arteries in the heart, brain or elsewhere. A *New England Journal of Medicine* study, also published in 1997, showed that heart patients with high homocysteine levels had higher mortality rates than patients with low homocysteine levels. And a study that year from the Netherlands, published in *Arteriosclerosis, Thrombosis and Vascular Biology,* determined that every 10 percent increase in homocysteine levels meant about a 10 percent increase in the risk of developing coronary disease.

The evidence was mounting, prompting some researchers to wonder out loud whether homocysteine was "the new cholesterol," an artery-clogging substance previously—and erroneously—considered harmless.

The B vitamin link

Meanwhile, scientists were also looking for a relationship between B vitamins—specifically folate (folic acid), B_6 and B_{12}—and coronary disease. In homocystinuria patients, doses of B vitamin supplements reduced homocysteine levels. Could B vitamin deficiency be linked to cardiac disease?

It seemed so. A 1996 Canadian study in *JAMA* found that participants who did not have diagnosed heart disease at the start of the study but who had the lowest folate levels were much more likely to die of coronary disease than those in the group with the highest levels of folate (who also began the study free of cardiac disease).

The Nurses' Health Study of more than 80,000 nurses found that the women who consumed the lowest amounts of folic acid and B_6 were more likely to develop heart disease, despite the fact that they had no known heart problems at the start of the study. The women who got the most folic acid and B_6 over the years cut their risk of heart disease in half.

A case-control study by Dr. Robinson and members of the European Concerted Action group, published in the Feb. 10, 1998, issue of *Circulation,* determined that lower levels of folate and B_6 conferred an increased risk of atherosclerosis. The study examined 1,550 patients under age 60 in 19 countries.

Results of a double-blinded, placebo-controlled study reported at the 1998 International Joint Conference on Stroke and Cerebral Circulation showed that a combination of folic acid, B_6 and B_{12} could lower homocysteine levels in patients who had had a stroke.

At the August 1998 Congress of the European Society of Cardiology in Vienna, it was reported that heart disease patients who are folate deficient are 1.7 times more likely to have a heart attack than those who have normal levels.

But findings from other, "prospective" studies (in which the research question is posed before the data are collected) have been less consistent. Some have shown a definite relationship between coronary artery disease and elevated homocysteine levels as well as an inverse correlation with B vitamins. Yet other large, well-designed studies—for example, The Atherosclerosis Risk in Communities (ARIC)—have not. In the July 21, 1998, issue of *Circulation,* ARIC authors stated that they could find no consistent relationship between homocysteine and the risk of disease.

The differences could be because of design problems or methodological limitations of the different studies, or even differences in tests used to measure homocysteine and sample size.

"It is perturbing that the prospective studies do not always bear out the findings of earlier case-control studies," Dr. Robinson says. "We need to determine whether there is a true cause-and-effect connection between heart disease and homocysteine.

"Of course, an association does not always prove causality. It's possible that what we are seeing when homocysteine levels are high is an 'epiphenomenon,' or a fellow traveler of vascular disease rather than a cause of it.

"The true question at this point in time," Dr. Robinson continues, "is if you treat the problem—high homocysteine—does the risk of cardiac disease disappear? This is what current trials are designed to find out."

What you can do

In general, doctors are loath to recommend any kind of treatment when a theory is still unproven. However, the intervention needed to keep homocysteine

---

What's a normal homocysteine level?

Before the dangers of cholesterol were understood, levels as high as 300 milligrams per deciliter (mg/dL) were considered safe. Today, normal is defined as under 200 in otherwise healthy people, and levels over 240 mg/dL call for medical treatment.

In a similar vein, the definition of normal levels of homocysteine is the subject of some debate. Different physicians believe "normal" is anywhere from five to 12 micromoles per liter.

"Studies show that the risk of cardiovascular disease rises as homocysteine levels go above 10 to 12," Dr. Robinson says. People who are vitamin deficient, taking certain drugs or in renal failure can have levels as high as 100 to 200.

Homocysteine levels are measured by a blood test, best done after fasting. Your physician won't necessarily test you for homocysteine, however, unless you are routinely seen at a teaching hospital where there is an academic interest in the question.

If you have been diagnosed with heart disease, or are at risk, you can request a homocysteine test, which may be covered by health insurance.

levels low—increasing your B vitamin intake—is so benign that many doctors are recommending it as a safe course of action until the study results become available in the next four to five years.

Dr. Robinson recommends starting with a heart-healthy diet that includes good sources of B vitamins. It's fairly easy to get enough B_6 and B_{12}—good sources include fish, poultry, lean meat, bananas, prunes, dried beans and whole grains.

It's a bit harder to reach the recommended dietary allowance (RDA) for folic acid, which was recently raised to 400 micrograms (mcg). Green leafy vegetables such as spinach and brussels sprouts, dried peas, beans, lentils and nuts are your best bets, in addition to some fortified cereals.

The government recently began fortifying breads and grains with folic acid, primarily to prevent birth defects that have been associated with folate deficiency. Check the nutrition label on foods you buy made with grain—there may be added folic acid.

Many doctors are advising their cardiac patients to take a multivitamin tablet daily to ensure adequate folic acid. "There's probably very little risk to taking a multivitamin supplement," Dr. Robinson says.

Warning

If you choose to supplement your diet with folic acid, it may be wise to also take 500 mcg of vitamin B_{12}. "Too much folic acid can mask a deficiency of B_{12} that is more common as we age," Dr. Robinson explains. "The deficiency may lead to nerve damage that could persist or worsen if undiscovered."

Alternatively, you could have your levels of B_{12} checked by your physician every six months. If they're normal, you would not need to add B_{12}.

Note: Even multivitamin pills should be taken under medical supervision if you have had a heart attack.

Soy: Cause for Joy?

By Jack Raso and Dr. Ruth Kava

The soybean, a legume that has for millennia been a staple in tropical and warm temperate regions of East Asia, has in the West recently been described as a superfood "leading the phytochemical revolution." Phytochemicals are diverse compounds whose common denominator is that plants produce them. The word usually refers to plant compounds termed "bioactive non-nutrients," and the vitamins that plants make are not conventionally referred to as phytochemicals. Ingesting phytochemicals, unlike ingesting vitamins and certain minerals, is not considered essential for maintaining human lives. But scientific findings tentatively suggest that habitual ample intakes of such compounds may contribute to disease prevention.

For example, such findings associate phenolic phytochemicals called "isoflavones" with the prevention of cancer, coronary heart disease (CHD), and osteoporosis. Isoflavones are a class of phytoestrogens, or "plant estrogens"—i.e., phytochemicals that have low estrogenic activity—and have been termed "dietary estrogens," "estrogeno-mimetics," and "estrogen mimics." Because of the isoflavone concentration in soy—which is greater than that in any of the other known edible-plant sources of these chemicals (chickpeas, for instance)—soybeans are exceptionally high in phytoestrogens. (Phytoestrogens also include certain "lignins"—noncarbohydrate dietary fibers.)

More than 2,500 varieties of soy are being cultivated. Soybeans are used to make many foods, including miso (a fermented paste), *natto* (soybeans that have been steamed, fermented, and mashed), soymilk, tempeh (fermented soy; also spelled "tempe"), tofu (bean curd), and certain meat substitutes and noodles. Miso, regular soymilk, roasted soy nuts, soy flour, tempeh, tofu, and textured vegetable protein (TVP) are rich in isoflavones. But soy oil, soy sauce, and some other soy products lack them.

Cholesterol reduction can result from ingesting as few as 25 grams of soy protein daily....

The most abundant isoflavone in soy is genistein, which has been the focus of most isoflavone research. Genistein and daidzein, another of the major isoflavones in soy, are structurally similar to the sex hormone estradiol—the main form of estrogen that the ovaries produce (and the form that occurs naturally in plants). Soybeans are the only significant dietary source of genistein and daidzein. Researchers attribute the healthful effects of consuming soybeans and soyfoods largely to the hormonal and other actions of these isoflavones and to the ability of soy protein to reduce cholesterol and low-density lipoprotein (LDL, or "bad") cholesterol in the blood.

But soybeans contain other compounds that might be preventive or have therapeutic utility in humans—for example, the Bowman-Birk inhibitor (BBI) and other protease* inhibitors; inositol hexaphosphate (IP6); and soaplike sugar derivatives called "saponins." The BBI may have utility in preventing and suppressing carcinogenesis. IP6—which is also a constituent of other legumes, rice, wheat bran, and virtually all mammalian cells—apparently can normalize various cancerous cells in mice. Saponins (many of which have a steroid portion) may have utility in preventing colon cancer and in reducing blood cholesterol. Moreover, soybeans are high in fiber (e.g., possibly anticarcinegenic lignins); folic acid; the trace element boron; and the essential minerals calcium, iron, magnesium, and zinc.

Heart Disease

About 34 million Americans have excessive cholesterol in their blood. That elevated plasma cholesterol is a major risk factor for CHD has been established. A decrease in plasma cholesterol of 1 percent decreases the risk of CHD by 2 percent.

---

* Proteases are enzymes that speed protein decomposition.

Cardiovascular disease (CVD)—which includes heart disease,* hypertension, and strokes—is the leading cause of death in the United States. But in Japan, for example, the incidence of CVD is low, and the difference in CVD incidence between the U.S. and Japan has been linked to dietary factors, such as soy-product consumption and daily calorie intake (which is lower in Japan than in the U.S.). The inhabitants of the Far East and Southeast Asia typically derive about 10 percent of their daily protein intakes from soybeans, whereas in the U.S. soybeans contribute minimally to such intake.

> ... [T]he daily calorie intake in countries characterized by high soyfood consumption is much less than that in the U.S.

In a study published in *The New England Journal of Medicine* in 1995, researchers compared data from 38 clinical trials performed over 25 years that had focused on the effects of soy protein consumption on blood lipid levels. They concluded that soy protein consumption can reduce plasma cholesterol by 9.3 percent. If this is so—and if a 1 percent reduction of plasma cholesterol reduces the risk of CHD by 2 percent—appropriate intakes of soy protein might reduce CHD risk by nearly 19 percent.

The cholesterol-lowering effect of soy protein seems independent of fat intake and is most pronounced in persons whose plasma cholesterol is elevated. Cholesterol reduction can result from ingesting as few as 25 grams of soy protein daily (as from one cup of soybeans, though 40 grams may be optimal for some persons), and this effect increases according to one's intake. The mechanism by which soy protein lowers blood cholesterol has not been elucidated but is an object of continuing scientific investigation. In any case, because soybeans have no cholesterol and are low in saturated fat and high in fiber (that soy fiber can reduce blood cholesterol has also been demonstrated), they are an appropriate food for most persons with heart disease.

In November 1998 the U.S. Food and Drug Administration proposed, pending public comments, to allow the labeling of foods that contain at least 6.25 grams of soy protein per serving as able—in the context of a diet low in saturated fat and cholesterol—to lower CHD risk.

Cancer

Cancer is the second leading cause of death in the U.S. In China, Japan, and other countries where soyfood intake is ample, the prevalence of breast, colon, and prostate cancers is much lower than that in the U.S. Scientific findings suggest that soy and soyfood consumption may be partly responsible for this low prevalence. But it is notable that the daily calorie intake in countries characterized by high soyfood consumption is much less than that in the U.S.

> The soy isoflavones diadzein and genistein are similar to ipriflavone, a synthetic drug used widely in Asia and Europe that tends to prevent decreases in bone mass.

Estrogen can promote tumors, and high estrogen levels increase one's risk of developing breast cancer. Because isoflavones bind to receptors to which estrogen would otherwise have bound, they can, theoretically, prevent or lessen interactions between estrogen and tumors.

Isolated isoflavones have appeared beneficial against cancer in *in vitro* tests and, at very high levels, in animal experiments. Thus, the hypothesis that soybeans and soyfoods are protective against cancer in humans deserves testing. But whether ingesting soybeans, soyfoods, or isolated isoflavones in adulthood lowers one's risk of developing cancer is far from settled. For example, some reports of laboratory studies indicate that genistein stops the growth of human breast-cancer cells, while others indicate it contributes to such growth. Factors, dietary (e.g., a relatively low daily calorie intake) and nondietary (e.g., relatively high activity), that tend to accompany the consumption of soybeans and soyfoods may well explain differences in cancer incidence. Lifestyles and overall diets in Japan, for example, differ considerably from those in Western countries.

Osteoporosis

Osteoporosis is a disease marked by a loss of bone mass that increases the risk of fractures. One of every five American women over age 65 has had at least one bone fracture. Diet and exercise affect bone mass and the risk of osteoporosis. The mineral chiefly responsible for maintaining bone mass is calcium. High protein intakes—because they retard the deposition of calcium in bone and promote the release of calcium therefrom and its removal from the body—can eventually cause a decrease in bone mass.

Soy protein is anabolically equivalent to animal protein (i.e., equivalent in its ability to maintain bodily tissues) in all humans except premature infants. But—like other vegetable proteins—soy protein does not induce as much urinary removal of calcium from the body as does animal protein. Moreover, whole soybeans and many soyfoods—for example, fortified soymilk, tempeh, tofu made with a

---

* "Heart disease" refers to any heart or coronary-artery condition that adversely affects circulation.

24. Soy: Cause for Joy?

> *The proportion of soy isoflavones, or of various soy constituents, may be crucial to the healthfulness of consuming soy.*

calcium-containing reagent (such as calcium sulfate), and TVP—are rich in calcium, and the human body absorbs soy calcium well.

The soy isoflavones daidzein and genistein are similar to ipriflavone, a synthetic drug used widely in Asia and Europe that tends to prevent decreases in bone mass. Animal-research findings suggest that genistein may also do so—at quantities attainable with conventional foods. Genistein binds almost as well as estrogen does to *ER beta*, the type of estrogen receptor that predominates in bone (and in the cardiovascular system). Evidence from research on the relationship between soy and osteoporosis suggests that daily ingestion of both soy protein and isoflavones at quantities comfortably attainable with conventional foods can favorably affect bone. But such evidence is insufficient for offering definitive nutritional advice.

Menopausal Problems

Menopause is the period during which ovarian production of estrogen diminishes and a woman naturally and permanently ceases menstruating. Menopausal estrogen reduction has both physical and psychological effects. Hot flashes and "night sweats," for instance, are commonly reported. But reports worldwide of how severe and how frequent such effects are, are inconsistent. For example, the likelihood of a menopausal Japanese being thus affected is apparently one third that of a menopausal American. The hypothesis that soy isoflavone consumption is partly responsible for this apparent difference deserves testing. The estrogenic activity of soy isoflavones might moderate the effects of the reduction in ovarian estrogen. But the scientific data concerning whether soy isoflavones can ease menopausal complaints are inconsistent, and the healthful menopausal effects found in isoflavone research have been moderate.

Caution Is Advisable

In the context of a healthful diet and lifestyle, consuming soybeans and traditional soyfoods can lower the risk of coronary heart disease, might contribute to preventing cancer and osteoporosis, and might ease menopausal complaints. Furthermore, evidence is lacking that ingesting isoflavones at quantities attainable with traditional soy products has adverse effects.

Nevertheless, caution is in order:

- Some soy products are high in fat and/or sodium and are therefore inappropriate as central dietary items for some persons with cardiovascular disease.
- Genistein can have toxic side effects at high intakes.
- Theoretically, isoflavones, because of their estrogenic activity, may have adverse side effects similar to those of ovarian estrogen.
- The human health repercussions of long-term consumption of isolated soy isoflavones (as pill ingredients, for instance), and that of soy protein isolates (which often contain isoflavones and other water-soluble soy constituents), are unknown. The proportion of soy isoflavones, or of various soy constituents, may be crucial to the healthfulness of consuming soy.

In 1996, at the Second International Symposium on the Role of Soy in Preventing and Treating Chronic Disease, noted soy researcher Kenneth D. Setchell, Ph.D., who identified phytoestyrogens in human blood and urine some 20 years ago, said in conclusion that "negative effects" are likely from high supplemental intakes of isoflavones and that "the potential for self-induced mega-dosing with [over-the-counter soy isoflavone preparations] should be a serious concern for the future."

Findings from research on the health effects of eating soy have enabled only very tentative conclusions. Pending further clinical-research data, we can prudently use soy as a preventive by consuming soybeans and soyfoods in the context of a diet distinguished by high intakes of varied plant foods.

JACK RASO, M.S., R.D., IS ACSH'S DIRECTOR OF PUBLICATIONS. RUTH KAVA, PH.D., R.D., IS ACSH'S DIRECTOR OF NUTRITION.

False alarms about food

Allergies and intolerances to food can make some people sick. But myths about food reactions may also harm your health—and your pocketbook.

A peanut-butter sandwich with a glass of milk is a classic American lunch. But the components of that meal are under attack. Because peanuts can cause fatal allergic reactions in susceptible individuals, some parents have called for peanut-free zones in school cafeterias—tables where peanut products would be banned, to shield allergic children from even the peanut dust that can send extra-sensitive individuals into shock. The Department of Transportation recently advocated similar zones around allergic airline passengers.

Meanwhile, many "holistic" or alternative publications, practitioners, and food or diet companies are breeding fear of milk and wheat. On the Internet, for example, an outfit called Alpha Nutrition offers a checklist of symptoms that supposedly indicate allergy to gluten, a protein in wheat and other grains, that would supposedly warrant ordering the company's gluten-free diet program. But those symptoms are so numerous and vague that virtually all people who read the list might conclude they're allergic.

Then there are the makers of *Dairy Ease* and *Lactaid*—drops or pills containing the enzyme that breaks down lactose, or milk sugar. Both advertise bloated estimates of how many people have trouble digesting the sugar. One even suggests a supposed way to test for lactose intolerance, which requires drinking so much milk that people who could consume a smaller amount with no problem at all would still test positive for the disorder.

Such publicity has created the impression that food reactions are far more prevalent and serious than they generally are. Unfounded fears of food can cause you needless inconvenience and expense, deprive you of needed nutrients, and expose you to unproven or even dangerous treatments. Here are six such myths—and the facts about what to do if you truly can't handle certain foods.

> **Many people mistakenly think they're allergic to foods.**

❶ **Myth: Food Allergies are common.**

Truth: Allergies to what you eat or drink are decidedly *un*common, particularly in adults. In one large survey, 16 percent of the respondents thought at least one member of their immediate family was allergic to at least one food. But research based on actual tests for the condition suggest a true prevalence of only about 2 percent of adults and 8 percent of young children; allergy to multiple types of food is even rarer.

That's fortunate, since genuine food allergy is a serious disorder, where the immune system mistakes a food for a dangerous invader. The resulting response may cause local symp-

25. False Alarms about Food

toms in the regions exposed to the food, such as swelling and discomfort in the lips, mouth, and throat, or upset stomach, gas, and diarrhea. It may also cause various systemic symptoms, such as runny nose, itching, rashes, and hives, or in more serious cases, wheezing and even potentially fatal reactions such as difficulty breathing or a drop in blood pressure.

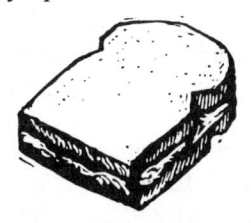

A few people develop an atypical food allergy variously known as gluten sensitivity, celiac disease, or sprue. In that condition, the protein gluten, which is found in wheat, rye, barley, and possibly oats, triggers an unusual immune response that damages the intestinal lining, potentially causing severe digestive symptoms and malnutrition. But despite the belief in widespread wheat allergies, gluten sensitivity afflicts fewer than 1 of every 250 Americans, according to one study.

One reason why so many people mistakenly think they're allergic to foods is that various other common problems—such as irritable bowel syndrome, gastritis, food poisoning, or just stress and anxiety—can cause similar digestive symptoms. But the one condition that people most often mistake for an allergy is food intolerance—a habitual reaction to food that doesn't involve the immune system at all and is virtually never life threatening.

Most food intolerances are simply digestive problems. For example, some people have particular difficulty breaking down high-fiber foods, such as bran, beans, and cruciferous vegetables (broccoli, brussels sprouts, cabbage, cauliflower, kale, and turnips). And some people have inadequate amounts of an enzyme needed to digest a particular nutrient, most often the milk sugar lactose.

The most common *non*digestive reactions to food include asthma attacks provoked by the sulfites and other sulfur-based preservatives in wine, dried fruits, shrimp, peeled or processed potatoes, and several other foods; and migraine headaches, set off by histamines, tyramines, or other chemicals in items such as alcohol, aged cheese, chocolate, cured meats, organ meats, nitrate preservatives, and certain fruits and vegetables. Less often, the histamines can cause rashes or wheezing, just as allergies can. (That's because histamines released by the body help produce allergic attacks.) But except for certain types of spoiled fish, food rarely if ever contains enough histamines to provoke a truly serious reaction.

Food intolerances, like food allergies, are far less common than many people think. In one study, for example, only about one in five people who claimed that they couldn't tolerate a specific food actually did react to that food when they didn't know what they were eating.

❷ **Myth: If I'm lactose intolerant, I can't consume any milk or milk products.**

Truth: Overall, roughly one out of ten white Americans and a much higher proportion of certain specific groups, such as African-Americans and Ashkenazi Jews, have a low level of the enzyme that breaks down lactose. But a recent study found that a group of people who had difficulty digesting lactose could still tolerate an 8-ounce glass of milk at breakfast and dinner. (Two small studies suggest that regularly consuming small amounts of milk may actually reduce lactose intolerance.) Further, people with the disorder may tolerate other dairy products better than they do milk. For example, aged or hard cheeses, such as Swiss or cheddar, contain little lactose; cottage cheese and ice cream contain more lactose than those cheeses but less than milk does. The bacteria in yogurt have already digested a portion of the lactose, and they help digest it further when you eat the food. (Look for the words "active" or "live" cultures on the label.) Chocolate milk is less likely to cause symptoms of intolerance than unflavored milk, for unknown reasons. And eating dairy foods together with other, solid foods can make the dairy items easier to tolerate.

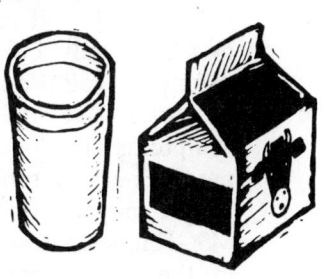

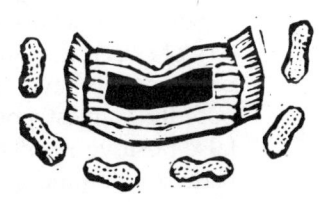

Of course, you could try lactose-free products if you don't mind the extra trouble or expense. Milk with no lactose typically costs about 70 percent more than regular milk. An often cheaper but less convenient alternative is to add enzyme drops to regular milk and let it stand in the refrigerator for 24 hours or more, which can eliminate anywhere from about two-thirds to nearly all of the lactose, depending on how many enzyme drops you use. The drops add about 30 to 90 percent to the cost of the milk. Taking enzyme tablets just before drinking milk digests only about half the lactose, at a cost of about 30 to 40 cents per glass, but the tablets can come in handy if you're eating out.

❸ **Myth: MSG in food often provokes reactions.**

Truth: The flavor enhancer monosodium glutamate, frequently used in Chinese food, has been accused of causing a wide range of symptoms, including headache, nausea, diarrhea, sweating, tingling, tightness or burning in the chest, and asthma. But research suggests that only 1 to 2 percent of Americans react to a typical dose of MSG, and those individuals develop only three of the mildest symptoms: tingling skin as well as the tightness or burning sensation in the chest. More people may react similarly to large doses of MSG, but such doses aren't likely to be found in the foods consumed in restaurants or bought off grocery shelves. In 1995, after reviewing the available evidence, the Food and Drug Administration reaffirmed that MSG belongs in the same category as salt and pepper—"generally recognized as safe."

❹ **Myth: Skin and blood tests can accurately determine whether you have a food allergy.**

Truth: A negative response to standard skin tests of a suspect food almost always rules out typical allergies. But more than half of people who have a positive response—a small red bump—do not experience symptoms when they actually eat the food. (Specialized antibody tests can indicate the likelihood of celiac disease, but only an intestinal biopsy can diagnose it definitely.)

Some physicians perform an extensive battery of skin tests—sometimes 100 or more—in patients who have vague symptoms that supposedly suggest possible food allergy. Since false-positive results are so common, such a battery will almost surely turn up some supposed allergies in patients with no real allergy. Skin tests should be done only to evaluate specific foods that you already suspect are causing some kind of allergic reaction. A positive result should be confirmed by a controlled oral "challenge" with the suspect food—provided the possible reaction won't be life threatening—under a doctor's supervision.

The radioallergosorbent test (RAST), a blood test for allergy, is slightly less sensitive than the standard skin tests. Two other blood tests, the food-immune-complex and IgG tests, assess aspects of the immune response to food, which lends them an aura of scientific plausibility. But just about everyone generates those response to foods, whether or not they're actually allergic—so just about everyone is likely to receive a positive diagnosis from those tests.

Another unproven test that appears to indicate food allergies in most if not all patients, whether or not they're actually sensitive to the suspect food, is symptom-provocation testing (sometimes called sublingual or subcutaneous provocation testing). The doctor places an extract of the food beneath the tongue or injects it under the skin, then watches for vague symptoms such as fatigue or chills, rather than merely placing the extract on the skin, pricking that spot, and looking for a skin reaction. Symptom-provocation tests are not only inaccurate but also far more likely than standard skin tests to provoke a dangerous reaction in someone who truly is allergic to a food.

❺ **Myth: Allergy shots are safe and effective for food allergies.**

Truth: While allergy, or "desensitization," shots work for allergies to inhaled substances such as pollen, no well-controlled study has ever validated that approach for foods. And the shots can provoke serious reactions, particularly in people with peanut allergies. The Food and Drug Administration has not approved such shots.

But some doctors use another treatment, called "neutralization" therapy, that's designed to let the person eat the provoking food, supposedly by preventing the reaction. The practitioner administers progressively smaller amounts of a food extract, until the patient no longer reacts. The patient then takes that "neutralizing" dose, usually by mouth, before or after eating the suspected food. But again, there's no reliable evidence that this implausible approach works. The one controlled trial done so far found that salt-water injections worked just as well as the neutralizing doses.

❻ **Myth: If my allergic reactions to a food are mild, I don't have to worry about having a serious reaction.**

Truth: People who've reacted mildly to a food can start having more serious reactions at any time. Those who've had only localized reactions confined to the site of contact with the food—such as swollen lips, diarrhea, or upset stomach—can develop systemic responses, such as hives or wheezing. And those who've had a systemic response are at risk for fatal reactions in the future.

So if you've had *any* allergic reaction to a food, even a mild one, you need to avoid the food entirely. That means you have to read all food labels scrupulously, know the many obscure ingredients made or derived from the food, and speak directly with the cook before ordering a meal. If you've ever had a systemic allergic reaction, you should carry a self-injecting device (*EpiPen, Ana-Guard*) loaded with the drug epinephrine, which can halt a dangerous allergic reaction.

If you know that you've inadvertently eaten a forbidden food, watch for the warning signs of a serious allergic reaction, including tingling or tightness in the throat, a voice change, increase pulse rate, sweating, wheezing, difficulty breathing, or feeling weak or faint. If you experience any of those symptoms, inject the epinephrine and get to a hospital immediately. In one study, most people killed by food-allergy reactions had either downplayed their symptoms or tried to treat them with antihistamines or asthma drugs alone.

Summing up

Both allergy and intolerance to food, including milk and MSG, are much less common than most people think. To determine whether you do react to suspect foods, consult an allergist. Avoid the food-immune-complex and IgG blood tests as well as symptom-provocation testing. Avoid dubious treatments, too, including food-allergy shots—which are not only unproven but also dangerous—and neutralization therapy.

If you are lactose intolerant, you can probably still tolerate modest amounts of milk as well as yogurt and certain cheeses. If you're truly allergic, avoid the food entirely, and if you've ever had a systemic reaction, carry an epinephrine injector.

Questions and Answers about Cancer, Diet and Fats

Research is evolving about the relationship of diet to cancer. Cancer is a very complex disease, having few definitive answers regarding its cause. Factors to be considered include:

- There are well over 100 different types of cancers, with many differing causes.
- The average diet contains a tremendous amount of different components, some of which may lower the risk of cancer, while others may raise it.
- Unlike heart disease in which blood cholesterol levels serve as an indicator of risk, there are no similar types of markers to indicate a cancer may be developing.
- Cancer takes a long time to develop, which makes it difficult to establish a cause and effect relationship.
- Because of the many questions about diet and cancer that remain unanswered, dietary recommendations should be based on the body of scientific evidence, not just one study. Research published in peer-reviewed journals is the most reliable source of emerging information about diet and cancer.

What can be done to help reduce my risk for developing cancer?

More than 100 types of cancers exist with as many different causes which are not yet completely understood. For that reason, there is no sure way to prevent cancer. But health experts agree there is one general approach to take to help reduce your risk for developing cancer: Adopt a healthy lifestyle that includes getting regular physical activity, eating a balanced diet and not smoking. A healthy lifestyle plays a major role in determining cancer risk.

How does diet affect cancer risk?

Several dietary factors appear to affect the risk of cancer. The type of food is one factor. Diets rich in plant foods such as whole grains, vegetables, fruits and beans may reduce risk for some types of cancer such as colorectal, oral and esophageal. In addition, some studies have linked a diet high in animal products such as red meat with an increase in cancer of the colon and prostate. Recent research, however, indicates the potential link between red meat and colon and prostate cancer can be explained by many other diet and lifestyle factors and needs to be investigated more thoroughly.

Obesity is another risk factor for cancer that is affected by diet. Consuming more calories than you need can lead to obesity. Physical activity has a doubled impact here—it not only helps reduce risk for obesity, it also independently helps reduce the risk of developing certain cancers.

What is the most important dietary step to help reduce risk of cancer?

The strongest evidence points to a well-balanced diet high in whole grains, vegetables, fruits and beans. These foods contain fiber, which is believed to reduce the risk of getting cancers of the rectum and colon. They are also rich in other substances including antioxidant vitamins and minerals and other phytochemicals that may play an important role in reducing cancer risk. For example, lycopene, a carotenoid found abundantly in tomato-based foods, has been found to have potent antioxidant properties that appear to be particularly effective against prostate cancer.

What role does dietary fat play in cancer risk?

The role of dietary fat in the development of cancer, if any, is still unclear. Epidemiological research, which can only propose but not prove associations, suggests high-fat diets may increase risk for some cancers in some people. But other influences, such as that people who eat high-fat diets tend to be heavier and eat more calories and fewer fruits and vegetables, may play a greater role in the development of cancer.

26. Questions and Answers about Cancer, Diet and Fats

According to the 1996 Dietary Guidelines of the American Cancer Society, high-fat diets have been associated with the development of colon, rectal and prostate cancers. However, increasing consumption of whole grains, vegetables, fruits, beans and other fiber-containing foods seems to be more important than decreasing fat intake to reduce the risk of cancers that have been associated with a high-fat diet. More research is needed to determine clearly whether fat plays a direct role in the development of these cancers.

Diets high in fat have not been shown to be a factor in cancers of the stomach, kidney, esophagus, and larynx.

Does fat intake affect risk of breast cancer?

Scientists are still trying to determine if dietary fat plays a role in breast cancer. Breast cancer is associated with circulating hormone levels throughout life, which are influenced by several factors including obesity and physical activity. A recent study of 90,000 women in the United States and Europe found only no significant association between diets high in dietary fat and breast cancer.

To lower risk of breast cancer, the American Cancer Society advises women to eat a diet rich in fruits and vegetables, be physically active, avoid obesity, and limit intake of alcoholic beverages.

Do the individual types of fats affect cancer risk?

The relationship of types of fat to cancer risk is being actively investigated, but it is not yet clear how saturated, monounsaturated or polyunsaturated fatty acids may affect cancer risk. Although several animal studies suggest polyunsaturated fats may increase tumor growth, no relationship has been found between polyunsaturated fats and cancer in humans. Likewise, studies in animals have found that omega-3 fatty acids suppress cancer formation, but there is no direct evidence for protective effects in humans at this time. The most recent review of the literature on trans fats and cancer concluded that there is no evidence that the intake of trans fats affects risk for cancer.

What advice do health experts give for cancer prevention?

Health experts advise a total approach to cancer prevention that includes getting enough physical activity, eating a healthful diet and not smoking.

The recommendations to help prevent chronic disease, including cancer, are embodied in the *Dietary Guidelines for Americans*, which are tenets for an overall healthful lifestyle for all:

- *Eat a variety of foods.* To make sure you get all of the nutrients and other substances needed for health, choose the recommended number of daily servings from each of the five major food groups displayed in the Food Guide Pyramid.
- *Balance the food you eat with physical activity—maintain or improve your weight.* If you are sedentary, try to become more active. If you are already very active, try to continue the same level of activity as you age. If your weight is not in the healthy range, try to reduce health risks through better eating and exercise habits.
- *Choose a diet with plenty of grain products, vegetables and fruits.* Eat more grain and whole-grain products (breads, cereals, pasta, rice), vegetables, fruits, beans, lentils and peas.
- *Choose a diet low in fat, saturated fat, and cholesterol.* Some dietary fat is needed for good health. But to keep fat intake in a healthful range, use fats and oils in moderation, and frequently choose lean and lower-fat foods. The Nutrition Facts label helps you choose foods lower in fat, saturated fat, and cholesterol.
- *Choose a diet moderate in sugars.* Use sugars in moderation—sparingly if your calorie needs are low. Read the Nutrition Facts label on foods you buy.
- *Choose a diet moderate in salt and sodium.* Read the Nutrition Facts label to compare and help identify foods lower in sodium within each group. Use herbs and spices to flavor food. Try to choose forms of foods that you frequently consume that are lower in sodium and salt.
- *If you drink alcoholic beverages, do so in moderation.* If you drink alcoholic beverages, do so in moderation, with meals, and when consumption does not put you or others at risk.

References

Giovannucci, E., Ascherio, A., Rimm, E.B., et al. *Intake of carotenoids and retinol in relation to risk of prostate cancer.* J Natl Cancer Inst, Dec 1995, 87(23): 1767–1776.

Guidelines on Diet, Nutrition, and Cancer Prevention: Reducing the Risk of Cancer with Healthy Food Choices and Physical Activity. Atlanta, GA: The American Cancer Society, 1996.

Ip, C. and Marshall, J. *Trans Fatty Acids and Cancer.* Nutrition Reviews, May 1996, 54: 5: 138–145.

U.S. Department of Agriculture and U.S. Department of Health and Human Services. *Nutrition and Your Health: Dietary Guidelines for Americans,* 4th ed. Home and Garden Bulletin 232. Washington, DC: Government Printing Office, 1995.

Willett, W.C., Hunter, D.J., Stampfer, M.J., et al. *Dietary fat and fiber in relation to risk of breast cancer.* An 8-year follow-up. J Amer Med Assoc, Oct. 21, 1992, 268(15): 2037–2044.

For more information contact: International Food Information Council 100 Connecticut Avenue, NW Ste. 430 Washington, DC 20036

Article 27

HOW TO GROW A HEALTHY CHILD

SUMMARY

Parents and other child care providers are understandably concerned about how best to feed their children and help them adopt healthful lifestyles to achieve optimal growth and development. This concern has been fueled by recent reports of children's failure to consume the recommended number of servings of foods from the five food groups and the unprecedented rise in overweight among the nation's youth.

Only 2% of children consume the recommended number of servings of foods presented in USDA's Food Guide Pyramid and 11% do not meet any of the recommendations according to a recent survey. Children's food intake patterns contribute to their low intake of essential nutrients including calcium and iron, as well as dietary fiber. Dairy foods, for example, are not only a major source of dietary calcium, but they also provide other essential nutrients important for bone and overall health. Children's low calcium intake increases their risk of osteoporosis in later years. Efforts are underway to motivate children and adolescents to improve their calcium intake by consuming three to four servings of dairy foods such as milk a day.

Meeting needs for iron during childhood is important to protect against iron deficiency anemia and its concomitant adverse effects on motor development and cognition. Likewise, consuming a sufficient intake of fiber-rich foods such as fruits, vegetables, and whole grains can help reduce children's risk of constipation, nutrient deficiencies, and obesity.

Overweight among children from preschool age through adolescence has risen dramatically in recent decades. As many as 25% of children are overweight or at risk of becoming overweight. Considering the adverse effects of childhood overweight, prevention is a priority. Scientists agree that the problem of childhood obesity cannot be solved without changing environmental factors, such as a sedentary lifestyle. Data from national surveys indicate that there has been a clear decline in the amount of time children spend being physically active.

Parents and other child care providers can play a critical role in influencing their children's food preferences, their food acceptance patterns, the overall nutritional quality of their diets, and their physical activity. However, parents need to understand that their well-intentioned efforts to encourage or restrict children's intake of specific foods may adversely affect the development of children's food preferences and disrupt children's ability to regulate their energy intake. Coercive strategies to control child feeding practices may lead to childhood overweight and eating problems. The optimal environment for child feeding is one in which parents provide a variety of healthful food choices but allow children to exert control over which of the foods offered, how much, and whether to eat. By consuming healthful diets and leading physically active lifestyles themselves, parents also serve as positive role models for their children.

INTRODUCTION

Children's diets do not meet recommendations presented in USDA's Food Guide Pyramid (1,2). As a result, many children fail to meet their needs for nutrients such as calcium, iron, and fiber.

Overweight among U.S. children from preschool through adolescence has increased dramatically in recent decades (3–8). As many as 25% of children are overweight or at risk of becoming overweight (3). Not only is overweight among children increasing, but it appears to be affecting younger and younger children, including preschoolers (5,6).

Understandably, these well-publicized facts have increased parents'/care providers' anxiety regarding how best to feed their children to achieve optimal growth and development. New research indicates that parents can influence their children's food preferences and food selections by the foods they make available, by their interactions with children in an eating setting, and by serving as role models (9). This *Digest* reviews children's eating patterns, the rising incidence of obesity among children, and strategies for parents and other child care providers to help ensure the health and well-being of children.

CHILDREN'S FOOD CONSUMPTION PATTERNS FALL SHORT OF RECOMMENDATIONS

The eating patterns of most U.S. children fall short of national recommendations, according to a recent survey of 3307 children ages 2 to 19 years (1,2). This survey compared children's food intake reported in USDA's 1989 to 1991 Continuing Survey of Food Intakes by Individuals (CSFII) with the recommended number of servings of foods in USDA's Food Guide Pyramid (10).

Only 2% of the children surveyed met all recommendations and 11% met none of the recommendations (1,2). Approximately 30% of the children met the recommendations for fruit and meat. A slightly higher percentage of children met the recommendations for grains (36%), vegetables

Percentage of U.S. Children Meeting USDA's Food Guide Pyramid Recommendations

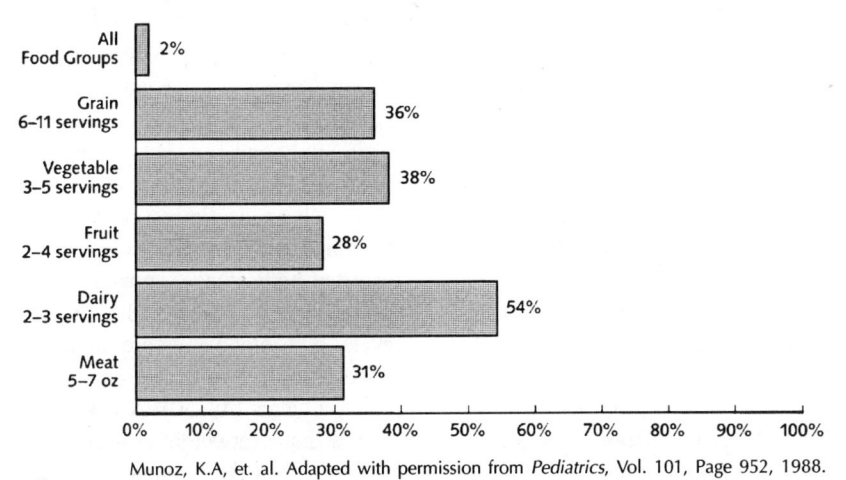

Food Group	Percentage
All Food Groups	2%
Grain 6–11 servings	36%
Vegetable 3–5 servings	38%
Fruit 2–4 servings	28%
Dairy 2–3 servings	54%
Meat 5–7 oz	31%

Munoz, K.A, et. al. Adapted with permission from *Pediatrics*, Vol. 101, Page 952, 1988.

(38%), and dairy (54%) (2,Figure). Children consumed 35% of their energy as fat and an average of 15% of calories as added sugars (1). The researchers found that children whose dietary pattern met all the Pyramid recommendations had nutrient intakes above the 1989 Recommended Dietary Allowances (RDAs) (11), whereas intakes of calcium, iron, zinc, vitamin B_6, and fiber were below the RDAs for children who met none of the Pyramid recommendations (1). Other surveys have found low intakes of calcium, iron, other nutrients, and fiber among many U.S. children (12–14).

A recent study involving 693 second- and third-grade students in New York City also found that children consumed fewer than the recommended number of servings of foods, particularly fruit, vegetables, and grains, in USDA's Food Guide Pyramid and the National Cancer Institute's "5 A Day for Better Health" program (15). Ten percent of second graders and seven percent of fifth grade students skipped breakfast (15). This finding supports observations from another recent survey indicating that many children skip breakfast (16). Skipping breakfast can compromise children's intake of essential nutrients such as calcium and may adversely affect cognitive function and performance at school (17–19).

Recent health professional and government organizations recommend

Only 2% of U.S. children ages 2 to 19 years have a perfect score when it comes to consuming diets meeting the recommended number of servings from the five food groups in USDA's Food Guide Pyramid.

that children about two years of age gradually adopt a diet that, by about 5 years of age, provides no more than 30% of calories from fat (20–23). Children currently consume about 35% of their calories from fat (1). Before two years of age when rapid growth and development require high energy intakes, children's fat intake should not be restricted (22,23). Fat in children's diets is an important source of energy and essential fatty acids. Restricting fat intake may compromise intake of foods that are good sources of essential nutrients such as calcium (24). Transitioning children to a lower fat diet therefore requires care to avoid excessive fat restriction (23).

Recognizing that some parents and their children may be overzealous in their effort to modify fat intake, health professional organizations advise against the use of low fat diets (20% of calories or less) for children

(22,25). The American Academy of Pediatrics (AAP) states that consuming less than about 30% of calories from total fat "is usually not necessary and, for some children and adolescents, may make it difficult to provide enough calories and minerals for optimal growth and development" (22). Clearly, recommendations to lower fat in children's diets must be counterbalanced by advice to assure the nutritional adequacy of such diets.

Children's high sugar intake is also of concern given that high sugar-containing foods often contain minimal amounts of essential nutrients and displace more nutrient dense foods (1,20,26). Excessive sugar intake, especially if consumed in a form that adheres to teeth, may also contribute to tooth decay (20). However, the suggestion that sugar intake causes hyperactivity and other behavioral disorders in children is not supported by scientific evidence (27). Moderation in sugar intake is recommended (20).

The fact that nearly half (46%) of children do not consume the recommended number of servings of milk and other dairy foods (1, 2) explains children's low intake of calcium. Surveys indicate that calcium is one of the nutrients most likely to be underconsumed by children (12,14,28). Data from USDA's 1994–96 CSFII indicate that seven out of ten girls ages 6 to 11 years and six out of ten boys of the same ages do not consume sufficient calcium in their diets (14). An even larger gap exists between calcium intake and calcium needs in older children (14). Low dietary intake of calcium may increase children's risk of bone fractures (29) and osteoporosis in later adult years (30–32).

Optimizing peak bone mass during growth is a recognized strategy to reduce future risk of osteoporosis. A daily intake of 800mg calcium/day is recommended for children ages 4 through 8 years, whereas 1300mg/day is recommended for older children (9 through 18 years) (30). Numerous scientific studies indicate that increasing calcium intake during childhood to levels of at least 1300mg/day and closer to the 1500mg/day as recommended by the National Institutes of Health (31) and supported by the American Medical Association (32) benefits children's bone health (33–38). Studies also demonstrate that intake of calcium-rich foods such as milk and yogurt favorably affects children's bones (34,39).

It is difficult to meet dietary calcium recommendations without consuming dairy foods (31,32,40). Milk and milk products are not only a rich source of calcium, but these foods also contribute a number of other essential nutrients important to children's growth and development. Unfortunately, consumption of fluid milk by children 5 years and under has decreased since the late 1970s, while intake of carbonated soft drinks and juices has increased (41). The AAP cautions that replacing milk in children's diets with juice can nega-

Intake of the recommended number of servings of milk and other dairy foods helps children meet their calcium needs. Dairy foods are not only calcium-rich foods, but they also provide other essential nutrients important for children's growth and development.

tively affect their nutritional intake (23). Efforts are underway to motivate children and adolescents to improve their calcium intake, such as by consuming three to four servings of dairy foods such as milk a day (42).

Children's failure to consume the recommended number of servings of foods as outlined in USDA's Food Guide Pyramid, especially iron-rich meats and iron-fortified cereals, may compromise their iron intake. Although iron deficiency has substantially decreased in the U.S., it is still relatively common (43-45). About 9% of U.S. children 1 to 3 years of age are iron deficient and 3% have iron deficiency anemia, the most severe form of iron deficiency (43). Among children older than 3 years, iron deficiency has declined to less than 1%, although it may be higher in children with low intakes of iron-rich foods (43). Iron deficiency contributes to developmental delays and behavioral disturbances (e.g., decreased motor activity, social interaction, and attention to tasks) in children (43,46).

Children also fail to consume adequate amounts of dietary fiber. A low intake of fiber-rich foods such as vegetables, fruits, and whole grain products may contribute to constipation, nutrient deficiencies, and increased risk of obesity and other diseases (47). Current dietary fiber recommendations for children are "age plus 5g/day" (47). Accordingly, minimal fiber intake recommendations range from 10g/day at age 5 to 20g/day at age 15 (47).

CHILDHOOD OBESITY RISING AT AN ALARMING RATE

Paralleling the rise in obesity among adults, overweight among children from preschool age through adolescence has increased dramatically since the mid-1960s (3–6). Approximately 11% of children and adolescents were overweight (95th percentile of body mass index or BMI) in 1988 to 1994 and an additional 14% were at risk of becoming overweight according to data from the National Health and Nutrition Survey (NHANES) III (3). Nationally representative surveys reveal that not only has the prevalence of overweight among children increased over the years, but that the heaviest children are getting heavier. Even among preschool children, overweight is becoming more prevalent (5,6). Based on NHANES data, more than 10% of children 4 to 5 years of age were overweight in 1988 through 1994 compared to less than 6% in 1971 through 1974 (5).

Excess body weight in childhood is of concern because of its immediate adverse effects and the potential increased risk of morbidity and mortality in adulthood (48–51). Overweight children face immediate psychosocial risks such as discrimination from peers and adults, social isolation, and distorted body image, as well as medical risks such as adverse lipoprotein levels, high blood pressure, abnormal blood glucose levels, sleep apnea, and joint problems (48–50). A major concern is that overweight children will become overweight adults with heightened medical risks (8,48–51).

What has caused this substantial rise in overweight among U.S. children? The reasons are complex and involve the interaction of genes with an environment that encourages excess energy consumption and a sedentary lifestyle (52). Physical inactivity appears to be a major factor contributing to overweight among children (23,53-56). Fewer than one in four children participate in 20 minutes of vigorous activity a day or get at least half an hour of any type of physical activity each day, according to a recent survey of 1,504 families (53). A variety of factors can influence children's physical activity behavior (54). Television, video games, and computers are often given as reasons for children's sedentary behavior (55). Parents who lead sedentary lifestyles tend to have children who are less physically active than children with physically active parents (54).

Treatment of overweight children consists of age-appropriate behavioral modification, nutrition, and physical activity (57). Interventions should modify children's eating and exercise behaviors without compromising their growth and development (20,57). Given the current high prevalence of overweight among children, the immediate and potential future health problems associated with overweight, and the concomitant health burden for the nation, efforts to prevent overweight should begin early in childhood (7,8,23).

WHAT'S A PARENT/CHILD CARE PROVIDER TO DO?

To help children develop a healthful lifestyle, parents/child care providers must understand factors shaping children's behavior such as their food preferences and acceptance patterns. Food acceptance patterns are unique to each child and are influenced by a variety of factors, some innate and others learned (9,58,59).

Children's unlearned food preferences include those for sweet and salty tastes and their rejection of sour and bitter tastes (9). Also, children are predisposed to be neophobic or reject new foods (9). Generally, about 5 to 10 exposures to a new food are necessary before it is accepted by a young child. This means that to turn an initially rejected new food into an accepted or preferred food, parents may need to provide young children with repeated opportunities to try this food by making it available and accessible (26). Also young children, even of elementary school age, are predisposed to regulate the energy density of their diet over a 24-hour period (9,60). However, there are individual differences in children's regulation of energy intake beginning as early as the preschool years. These differences are explained by learned food acceptance preferences which in turn appear to be influenced by parents' child-rearing practices.

Physiological consequences of eating can influence children's food acceptance patterns. If eating a food, such as a high-energy food, is followed by positive feelings of satiety, especially when the child is hungry, a learned preference for high-energy foods develops. In contrast, if consumption of a food is followed by illness (emesis), the child will likely develop a conditioned aversion to that food. Repeated positive experiences with foods high in energy can increase children's preferences for these foods, especially in families which make these foods readily available (61). A study of 3- to 5-year old children demonstrated that children with a conditioned preference for high energy foods were fatter, consumed higher fat diets, and had parents with the highest body mass (61). Children's learned preferences for high energy foods, especially when supported by an environment in which such foods are readily available, predicts their food choices (61).

Parents, by their behavior, serve as role models for the developing child. The food selection patterns and eating behavior of parents can influence children's food preferences (9). For example, well-intentioned parents who are concerned about either their own and/or their children's weight and diets may exert a high degree of control over what and how much their children eat. This parental influence can affect children's food preferences, often with negative and unintended results. Coercive strategies intended to encourage young children to consume a particular food (e.g., fruit, vegetable) may increase their dislike for that food, and limiting children's access to "preferred" foods (e.g., sweets, high fat foods) may actually promote overconsumption of these foods, especially for girls (9,59). Controlling child feeding practices that encourage or restrict children's food intake can also disrupt children's ability to regulate their energy intake and the amount of food consumed. This in turn increases the child's risk for overweight. Restricting children's intake of less nutritious foods, or offering them only in social contexts such as holiday celebrations, sends mixed messages to children and fosters the misperception that there are "good" and "bad" foods.

If the rise in childhood obesity is not curtailed, scientists predict that today's children will grow into the most obese generation of adults in U.S. history.

So what's a parent to do? Parents and other child care providers should provide children with a variety of healthful foods in a supportive environment, but let children decide for themselves when and how much they will eat (9,59,62). Child health experts believe that this feeding strategy will foster children's responsiveness to their internal cues of hunger and satiety and to the energy density of their diet. Parents' messages to their children should be food-based, rather than nutrient-based, and avoid categorizing foods as either "good" or "bad" (55).

Parents can serve as positive role models to encourage healthful diets and a physically active lifestyle that will promote normal growth and development during childhood (23,53–55). By following a middle ground, being neither too restrictive nor too permissive, parents can help foster a healthful lifestyle for both themselves and their children (23,55).

REFERENCES

1. Munoz, K.A., S.M. Krebs-Smith, R. Ballard-Barbash, et. al. Pediatrics *100*: 323, 1997.
2. Munoz, K.A., S.M. Krebs-Smith, R. Ballard-Barbash, et. al. Pediatrics *101*, 952, 1998.
3. Troiano, R.P., and K.M. Flegal. Pediatrics *101s*: 497, 1998.
4. Division of Health Examination Statistics, National Center for Health Statistics, Division of Nutrition and Physical Activity, National Center for Chronic Disease Prevention and Health Promotion, CDC. MMWR *46(9) (March 7)*: 199, 1997.
5. Ogden, C.L., R.P. Troiano, R.R. Briefel, et. al. Pediatrics 99: e1, 1997. (http://www.pediatrics.org/cgi/content/full/4/e1)
6. Mei, Z., K.S. Scanlon, L.M. Grummer-Strawn, et. al. Pediatrics *101*: e12, 1997.
7. Christoffel, K.K., and A. Ariza. Pediatrics *101*: 103, 1998.
8. Hill, J.O., and F.L. Trowbridge. Pediatrics *101s*: 570, 1998.
9. Birch, L.L., and J.O. Fisher. Pediatrics *101s*: 539, 1998.
10. U.S. Department of Agriculture, Human Nutrition Information Service. *The Food Guide Pyramid.* Home and Garden Bulletin No. 252. Washington, DC: U.S. Government Printing Office, 1992.
11. Commission on Life Sciences, National Research Council. *Recommended Dietary Allowances, 10th Edition.* Food and Nutrition Board. Washington, DC: National Academy Press, 1989.
12. Alaimo, K., M.A. McDowell, R.R. Briefel, et. al. Dietary intake of vitamins, minerals, and fiber of persons ages 2 months and over in the United States: Third National

> *Parents and other child care providers should serve children a variety of foods from the basic food groups. However, it is the child's responsibility to decide which of the foods offered, how much, and even whether to eat.*

Health and Nutrition Examination Survey, Phase 1, 1988–1991. Advance Data from Vital and Health Statistics: No. 258. Hyattsville, MD: National Center for Health Statistics, 1994.
13. U.S. Department of Health and Human Services, Public Health Service, Centers for Disease Control and Prevention, National Center for Health Statistics. *Healthy People 2000 Review 1995–96.* DHHS Publ. No. (PHS) 96-1256. Hyattsville, MD. November 1996.
14. U.S. Department of Agriculture, Food Surveys Research Group. *Data Tables: Results from USDA's 1994–96 Continuing Survey of Food Intakes by Individuals and 1994–96 Diet and Health Knowledge Survey.* Riverdale, MD: ARS, USDA. December 1997.
16. Melnik, T.A., S.J. Rhoades, K.R. Wales, et. al. J. Am. Diet. Assoc. 98: 159, 1998.
17. Dairy Management Inc. Children's Breakfast Survey. Interviews with boys and girls ages 8–13. Prepared by McDonald Research, Inc. Skokie, IL, May 1997.
18. Pollitt, E., and R. Mathews. Am. J. Clin. Nutr. 67: 804s, 1998.
19. Ortega, R.M., A.M. Requejo, A.M. Lopez-Sobaler, et. al. J. Am. Coll. Nutr. 17: 19, 1998.
20. Miller, G.D., T. Forgac, T. Cline, et. al. J. Am. Coll. Nutr. 17: 4, 1998.
21. U.S. Department of Agriculture, U.S. Department of Health and Human Services. *Nutrition and Your Health: Dietary Guidelines for Americans.* 4th ed. Home and Garden Bulletin No. 232, 1995.
22. American Heart Association, Nutrition Committee. Circulation 94: 1795, 1996.
23. American Academy of Pediatrics, Committee on Nutrition. Pediatrics 101: 141, 1998.
24. Kleinman, R.E. (Eds). *Pediatric Nutrition Handbook.* 4th edition. Elk Grove Village, IL: American Academy of Pediatrics, 1998.
25. Johnson, R.K., and M.Q. Wang. Am. J. Health Studies 13(4): 174, 1997.
26. Lichtenstein, A.H., and L.V. Horn for the Nutrition Committee, American Heart Association. Circulation 98: 935, 1998.
27. Sullivan, S.A., and L.L. Birch. Development. Psychol. 26: 546, 1990.
28. White, J.W., and M. Wolraich. Am. J. Clin. Nutr. 62s: 242, 1995.
29. Lin, B.-H., J. Guthrie, and J.R. Blaylock. The diets of America's children. Agricultural Economic Report No. 746. Washington, DC: Center for Nutrition Policy and Promotion. December 1996.
30. Goulding, A., R. Cannan, S.M. Williams, et. al. J. Bone Miner. Res. 13: 143, 1998.
31. Institute of Medicine. *Dietary Reference Intakes for Calcium, Phosphorus, Magnesium, Vitamin D, and Fluoride.* Standing Committee on the Scientific Evaluation of Dietary Reference Intakes. Food and Nutrition Board. Washington, DC: National Academy Press, 1997.
32. U.S. Department of Health and Human Services, Public Health Service, National Institutes of Health. Consensus Development Conference Statement. Optimal Calcium Intake 12(4): 1, 1994.
33. Council on Scientific Affairs, American Medical Association. Arch. Fam. Med. 6: 495, 1997.
34. Johnston, C.C. Jr., J.Z. Miller, C.W. Slemenda, et. al. N. Engl. J. Med. 327: 82, 1992.
35. Chan, G.M., K. Hoffman, and M. McMurray. J. Pediatr. 126: 551, 1995.
36. Lloyd, T., M.B. Andon, N. Rollings, et. al. JAMA 270: 841, 1993.
37. Bonjour, J.P., A.L. Carrie, S. Ferrari, et. al. J. Clin. Invest. 99: 1287, 1997.
38. Jackman, L.A., S.S. Millane, B.R. Martin, et. al. Am. J. Clin. Nutr. 66: 327, 1997.
39. Nowson, C.A., R.M. Green, J.P. Hopper, et. al. Osteop. Int. 7: 219, 1997.
40. Cadogan, J., R. Eastell, N. Jones, et. al. Br. Med. J. 314: 1255, 1997.
41. Neumark-Sztainer, D., M. Story, L.B. Dixon, et. al. J. Nutr. Educ. 29: 12, 1997.
42. U.S. Department of Agriculture, Agricultural Research Service. *What We Eat in America 1994–96. Results from the 1994–96 Continuing Survey of Food Intakes by Individuals.* December 1997.
43. National Institute of Child Health and Human Development, National Institutes of Health, U.S. Department of Health and Human Services Childhood and Adolescent Nutrition. *Why Milk Matters Now For Children and Teens.* Rockville, MD: NICHD Clearinghouse, 1998.
44. CDC, U.S. Department of Health and Human Services. MMWR 46 (No. RR-3): 1, 1998.
45. Beard, J.L., H. Dawson, and D.J. Pinero. Nutr. Rev. 54(10): 295, 1996.
46. Looker, A.C., P.R. Dallman, M.D. Carroll, et. al. JAMA 277: 973, 1997.
47. Center on Hunger, Poverty, and Nutrition Policy. Tufts University School of Nutrition. *Statement on the Link Between Nutrition and Cognitive Development in Children.* 2nd edition. Medford, MA: Tufts University, 1995.
48. Williams, C.L. J. Am. Diet. Assoc. 95: 1140, 1995.
49. Dietz, W.H. J. Nutr. 128: 411s, 1998.
50. Dietz, W.H. Pediatrics 101s: 518, 1998.
51. Dwyer, J.T., E.J. Stone, M. Yang, et. al. Am. J. Clin. Nutr. 67: 602, 1998.
52. Whitaker, R.C., J.A. Wright, M.S. Pepe, et. al. N. Engl. J. Med. 337 (13): 869, 1997.
53. Rosenbaum, M., and R.L. Leibel. Pediatrics 101s: 525, 1998.
54. International Life Sciences Institute. *Improving Children's Health Through Physical Activity: A New Opportunity.* A Survey of Parents and Children about Physical Activity Patterns. July 1997.
55. Kohl, H.W., III, and K.E. Hobbs. Pediatrics 101s: 549, 1998.
56. Andersen, R.E., C.J. Crespo, S.J. Bartlett, et. al. JAMA 279: 938, 1998.
57. Goran, M.I., B.A. Gower, T.R. Nagy, et. al. Pediatrics 101s: 887, 1998.
58. Epstein, L.H., M.D. Myers, H.A. Raynor, et. al. Pediatrics 101s, 554, 1998.
59. Birch, L.L. J. Nutr. 128: 407s, 1998.
60. Johnson, S.L., and L.L. Birch. Pediatrics 94: 653, 1994.
61. Johnson, S., and J. Hill. FASEB J. March: abst. #2020, 1998.
62. Fisher, J.A., and L.L. Birch. J. Am. Diet. Assoc. 95: 759, 1995.
63. Satter, E.M. J. Am. Diet. Assoc. 96: 860, 1996.

ACKNOWLEDGMENTS

National Dairy Council® assumes the responsibility for this publication. However, we would like to acknowledge the help and suggestions of the following reviewers in its preparation:

■ S.L. Johnson, Ph.D.
Instructor Fellow,
Health Science Center
Center for Human Nutrition
University of Colorado
Denver, CO

■ M.F. Picciano, Ph.D.
Professor, Department of Nutrition
Pennsylvania State University
University Park, PA

The *Dairy Council Digest*® is written and edited by Lois D. McBean, M.S., R.D.

A Focus on Nutrition for the Elderly: It's Time to Take a Closer Look

Longevity trends, combined with the swelling wave of aging "baby boomers," are contributing to an explosive growth in the U.S. elderly population, aged 65 and over, which has grown 11-fold during the 20th century[1]. By 2050 about 19 million Americans (24 percent of elderly Americans) will be aged 85 and over[1]. Older people may not know that their nutrient requirements can change from their younger years. The process of aging can introduce other factors—chronic disease, physical disabilities, poor economic status, social isolation, prescription medications, and altered mental status that may cause poor eating habits that do not meet an older person's current nutrient needs. The elderly face the challenge of choosing a nutrient dense diet, one that provides an adequate intake of nutrients at a time when their activity levels and energy needs decline. Assessing the diet quality of the elderly is critical to addressing issues relevant to their health and nutritional status.

This *Nutritional Insight* summarizes the overall diet quality of three age groups of independent, free-living elderly Americans—the young-old, 65–74 years; the old, 75–84 years; and the oldest-old, 85 + years— using the Healthy Eating Index (HEI)[2]. Data from USDA's Continuing Survey of Food Intakes by Individuals (CSFII) 1994–96, a nationally representative survey containing information on people's consumption of foods and nutrients, were used in the analysis. Scores for the elderly groups are compared with the overall HEI for "pre-elderly" adults aged 45–64.

About the Healthy Eating Index

The HEI is a summary measure of people's overall diet quality. It is an excellent tool both for assessing the quality of Americans' diets and for understanding better the influence of food choices on Americans' health. The HEI is expressed as one score on a scale of 1–100 but is comprised of the sum of 10 components. Each component score can range between 0 and 10. Components 1–5 measure the degree to which a person's diet conforms to the serving recommendations from the USDA Food Guide Pyramid's five major food groups: Grains, vegetables, fruits, milk, and meat. A high score for these components is reached by maximizing consumption of recommended amounts. Components 6–9 measure compliance of total fat and saturated fat intake according to the *Dietary Guidelines for Americans* and of cholesterol and sodium from the *Daily Values* listed on the Nutrition Facts Label. A high score is reached by consuming at or below recommended amounts. The last component evaluates variety in the diet. A person consuming 8 or more different foods each day will score 10 points. A summary HEI score above 80 implies a "good" diet; a score between 51–80 implies a diet that "needs improvement"; and a score less than 51 implies a "poor" diet.

Overall HEI Snapshot

The CSFII 1994–96 data show the average HEI score for elderly persons 65 + years old is 67.2 out of a possible score of 100. The average HEI score for the pre-elderly group aged 45–64 is 63.4. Both fall midway in the "needs improvement" range.

Among the three elderly groups, as age increases, those with an overall diet quality of "good" remain consistent at around 20–21 percent (fig. 1). Most movement in diet quality occurs between the "needs improvement" and "poor" ratings. The data indicate that with an increase in age there is a slight, but gradual, increase in the percentage of elderly with a "poor" diet (12 to 15 percent). In comparison, fewer individuals in the pre-elderly group (aged 45–64) achieve a "good" diet, and more of them have a diet rated as "needs improvement" or "poor." However, the elderly people's mean HEI scores decrease as income levels decrease, indicating a greater risk for a poor diet quality among lower socio-economic groups.

Figure 1. Overall diet quality, older age groups

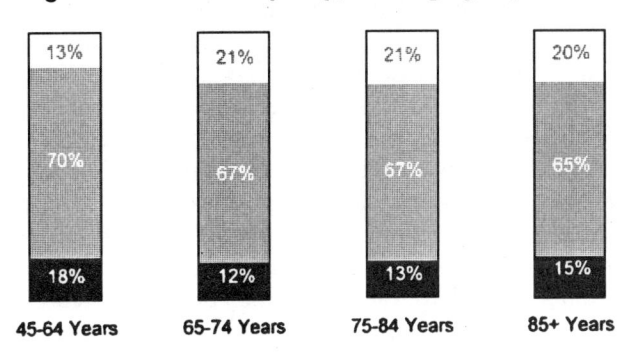

Age Group	Poor (HEI < 51)	Needs Improvement (HEI 51–80)	Good (HEI > 80)
45–64 Years	18%	70%	13%
65–74 Years	12%	67%	21%
75–84 Years	13%	67%	21%
85+ Years	15%	65%	20%

Looking Closer at the Components

A closer look at the HEI component scores reveals more pronounced differences between age groups (fig. 2). Among the three elderly age groups, the median scores for each of five components—total fat, saturated fat, cholesterol, sodium, and variety—are 8.0 or better. Despite good scores, the pre-elderly group's component scores were not as high as the elderly groups' scores in three of those same five components. A high score for total fat, saturated fat, cholesterol, and sodium is reached by consuming at or below recommended amounts: thus interpretation of these high scores may be deceiving. A review of CSFII food energy intake data showed that an elderly person's caloric intake declines by as much as 500 calories between ages 65 and 85. Therefore, although the score is high, without further study, it is not possible to know whether reduced food intake is keeping the intake of these components low, or whether the elderly are receiving well-balanced nutrition assistance.

The fruits and milk components had the lowest HEI scores for all age groups. Median fruit scores for the three elderly age groups ranged from 4.6 to 4.9. A slight decrease is noted with advancing age. Median fruit scores for the pre-elderly age group hovered around 3.1, much lower than even the lowest fruit score of the three elderly age groups. Milk component median scores "see-sawed" tightly with advancing age.

In terms of age group, the HEI component scores of the younger, pre-elderly group lagged behind those of the elderly age groups in 3 of the 10 food components (fruit, total fat, and sodium), but they either met or exceeded the elders' scores in 6 other components (grains, vegetables, milk, meat, saturated fat, and variety). All ages studied have a median score of 10.0 for cholesterol.

As Aging Advances

A noticeable, but not extreme, decline in the overall diet quality of Americans aged 65 and over is indicated in Figure 1. This trend, however, is more clearly observed by looking at their median HEI component scores in Figure 2. Only milk, total fat, and sodium scores deviated from this trend. Milk and total fat component scores vacillated from 4.3 to 5.0 and from 7.4 to 8.4, respectively, among all age groups studied. Sodium component scores showed a reverse trend—the older the group, the higher the component score. Until age 85, the groups' median variety score remained at a constant 10.0. After age 85, the group's score dropped dramatically to 8.0.

Figure 2. Median HEI component scores

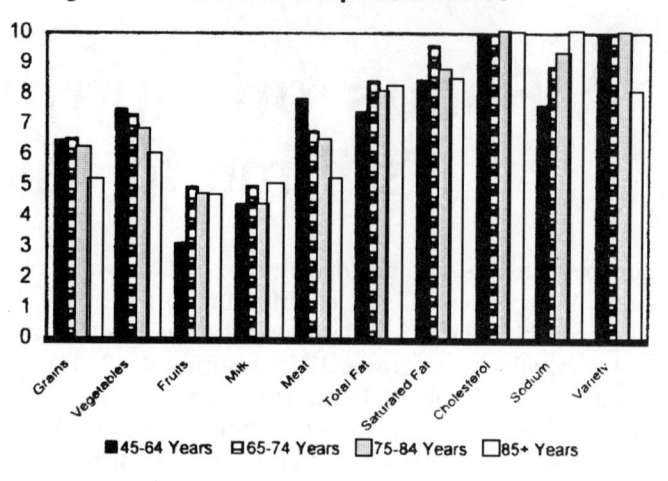

■ 45-64 Years ▨ 65-74 Years ☐ 75-84 Years ☐ 85+ Years

Conclusions

The overall diet quality of the elderly seems to be better than for their pre-elderly counterparts, but it still falls into the "needs improvement" category. The data indicate the elderly are consuming enough different foods (i.e., variety). However, research efforts and nutrition education strategies should target the quantity and nutrient density of foods the elderly consume, because both quantity and nutrient density are integral to meeting the recommended intake levels of the five major food groups. Inadequate intake of the milk and fruits components, in particular, needs addressing. In addition to eating patterns and income status, poor HEI scores also may be affected by other influential risk factors, such as physical limitations, depression, and non-participation in nutrition programs. Such factors should be considered when conducting research and developing nutrition communications that lead to successful aging.

The United Nations International Year of the Older Person is being celebrated during 1999. Its theme "Healthy Aging, Healthy Living—Start Now!" is indicative that it is time to focus more of our nutrition research, nutrition policy development, and nutrition promotion efforts on the elderly now and into the next millennium.

Contributors: Nancy W. Gaston, M.A., R.D., Anne Mardis, M.D., M.P.H., Shirley Gerrior, Ph.D., R.D., Nadine Sahyoun, Ph.D., R.D., and Rajen S. Anand, Ph.D.

References

1. U.S. Department of Commerce. Economics and Statistics Administration (visited 1998, December 9). U.S. Census Bureau the Official Statistics Statistical Brief, "Sixty-five plus in the United States," May 1995 [WWW document]. URL http://www.census.gov/socdemo/www/agebrief.html.

2. Bowman, S.A., Lino, M., Gerrior, S.A., and Basiotis, P.P. 1998. The Healthy Eating Index: 1994–96. U.S. Department of Agriculture, Center for Nutrition Policy and Promotion. CNPP-5. Available at http://www.usda.gov/cnpp

PHYSICAL ACTIVITY AND NUTRITION: A WINNING COMBINATION FOR HEALTH

INTRODUCTION

Health professionals and the federal government recognize the importance of regular physical activity and a healthful diet to reduce the risk of major chronic diseases and improve well-being (1–9). In recent years, scientific evidence of the health benefits of being physically active, from early childhood throughout later adult years, has led to specific recommendations and/or practical suggestions to increase physical activity (2, 4–8).

Regardless of age, everyone benefits from a physically active lifestyle. Compared to their sedentary peers, physically active children tend to be at lower risk of overweight (10) and are more likely to become physically active adults (11). For adults, regular physical activity, along with a healthful diet, helps to reduce the risk of major chronic diseases such as cardiovascular disease, hypertension, obesity, adult-onset diabetes mellitus, osteoporosis, and some cancers (1–3, 5–9).

Improved mental health or psychological well-being is another benefit of physical activity (6). For older adults, regular physical activity improves muscle strength, functional mobility/independence, and quality of life (12, 13). A physically active lifestyle also delays all-cause mortality (6, 14–16).

Despite a growing consensus and awareness of the substantial health benefits of regular physical activity, many Americans lead relatively sedentary lifestyles (2, 6, 10, 17–20). According to the Surgeon General's Report on Physical Activity and Health (6), only 22% of adults in the U.S. engage in physical activity sufficient to derive health benefits; 53% are somewhat active but not active enough to derive health benefits; and 25% are completely sedentary. Children also lead relatively sedentary lifestyles (6, 10). Only 22% of children participate in 30 minutes of vigorous activity a day and one in four children receives no physical education in school, according to a recent survey of 1,504 families with children in grades 4–12 (10).

The current levels of physical activity among both young and old make it unlikely that many of the federal government's *Healthy People 2000* objectives for physical activity will be achieved (18, 19). Americans give several reasons for their relatively sedentary lifestyles. These include lack of time, injury or other physical difficulties, inclement weather, a dislike for exercise, fear of crime in their neighborhoods, and our "information age" which fosters time spent in front of the computer, television, and video screen (2).

This *Digest* reviews recent research findings supporting the beneficial role of regular physical activity and a healthful diet throughout life, from early childhood through later adult years. Also presented are current recommendations for physical activity offered by various health organizations.

CHILDHOOD AND ADOLESCENCE

Regular physical activity benefits children and adolescents by improving their strength and endurance, helping to control body weight, building healthy bones, and reducing anxiety and stress (21). A growing proportion of children and adolescents in the U.S. are overweight (22–25). Approximately 14% of children aged 6 to 11 years and 12% of adolescents aged 12 to 17 years are overweight (22). Not only is overweight highly preva-

> *Physical inactivity is a major public health concern in the U.S. In general, females are less physically active than males and physical activity declines with age.*

lent among young people, but this condition has continued to rise over the years (22) and affect younger and younger children (24, 25). This situation, coupled with recognition that overweight in children and adolescents may increase the likelihood of adult morbidity and mortality (26), has drawn attention to contributing factors (23, 27).

Physical inactivity is regarded as a major contributing factor to overweight among children and adolescents (6, 10, 23). Because childhood and adolescence can set the stage for lifelong physical activities (11), parents, care providers, teachers, athletic coaches, and others are urged to encourage children to become more physically active (5, 6, 10, 21). Care should be taken to ensure that efforts to prevent overweight in children do not compromise children's growth and development (5).

Physical activity and nutrition, especially adequate calcium intake, play an important role in the development of genetically-determined bone mass (6, 28–31). Maximizing peak bone mass, which occurs between ages 19 and 30 years depending on specific bones, and reducing bone loss in later years lower the risk of osteoporosis. Physical activity during childhood can strengthen bones and contribute to increased peak bone mass in adulthood (6, 28–31). In a prospective study of 470 healthy children ages 8 to 16 years, weight-bearing physical activity and a high calcium intake increased forearm trabecular bone mineral density (30). A study of over 200 women ages 18 to 31 years found that those who were more physically active during their high school years exhibited higher hip bone density, total body and spine bone mineral content, and total body bone mineral density than their less physically active counterparts (31).

Physical activity during childhood and adolescence may favorably influence blood lipid profiles (6, 32). The Cardiovascular Risk in Young Finns Study involving more than 2,300 children and young adults links higher levels of physical activity with increased blood levels of high density lipoprotein (HDL) cholesterol in males and lower triglyceride levels in females (32).

Regular physical activity also reduces anxiety and stress, increases self-esteem (21), and allows an increase in caloric intake without weight gain which enables an individual to increase food choices and improve nutrient intake. A recent cross-sectional study of nearly 500 low-income children 9 to 12 years of age in Montreal found that children who were more physically active consumed more calories, calcium, iron, zinc, and fiber, but did not gain more weight than their inactive peers (33).

ADULTHOOD

Cardiovascular Disease. Numerous studies have established that physical activity reduces the risk of cardiovascular disease, particularly among previously inactive individuals (1, 6, 8, 34, 35).

Regular physical activity and a healthful diet throughout life reduce the risk of major chronic diseases and improve overall health and well-being.

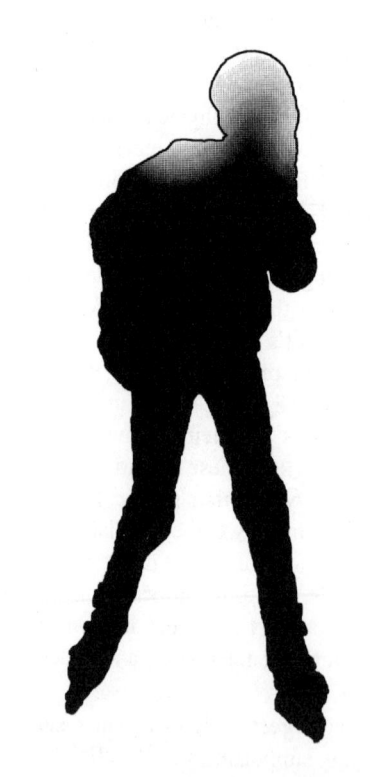

Physical activity exerts its beneficial effect on cardiovascular health through a variety of direct and indirect mechanisms. Physical activity favorably influences the blood lipid profile, specifically raising HDL cholesterol and lowering elevated blood levels of total and low density lipoprotein (LDL) cholesterol and triglyceride levels (6–8, 35–37). In addition, physical activity increases lipoprotein lipase, an enzyme that removes cholesterol and free fatty acids from the blood, decreases plasma viscosity thereby influencing blood flow, and favorably affects blood clotting and fibrinolytic mechanisms (1, 6, 7, 38). Physical activity may also reduce risk of cardiovascular disease by its beneficial effects on other cardiovascular disease risk factors such as high blood pressure, obesity, and adult-onset diabetes mellitus (6, 7, 35). The cardiovascular benefits of regular physical activity have been demonstrated in both males and females (36, 38–41), as well as in patients with cardiovascular disease or individuals at high risk of developing this disease (42).

To reduce the risk of heart disease, the NIH Consensus Panel on Physical Activity and Cardiovascular Health (7) recommends that children and adults participate in moderate intensity physical activity for at least 30 minutes on most, and preferably all, days of the week. The American Heart Association recommends that adults should also participate in resistance exercise (e.g., lifting weights) for a minimum of two days a week (8).

Hypertension. Physical inactivity contributes to high blood pressure, an established risk factor for cardiovascular disease (6, 8, 39, 43). Sedentary normotensive individuals exhibit a 20% to 50% higher risk of developing hypertension than do their more physically active counterparts (43). Moderately intense physical activity such as brisk walking for 30 to 45 minutes on most days of the week can lower blood pressure (43).

Overweight. Paralleling the trend observed among children, the prevalence of overweight among U.S. adults has markedly increased, specifically from about 25% between 1960 and 1980 to 33% in 1988–91 (18, 44). Physical inactivity is an important contributor to the rise in overweight among U.S. adults (6, 45).

Studies report lower body weight, body mass index, or skinfold measures among physically active adults than among their sedentary counterparts (3, 5–7, 39). Regular physical activity contributes to weight maintenance and/or reduction by increasing caloric expenditure (1, 6, 46). Research indicates that physical activity does not necessarily produce a compensatory increase in appetite or energy intake (6, 47).

As a component of a weight reduction program, physical activity favors the loss of body fat and helps to preserve lean body tissue (6, 46, 48). Minimizing lean tissue loss helps to protect against a decrease in metabolic rate which can increase the propensity to regain weight (48). Physical activity in conjunction with moderate energy restriction may also enhance dietary compliance (49), help to maintain weight loss (6, 7, 50, 51), and improve maximal oxygen consumption or functional capacity (52).

The 1995 *Dietary Guidelines for Americans* (5) recognizes the importance of physical activity, along with a healthful diet, to maintain a healthy body weight. These guidelines call for 30 minutes or more of moderate physical activity on most, and preferably all, days of the week. Health professional organization such as The American Dietetic Association support this position (3).

Diabetes Mellitus. The goals of managing adult-onset or non-insulin dependent diabetes mellitus (NIDDM) include achieving and maintaining normal blood glucose, lipid, and blood pressure levels (1, 53). Although there are few data regarding the effects of combined dietary modification and physical activity on NIDDM, regular physical activity is recommended to help achieve and maintain normal blood glucose levels and a reasonable body weight (1, 6, 53). Epidemiological data indicate a protective effect of physical activity against developing NIDDM (6, 54, 55). The benefits of physical activity appear to be most pronounced for individuals at high risk for developing NIDDM (1, 55).

Cancer. Epidemiological studies provide fairly consistent support for a protective effect of regular physical activity against colon cancer, the third most common cancer among adults (6, 9). Physical activity may reduce colon cancer risk by stimulating colon peristalsis, thereby speeding up the movement of dietary factors, bile acids, and carcinogens through the gastrointestinal tract. Physical activity may also favorably affect the immune system (9, 56), alter prostaglandin synthesis (6), and, in association with a lower body mass, create a metabolic environment less conducive to the growth of cancer (9).

"Successful weight management for adults requires a life-long commitment to healthful behaviors emphasizing eating practices and daily physical activity that are sustainable and enjoyable," states the American Dietetic Association (3).

Although less consistent than for colon cancer, epidemiological findings indicate that regular physical activity may reduce the risk of breast cancer, especially in premenopausal or younger women (6, 9, 57, 58). Evidence is too limited or inconsistent to support conclusions regarding the effect of physical activity on other cancers (6, 9).

Osteoporosis. Throughout life, regular weight-bearing physical activity helps to maintain the normal structure and functional strength of bone (1, 6). Increasing peak bone mass reached by age 30 and protecting against bone loss in later years reduces the risk of osteoporosis, a debilitating bone-thinning disease affecting 20 million women and 7 to 12 million men in the U.S. (59).

Numerous studies indicate that regular weight-bearing physical activity, especially throughout life, helps to protect against osteoporosis (6, 60–65). However, physical activity alone is insufficient to protect against this disease (66). In addition to physical activity, diet (especially adequate calcium and vitamin D intake), and hormonal status (estrogen) contribute to skeletal health (66).

Increased physical activity and calcium intake have been demonstrated to increase bone density and decrease bone loss at various skeletal sites (61, 67–70). A review of 17 trials found that physical activity exerted beneficial effects on bone mineral density at the lumbar spine at high calcium intakes (i.e., > 1,000 mg/day), but not at calcium intakes less than 1,000 mg/day (67). Other studies indicate independent effects of physical activity and dietary calcium on bone health (61, 69, 70). In a recent investigation involving 422 women ages 25 to 65 years in Finland, both high physical activity and high calcium intake (i.e., 1,475 mg/day versus 638 mg/day) were associated with higher total bone mineral content than in participants who were less physically active and consumed lower amounts of calcium (70).

Weight-bearing aerobic activities such as walking, tennis, and low impact aerobics, as well as high-intensity strength training, improve bone density (6, 68). When 39 post-menopausal, sedentary women participated in either high-intensity strength training exercises two days a week for one year or remained sedentary, bone density in the exercise group increased by an average of 1.5%, whereas it declined by about 2% in the sedentary women (68). The high-intensity strength training not only helped to preserve bone density, but it also increased muscle strength and balance, all of which can reduce the risk of future osteoporotic fractures (68).

Clearly, regular weight-bearing exercise benefits bone health at all ages. Because the benefits of weight-bearing exercise are site specific, it is best to participate in a variety of physical activities.

LATER ADULT YEARS

Physical activity is especially important for older adults because of their often low functional status and high incidence of major chronic diseases (6, 12, 71, 72). A recent cross-sectional study involving over 2,000 adults 65 years of age and older associated high intensity physical activity with lower blood insulin, triglyceride, and fibrinogen levels, reduced obesity, higher HDL cholesterol levels, and reduced risk of heart attacks and heart injury (72). Similarly, physical activity in later adult years positively affects multiple risk factors for osteoporotic fractures (i.e., skeletal fragility, muscle weakness, and deteriorating balance) (6, 8, 68).

Physical activity in later adult years may help improve muscle strength, aerobic endurance, functional capacity, gait, joint flexibility, balance, reaction time, and overall quality of life (6, 8, 12, 13, 68). Reduced muscle strength is a major cause of disability among older adults (12). Resistance or strength training has been demonstrated to be beneficial for even frail, institutionalized elderly adults aged 72 to 98 years (13). Also, the increased energy needs resulting from a more physically active lifestyle may allow older adults to improve their overall nutritional intake when energy needs are met by nutrient-dense foods.

RECOMMENDATIONS FOR A PHYSICALLY ACTIVE LIFESTYLE

There is a general consensus among medical and physical activity experts that all Americans, children and adults, should participate in about 30 minutes of moderate intensity physical activity on most, and preferably all, days of the week (2, 5–8). It is now widely recognized that moderate intensity activity equivalent to brisk walking at 3 to 4 mph, and not necessarily a structured, vigorous exercise program, confers health benefits. Resistance or strength exercise at a moderate intensity for two to three days a week is also recommended, especially for older adults (8, 13, 61, 68, 73).

Motivating sedentary individuals to become more physically active is a major challenge (35, 74). The key to encouraging individuals to lead more physically active lifestyles is to help them identify activities that they enjoy, feel competent and safe doing, and fit into their schedules and budgets (8, 35).

Physical activity alone is not the answer to health. Rather, physical activity should be combined with a healthful diet made up of a variety of foods in moderation from the major

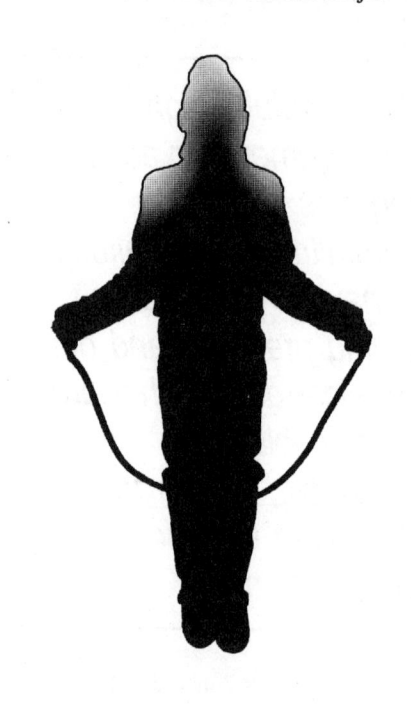

All Americans, children and adults, are encouraged to participate in about 30 minutes of moderate intensity physical activity on most, and preferably all, days of the week.

food groups (3, 5). To help the public put food, nutrition, and physical activity messages into action, the Dietary Guidelines Alliance (4) has implemented a campaign called "It's All About You." This campaign provides action tips for the following five supporting messages: "Be Realistic," "Be Adventurous," "Be Flexible," "Be Sensible," and "Be Active" (4). The "Be Active" message encourages the public to think fun and remember that small amounts of physical activity add up over time (4).

REFERENCES

1. Blair, S.N., E. Horton, A. S. Leon, et. al. Med. Sci. Sports Exerc. 28 (3): 335, 1996.
2. Pate, R. R., M. Pratt, S. N. Blair, et. al. JAMA 273: 402, 1995.
3. The American Dietetic Association. J. Am. Diet. Assoc. 97: 71, 1997.
4. The Dietary Guidelines Alliance. *Reaching Consumers With Meaningful Health Messages. A Handbook for Nutrition and Health Communicators.* A project of the Dietary Guidelines Alliance, 1996.
5. U.S. Department of Agriculture and U.S. Department of Health and Human Services. *Nutrition and Your Health: Dietary Guidelines for Americans.* 4th edition. Home & Garden Bulletin No. 232. Washington, DC: U.S. Government Printing Office, 1995.
6. U.S. Department of Health and Human Services. *Physical Activity and Health: A Report of the Surgeon General.* Atlanta, GA: U.S. Department of Health and Human Services, Centers for Disease Control and Prevention, National Center for Chronic Disease Prevention and Health Promotion, 1996.
7. NIH Consensus Development Panel on Physical Activity and Cardiovascular Health, JAMA 276: 241, 1996.
8. Fletcher, G. F., G. Balady, S. N. Blair, et. al. Circulation 94: 857, 1996.
9. World Cancer Research Fund in association with American Institute for Cancer Research. *Food, Nutrition and the Prevention of Cancer: a Global Perspective.* Washington, DC: American Institute for Cancer Research, 1997.
10. International Life Sciences Institute. *Improving Children's Health Through Physical Activity: A New Opportunity.* A Survey of Parents and Children About Physical Activity Patterns. July 1997.
11. Telama, R., L. Laakso, X. Yang, et. al. Am. J. Prev. Med. 13: 317, 1997.
12. Evans, W. J., and D. Cyr-Campbell. J. Am. Diet. Assoc. 97: 632, 1997.
13. Fiatarone, M. A., E. F. O'Neill, N. D. Ryan, et. al. N. Engl. J. Med. 330: 1769, 1994.
14. Paffenbarger, R.S., Jr., J. B. Kampert, I. -M. Lee, et. al. Med. Sci. Sports Exerc. 26 (7): 857, 1994.
15. Kushi, L. H., R. M. Fee, A. R. Folsom, et. al. JAMA 277: 1287, 1997.
16. Kujala, U. M., J. Kaprio, S. Sarna, et. al. JAMA 279: 440, 1998.
17. The American Dietetic Association. *Nutrition Trends Survey 1997.* September 1997.
18. Federation of American Societies for Experimental Biology, Life Sciences Research Office. Prepared for the Interagency Board for Nutrition Monitoring and Related Research. *Third Report on Nutrition Monitoring in the United States: Executive Summary.* Washington, DC: U.S. Government Printing Office, December 1995.

29. Physical Activity and Nutrition

19. National Center for Health Statistics. *Healthy People 2000 Review, 1995–96.* Hyattsville, MD: Public Health Service, 1996.
20. U.S. Department of Agriculture, Agricultural Research Service. Data tables: results from USDA's 1996 Continuing Survey of Food Intakes by Individuals and 1996 Diet and Health Knowledge Survey, [Online]. ARS Food Surveys Research Group. December, 1997. Available (under "Releases"): http://www.barc.usda.gov/bhnrc/foodsurvey/home.htm[February 25, 1988].
21. Centers for Disease Control and Prevention, U.S. Department of Health and Human Services, National Center for Chronic Disease Prevention and Health Promotion. *CDC's Guidelines for School and Community Programs to Promote Lifelong Physical Activity Among Young People.* March 1997.
22. Division of Health Examination Statistics, National Center for Health Statistics, Division of Nutrition and Physical Activity, National Center for Chronic Disease Prevention and Health Promotion, DCD. *MMWR 46 (9) (March 7):* 199, 1997.
23. Bar-Or, O., J. Foreyt, C. Bouchard, et. al. Med. Sci. Sports Exerc. *30:* 2, 1998.
24. Ogden, C. L., R. P. Troiano, R. R. Briefel, et. al. Pediatrics *99 (4):* e[1], 1997.
25. Mei, Z., K. S. Scanlon, L. M. Grummer-Strawn, et. al. Pediatrics *101 (1):* e12, 1997.
26. Dietz, W. H. J. Nutr. *128:* 411s, 1998.
27. Christoffel, K. K., and A. Ariza. Pediatrics *101:* 103, 1998.
28. Vuori, I. Nutr. Rev. *54 (4):* 11s, 1996.
29. Dyson, K., C. J. R. Blimkie, K. S. Davison, et. al. Med. Sci. Sports Exerc. *29 (4):* 443, 1997.
30. Gunnes, M., and E. H. Lehmann. Acta Paediatr. *85:* 19, 1996.
31. Teegarden, D., W. R. Proulx, M. Kern, et. al. Med. Sci. Sports Exerc. *28:* 105, 1996.
32. Raitakari, O. T., S. Taimela, K. V. K. Porkka, et. al. Med. Sci Sports Exerc. *29 (8):* 1055, 1997.
33. Johnson-Down, L., J. O'Loughlin, K. G. Koski, et. al. J. Nutr. *127:* 2310, 1997.
34. Blair, S. N., J. B. Kampert, H. W. Kohl, III, et. al. JAMA *276:* 205, 1996.
35. Clark, K. L., In: *Cardiovascular Nutrition. Strategies and Tools for Disease Management and Prevention.* P. Kris-Etherton and J. H. Burns (Eds). Chicago, IL: The American Dietetic Association, 1998, p. 27.
36. Marragat, J., R. Elosua, M. -I. Covas, et. al. Am. J. Epidemiol. *143:* 562, 1996.
37. Leaf, D. A., D. L. Parker, and D. Schaad. Med. Sci. Sports Exerc. *29 (9):* 1152, 1997.
38. Koenig, W., M. Sund, A. Doring, et. al. Circulation *95:* 335, 1997.
39. Pols, M. A., P. H. M. Peeters, J. W. R. Twisk, et. al. Am. J. Epidemiol. *146:* 322, 1997.
40. Folsom, A. R., D. K. Arnett, R. G. Hutchinson, et. al. Med. Sci. Sports Exerc. *29 (7):* 901, 1997.
41. Mensink, G. B. M., D. W. Heerstrass, S. E. Neppelenbroek, et. al. Med. Sci. Sports Exerc. *29 (9):* 1192, 1997.
42. Niebauer, J., R. Hambrecht, T. Velich, et. al. Circulation *96:* 2534, 1997.
43. The Sixth Report of the Joint National Committee on Prevention, Detection, Evaluation, and Treatment of High Blood Pressure. Arch. Intern. Med. *157:* 2413, 1997.
44. Kuczmarski, R., K. M. Flegal, S. M. Campbell, et. al. JAMA *272:* 205, 1994.
45. National Institute of Diabetes and Digestive and Kidney Diseases, National Institutes of Health. *Physical Activity and Weight Control.* NIH Publ. No. 96-4031, April 1996.
46. Hill, J. O., and R. Commerford. Int. J. Sports Nutr. *6:* 80, 1996.
47. King, N. A., A. Tremblay, and J. E. Blundell. Med. Sci. Sports Exerc. *29:* 1076, 1997.
48. Pritchard, J. E., C. A. Nowson, and J. D. Wark. J. Am Diet. Assoc. *97:* 37, 1997.
49. Racette, S. B., D. A. Schoeller, R. F. Kushner, et. al. Am. J. Clin. Nutr. *62:* 345, 1995.
50. Grodstein, F., R. Levine, L. Troy, et. al. Arch. Intern. Med. *156:* 1302, 1996.
51. Schoeller, D.A., K. Shay, and R. F. Kushner. Am. J. Clin. Nutr. 66: 551, 1997.
52. Kraemer, W. J., J. S. Volek, K. L. Clark, et. al. J. Appl. Physiol. *83(1):* 270, 1997.
53. American Diabetes Association. Diabetes Care *21 (suppl. 1):* 32, 1998.
54. Burchfiel, C. M., D. S. Sharp, J. D. Curb, et. al. Am. J. Epidemiol. *141:* 360, 1995.
55. Lynch, J., S. P. Helmrich, T. A. Lakka, et. al. Arch. Intern. Med. *156:* 1307, 1996.
56. Hoffman-Goetz, L. Nutr. Rev. *56(s):* 126, 1998.
57. Thune, I., T. Brenn, E. Lund, et. al. N. Engl. J. Med. *336 (18):* 1269, 1997.
58. Gammon, M. D., E. M. John, and J. A. Britton. J. Natl. Cancer Inst. *90:* 100, 1998.
59. Looker, A. C., E. S. Orwoll, C. C. Johnston, Jr., et. al. J. Bone Miner. Res. *12 (11):* 1761, 1997.
60. American College of Sports Medicine. Med. Sci. Sports Exerc. *27 (4):* i, 1995.
61. Nelson, M. E., E. C. Fisher, F. A. Dilmanian, et. al. Am. J. Clin. Nutr. *53:* 1304, 1991.
62. Etherington, J., P. A. Harris, D. Nandra, et. al. J. Bone Miner. Res. *11 (9):* 1333, 1996.
63. Alekel, L., J. L. Clasey, P. C. Fehling, et. al. Med. Sci. Sports Exerc. *27 (11):* 1477, 1996.
64. Taffe, D. R., T. L. Robinson, C. M. Snow, et. al. J. Bone Miner. Res. *12 (2):* 255, 1997.
65. Dook, J. E., C. James, N. K. Henderson, et. al. Med. Sci. Sports Exerc. *29 (3):* 291, 1997.
66. Heaney, R. P. Nutr. Rev. *54 (4):* 3s, 1996.
67. Specker, B. L. J. Bone Miner. Res. *11 (10):* 1539, 1996.
68. Nelson, M. E., M. A. Fiatarone, C. M. Morganti, et. al. JAMA *272:* 1909, 1994.
69. Suleiman, S., M. Nelson, F. Li, et. al. Am. J. Clin. Nutr. *66:* 937, 1997.
70. Uusi-rasi, K., H. Sievanen, I. Vuori, et, al. J. Bone Miner. Res. *13 (1):* 133, 1998.
71. Evans, W. J. Nutr. Rev. *54 (1):* 35s, 1996.
72. Siscovick, D. S., L. Fried, M. Mittelmark, et. al. Am. J. Epidemiol. *145 (11):* 977, 1997.
73. Nelson, M. E., and S. Wernick. *Strong Women Stay Young.* New York: Bantam Books, 1997.
74. Andersen, R. E., S. N. Blair, L. J. Cheskin, et. al. Ann. Intern. Med. *127:* 395, 1997.

ACKNOWLEDGMENTS

National Dairy Council® assumes the responsibility for this publication. However, we would like to acknowledge the help and suggestions of the following reviewers in its preparation:

■ Kristine L. Clark, Ph.D., R. D
Director, Sports Nutrition Program
Assistant Professor of Nutrition
Center for Sports Medicine Pennsylvania State University University Park, PA

■ Miriam E. Nelson, Ph.D.
Associate Chief, Human Physiology Laboratory at the Jean Mayer USDA
Human Nutrition Research Center on Aging
Tufts University Boston, MA

The *Dairy Council Digest*® is written and edited by Lois D. McBean, M. S., R. D.

Article 30

STRAIGHT TALK ON THE MEDICAL HEADLINES

Alcohol and Health

THE STORY

Fountain of youth: A drink a day can help you live longer—Boston Herald, Dec. 11, 1997

Studies confirm relationship of alcohol to breast cancer—New York Times, Feb. 18, 1998

Which of these is the truth: Is alcohol a life-extending elixir or a soothing poison? It's actually a combination of these, depending on how much you drink, your general health, and personal risk factors for a host of health problems, including heart and liver disease, many cancers, and alcoholism.

In the United States, public health campaigns have traditionally urged people to avoid alcohol or cut back on their drinking. And rightly so—heavy drinking is the second leading cause of preventable death in the US, right behind cigarette smoking. Alcohol is implicated in up to half of all fatal traffic accidents. Heavy drinking clearly contributes to liver disease, a variety of cancers, a weakening of the heart muscle, high blood pressure, strokes, and depression, and can take a terrible toll on families and relationships. Even moderate drinking interferes with a host of medications or magnifies their negative side effects.

A new countermovement, though, is touting the apparent benefits of a drink a day on the heart and circulatory system. These recommendations are spurred by studies from around the world showing that alcohol offers some protection against heart disease, the leading cause of death in the US and other developed countries.

The latest, and largest, of these was published in the December 11, 1997 *New England Journal of Medicine.* Researchers from the American Cancer Society, the World Health Organization, and Oxford University looked at causes of death and death rates in half a million men and women, all of whom had answered a questionnaire in 1982 about their drinking, smoking, and other habits. Over the following 10 years, moderate drinkers—those who had a drink a day—were 20 percent less likely to die than people who didn't drink at all, thanks to substantial reductions in death from heart disease.

The overall picture masks some important trends. Even though moderate drinking was associated with an overall lower death rate from heart disease, alcohol's protective effect was relatively small among those at low risk for heart disease and more powerful among those at high risk for it. As expected, deaths from alcoholism; cirrhosis of the liver; cancers of the liver, mouth, throat, larynx, or esophagus; and injuries or accidents were highest among the heaviest drinkers. And when the researchers looked at causes of death for women, they found a greater risk of dying from breast cancer among women who reported having at least one drink a day compared with nondrinkers.

Other researchers found a similar connection between drinking and breast cancer in an analysis of six long-term studies that included more than 300,000 women, published in the February 18 *Journal of the American Medical Association.* Among women who averaged one or fewer drinks a day, the breast cancer risk was 9 percent higher than it was among nondrinkers. (This doesn't mean that 9 percent of women who have a drink a day will develop breast cancer. Rather, it's the difference between 11 of every 10,000 women developing breast cancer—the current US risk—and 12 of every 10,000 developing the disease.) Among those who reported having two to five drinks a day, breast cancer rates rose by 41 percent.

A study of more than 5,000 Italian women, published in the March 4 *Journal of the National Cancer Institute,* also found a connection between increasing amounts of alcohol and breast cancer. The researchers calculated that more than 20 grams of alcohol (slightly more than one drink) a day and little physical activity accounted for about 20 percent of breast cancers; and more than 40 percent among premenopausal women.

Parallel lines of research are showing that we can't view alcohol as all bad or all good. Finding your own balance of benefits and risks may be challenging, but it's well worth the effort.

—*The Editors*

THE PHYSICIAN'S PERSPECTIVE

Charles H. Hennekens, MD
Associate Editor

Given the way medical science works, and the way the media interact with scientists, you will probably see more conflicting headlines about alcohol and health in the months to come. Most studies, and the news reports that follow them, examine a single connection—alcohol and heart disease, alcohol and breast cancer, alcohol and mortality. While such narrowly focused studies clearly advance what we know about the impact of alcohol on the body, they don't reflect the broader reality. The alcohol you consume in a glass of wine, beer, or spirits alters mood and metabolism, and influences a variety of organs, including your brain, stomach, intestines, liver, and many glands. The complexity of alcohol's effects make it difficult to untangle its benefits from its risks.

Small amounts of alcohol offer some people subtle physical benefits. A drink before a meal can improve one's appetite and aid digestion, and may also keep bowel movements regular. Furthermore, many people look forward to having a drink at the end of a long, stressful day or enjoy the occasional drink with friends—emotional or psychic benefits that may improve health and well-being.

The scientific jury is still out on the degree to which light to moderate amounts of alcohol may benefit the heart, despite what the headlines may claim. A number of large, carefully constructed studies support the hypothesis that drinking small to moderate amounts of alcohol helps prevent the development of coronary heart disease. We think that alcohol itself is playing this role by raising levels of protective HDL cholesterol or by preventing the formation of small clots that can block blood vessels in the heart. It may, however, be something about people who drink in moderation that is the real cause. For example, according to a large national survey on American eating habits, moderate drinkers are more likely than nondrinkers or heavy drinkers to exercise, watch their diets, and get adequate sleep, each of which may have an independent and beneficial impact on heart disease.

Moderate drinking carries risks as well as benefits. It may interrupt sleep, or degrade the quality of sleep. It is notorious for impairing judgment. And even modest amounts of alcohol can interact with medications in harmful ways. Some antidepressants, sedatives, painkillers, and anticonvulsants can amplify the effects of alcohol, causing inebriation at lower intakes. Alcohol can also amplify the harmful side effects of some medications. Finally, research has consistently shown that moderate drinking increases the likelihood of dying from liver disease, strokes caused by bleeding inside the brain, breast cancer, and suicide and accidental deaths.

One thing is clear: Assumptions that the average person should begin to have a drink a day are premature, or even misguided. None of us is the mythical average person. Each of us has a unique personal and family history, as well as habits that predispose us to or protect us from diseases. So alcohol offers each of us different risks and benefits.

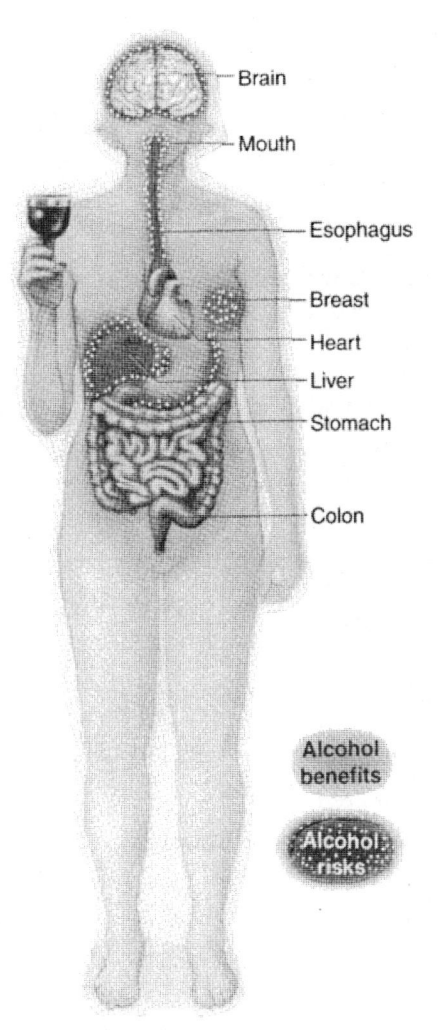

Alcohol offers abundant risk and no net benefit for pregnant women, recovering alcoholics, people with a family history of alcohol abuse, anyone with liver disease or a weakening of the heart muscle (cardiomyopathy), and anyone taking medications that may interact with alcohol.

Assuming that you don't fall into any of those categories, the balance between risk and benefit is harder to calculate. Let me give several examples. A 23-year-old man reaps no net benefit from a drink or two a day, because he is at very low risk for developing heart disease and is at high risk for accidental, often alcohol-related, injury or death. Furthermore, there's no getting an early start since any possible "heart benefits" of alcohol aren't stored up for the future. A 55-year-old man who has high cholesterol levels and whose mother died of a heart attack may benefit from a drink a day, assuming he doesn't fall into any of the categories mentioned above. For a 55-year-old woman with high cholesterol and a family history of breast cancer, the risk-benefit calculation is more complicated. Heart disease kills five to six times more women each year than breast cancer, 236,000 compared with 44,000. And the increase in breast cancer associated with a drink a day or less is small. So on the face of it, the occasional drink may offer a net benefit. But a woman who is more afraid of developing breast cancer than heart disease may want to choose to avoid alcohol.

The health benefits of an alcoholic drink a day are substantially smaller than those offered by exercise and eating right. So a healthy lifestyle offers you the best chance of avoiding disease and living longer. You can best determine whether or not the occasional drink should be part of that healthy lifestyle by talking with your physician and taking an inventory of your health and health risks.

If you decide that it should, the key word must be moderation. Given the complexity of alcohol's physiological, metabolic, and psychological effects, the difference between a little bit of alcohol and a lot may be the difference between preventing disease and premature death, and causing it.

Unit 4

Unit Selections

31. **Weight Control: Challenges and Solutions,** Dairy Council Digest
32. **Childhood Obesity and Family SES Racial Differences,** Patricia B. Crawford, Allison Drury, and Sheila Stern
33. **NIH Guidelines: An Evaluation,** Frances M. Berg
34. **The Great Weight Debate,** Consumer Reports on Health
35. **Exploding the Myth: Weight Loss Makes You Healthier,** Paul Ernsberger
36. **Simplifying the Advice for Slimming Down,** Tufts University Health & Nutrition Newsletter
37. **The History of Dieting and Its Effectiveness,** Wayne C. Miller
38. **Dieting Disorder,** David Rosen
39. **The Effects of Starvation on Behavior: Implications for Dieting and Eating Disorders,** David M. Garner

Key Points to Consider

❖ How does concern about your weight affect your life and that of your friends? Analyze your attitudes and behavior and describe what, if any, changes in these are appropriate.

❖ What are the issues of benefit and risk that one should consider before deciding to go on a diet?

❖ Find a description of a new trendy diet and evaluate it for effectiveness and safety.

❖ Which of the many products with fat and sugar substitutes do you like? What is your purpose in using them? Do you reduce total calories by using these products?

❖ Do you think weight reduction should be a national goal? Why or why not? What population groups would you target and what strategies would you use?

DUSHKIN ONLINE Links — www.dushkin.com/online/

23. **American Anorexia Bulimia Association**
    http://www.aabainc.org/home.html
24. **Calorie Control Council**
    http://www.caloriecontrol.org
25. **Eating Disorders: Body Image Betrayal**
    http://www.geocities.com/HotSprings/5704/edlist.htm
26. **Shape Up America!**
    http://www.shapeup.org

These sites are annotated on pages 4 and 5.

Fat and Weight Control

> If you wish to grow thinner, diminish your dinner,
> And take to light claret instead of pale ale; Look
> down with an utter contempt upon butter, And
> never touch bread till it's toasted—or stale.
>
> —H.S. Leigh, *A Day for Wishing*

At the beginning of this century, in 1903, it was news when President William Howard Taft, then 335 pounds, got stuck in the White House bathtub and vowed to lose weight. Perhaps this event signaled a change in cultural attitude, for the first diet pills were prescribed in 1910, and the term "ideal weight" was coined by insurance companies in 1923. These same insurance companies charged higher rates to their heavy clients. Subsequently, a series of substances were promoted as diet aids, beginning in the 1920s with the suggestion to "Reach for a Lucky (cigarette) instead of a sweet." In the 1930s and 1940s Benzedrine was followed by amphetamines as drugs that reduce appetites. Overeaters Anonymous, organized in 1960, led the way for other weight-loss organizations. Cyclamates and aspartame, both low-cal sweeteners, followed saccharin, which was already on the market. Now, at the turn of a new century, many lower fat and reduced-calorie food items are available and we are learning about hormones and neurotransmitters that govern weight.

Clearly thin is still in. For most of today's society, it is the willowy person who is seen as beautiful, socially acceptable, and appealing to the opposite sex. Many of us with bulges and bumps will knead and pound, use saunas, and starve ourselves—anything to lose a pound. In some cases, the price has been high. The once-popular combination drug fen-phen is now off the market due to a possible link to serious heart valve damage.

Inevitably, a discussion of weight turns to definitions. When is a person overweight? How much can one weigh and still be healthy? There is considerable scientific support for a causative connection between obesity and increased risks of numerous degenerative diseases such as diabetes, hypertension, and gallstones. The federal government, in the newest set of weight guidelines, has defined obesity as a body mass index (BMI) of 25 or greater. However, a candid observer might argue that nobody agrees on appropriate weights and that recommendations bounce up and down like a yo-yo. There is truth in this observation. Included in this edition are articles which challenge NIH's (National Institutes of Health) definition of obesity and its arguments that weight loss makes one healthier. There also is evidence of lower correlation between higher weights and health risks as people get into their seventies.

But weights continue to go up. It is generally conceded that, in affluent nations, obesity has become an epidemic and may become the biggest health problem of the next century. Using the new NIH guidelines, half our population is overweight, but even when other guidelines are used, the figures are high. In despair, many of us on the plus side of accepted weight guidelines have asked, "What is a body to do?" We briefly hoped that the discovery of the protein leptin would provide a real breakthrough to appetite control, but such is not yet the case.

Surveys indicate that 54 million Americans, or 27 percent of the population, will go on a diet this year. As many as half of adult women and a quarter of adult men are dieting at any given time. Even more dramatic is the high number of grade school and adolescent girls who have reported weight loss attempts, often at the behest of their mothers. Dieters will try different methods, often joining a locally available weight-loss program such as Weight Watchers or Nutri/System. Articles are included that attempt to identify what has worked for successful weight losers.

Some of us have given up repetitive dieting and have realized the necessity for a permanent lifestyle change if lower weights are to be achieved and maintained. It is difficult to keep that focus, however, as we rely more and more on food prepared away from home. The National Restaurant Association reports that, on a typical day, nearly half of all adults dine in a restaurant, where portion sizes are getting larger and where we often give ourselves permission to eat anything and everything. Taste remains the biggest factor affecting what we purchase to eat, even though a high percentage of the population claims to be eating more healthily than in earlier years.

For a long time we have believed that reducing fat intake would result in lower weight. According to surveys, people are eating lighter versions of favorite foods. Furthermore, we're making progress toward the recommended 30 percent of total calories or less from fat, for the percentage of calories attributed to fat is now between 33 and 34 percent, down from 40 percent a decade ago. Some of this reduction is merely an illusion. Because we have simultaneously kept total fat the same and increased the number of calories consumed, the percentage of fat calories has declined.

If there is a magic word used with weight loss, it is exercise, and its significance can hardly be overstated. The one simple thing about weight gain is that it represents an energy imbalance, an intake of more calories than the body uses. One solution, then, is to increase activity, a subject addressed in unit 3. Indeed, a study at Johns Hopkins University showed that children who watch at least 4 hours of television daily are fatter than those who watch less and are presumably more active. Two-thirds of teenagers get minimum amounts of exercise, and a fifth of girls get no exercise at all. Even larger numbers of adults are inactive. We might ask what happened to physical education in the schools.

An article on eating disorders and one on the effects of starvation are included in this unit. It is ironic, in a country with the highest prevalence of obesity, that we are simultaneously very concerned about the millions who subject themselves to starving. Health professionals are very concerned that our exaggerated focus on slimness and dieting has encouraged, if not caused, many young people to develop eating disorders. With their high morbidity and mortality rates, eating disorders often are not diagnosed because the behaviors seem culturally normal. It may be no surprise that anorexia nervosa is seven times more common in strict ballet schools as compared to the rest of the population and that half of these young women are amenorrheic. Almost 20 percent of high school wrestlers exhibit eating-disordered behaviors during wrestling season as well. And, unlike the stereotype of the upper class suburban white girl, eating disorders are also common among inner-city African Americans.

Article 31

WEIGHT CONTROL: CHALLENGES AND SOLUTIONS

SUMMARY

More than half of all adult Americans (55%), or an estimated 97 million, is overweight or obese, according to new standards set by a U.S. federal government expert panel. Overweight/obesity among both adults and children has risen at an alarming rate over the past two decades. This situation is of great concern considering the health, psychological, and economic burden imposed by obesity. This chronic disease costs the nation nearly $100 billion/year.

A myriad of genetic and environmental factors influences the development of obesity. The recent rise in this disease is attributed to our environment which favors overconsumption of energy-dense foods and limits or discourages physical activity.

Traditionally, treatment for obesity has been disappointing with few obese/overweight adults achieving long-term success. To help improve treatment outcome, the government expert panel recently issued evidence-based clinical guidelines to identify, evaluate, and treat overweight and obese adults. The decision to treat should be based on an individual's degree of overweight, risk of weight-related diseases, and motivation to follow a weight loss regimen.

The expert panel recommends a weight loss of 1 to 2 pounds per week to reach a 10% reduction in body weight after the first six months of treatment. Thereafter, weight loss should continue, if warranted, or a weight maintenance program should be followed. A combination of diet therapy (i.e., a 500 to 1000 kcal/day deficit), increased physical activity (i.e., at least 30 minutes per day), and behavior modification is the most successful strategy for weight loss and

The American Heart Association has upgraded obesity from a contributing to an independent risk factor for coronary heart disease.

maintenance. The weight loss diet should be individually planned, meet nutritional needs, and not contribute to other health problems such as osteoporosis. Because weight loss diets are associated with decreased bone density and increased risk of hip fractures, individuals following such diets should consume at least recommended intakes of calcium from calcium-rich foods, such as dairy foods. Prevention, starting in childhood and continuing throughout life, is by far the best treatment for overweight/obesity

Weight control is clearly a public health challenge. Health professionals, by working together, are taking steps to solve the obesity crisis in this nation. Important in this regard is shifting the public's concept of obesity from a purely cosmetic condition to a chronic disease with related comorbidities. Also, realistic weight loss and maintenance targets must replace the public's obsession with attaining an "ideal" body weight. Even moderate weight loss, if maintained, can lead to significant improvements in overall health.

THE EPIDEMIC OF OVERWEIGHT/OBESITY

Obesity threatens to become the leading health problem of the 21st century unless actions are taken to prevent this chronic disease. The prevalence of overweight/obesity among U.S. adults has reached epidemic proportions (1-3). An estimated 97 million adults, or about 55% of the population, is overweight or obese, according to new standards set by the U.S. government (1). Overweight is defined as a body mass index (BMI) (weight in kilograms divided by the square of height in meters) of 25 to 29.9; obesity as a BMI of 30 to 39.9; and extreme obesity as a BMI of 40 or more (1).

The problem of overweight/obesity pervades both genders and all ages, races, and ethnic groups (1). Overweight/obesity is particularly high among some minority groups, as well as people with low incomes and less education. An epidemic of obesity is also occurring among U.S. children and adolescents (4–6). As many as 11 to 25% of U.S. children and adolescents are overweight or at risk of becoming overweight (4). Considering that childhood obesity, particularly during adolescence, likely continues into adulthood (7,8), the future prevalence of adult obesity can be expected to be even greater if childhood obesity is not prevented (1). Obesity is not just a national epidemic, but a worldwide crisis (9).

In addition to its high prevalence in the U.S., overweight/obesity has risen dramatically in recent decades. Among children and adolescents, the prevalence of obesity has more than doubled during the past two decades (4,5). A similar trend is described for adults (10,11). The World Health Organization describes obesity as an "escalating epidemic" and "one of the greatest neglected public health problems of our time" (12). The public health challenge of reducing the prevalence of obesity in the U.S. has been acknowledged by several government agencies, as well as health professional organizations (1,13–16).

Despite progress in our understanding of overweight/obesity, weight control remains a formidable challenge. This *Digest* reviews the health and economic consequences, contributing factors, treatment approaches for adults, and prevention of overweight/obesity.

HEALTH AND ECONOMIC CONSEQUENCES

Overweight and obese adults with a BMI of 25 or greater are at risk of morbidity from coronary heart disease, dyslipidemia (e.g., low high density lipoprotein [HDL] cholesterol, high triglyceride, and high low density lipoprotein [LDL] cholesterol levels), stroke, hypertension, Type 2 diabetes mellitus, gallbladder disease, some cancers (e.g., endometrial, breast, prostate, colon), osteoarthritis, sleep apnea, and respiratory problems (1,12,17–22). Both gain in body fatness during adulthood and increased abdominal fat (i.e., waist circumference) are important determinants of cardiovascular disease (19,23,24). Obese individuals may also face social and psychological burdens, such as discrimination (2). In addition, obesity is associated with increased all-cause mortality (1,25). The American

The first federal guidelines on identifying, evaluating, and treating overweight and obesity in adults were recently released.

Heart Association has upgraded obesity from a contributing to an independent risk factor for coronary heart disease.

Obesity-related diseases as well as concern about weight control exact a heavy economic toll. Health risks associated with obesity are responsible for medical care and disability costs (1). Total costs attributable to obesity-related diseases amounted to nearly $100 billion in 1995 (1,26). In addition, personal costs related to weight control such as health clubs, weight loss programs, and exercise equipment are appreciable (19,27). Americans spend about $40 billion a year on weight loss treatments, mostly diets and diet foods (27).

WHAT CAUSES OVERWEIGHT/OBESITY?

Obesity develops when energy intake exceeds energy expenditure. Despite this seemingly simplistic statement, much remains to be learned about the basic causes of obesity (19). The etiology of obesity is multifactorial. Genetic, molecular, cellular, metabolic, physiologic, cultural, behavioral, and social factors are all believed to play an interactive role in the development of obesity (1,3,11,16,28,29).

Genetics determines about 25 to 40% of the variability in body mass or fat among family members (1,11,29). Among identical twins reared apart, the contribution of genetics to body fatness is even greater (i.e., about 70%). In recent years, a number of candidate genes and potential pathways for their contribution to obesity have been identified (1,11,16,19,30–32). For example, mutations in genes for leptin (i.e., an appetite-suppressant hormone) and its receptor have been cloned in obese rodents, as well as in some humans (33). With the rare exception, multiple genes appear to contribute to or increase the likelihood of becoming obese (1,19,30,32). The impact of genetics on individual susceptibility to obesity is generally attenuated or exacerbated by nongenetic or environmental factors (1).

The dramatic rise in obesity over the past two decades cannot be explained by genetics given that our genes have not substantially changed during this time (11,34). Rather, environmental factors related to overconsumption of food and decreased physical activity offer a more reasonable explanation for the obesity epidemic (1,29,34,35). Not only are there more frequent opportunities to consume large quantities of palatable, energy-dense foods, but our environment limits or discourages physical activity (34,35).

Of all the dietary variables linked to body fatness, dietary fat has received the most attention. Whether or not a high dietary fat intake is a contributor to the high prevalence of overweight/obesity in our society is currently debated (36–39). Dietary fat is believed to favor obesity because of its high energy density and its palatability which encourages overconsumption (11,34,40). It appears that the primary impact of dietary fat is to increase energy intake, and the effects of dietary fat that are independent of energy intake appear to play a minor role in body fatness (28,37,41–43).

While short-term laboratory studies in human subjects indicate that high fat diets can promote positive fat balance, there is a lack of accurate long-term data to substantiate this finding. There are no good long-term studies of dietary fat intake and weight gain and few studies of weight loss following reductions in dietary fat. In general, reducing dietary fat intake produces a very modest reduction in body weight that varies directly with the amount of dietary fat reduction (37,43,44). If the impact of a low fat diet is to reduce the chances of overeating, such a modest effect would be expected. It is clear that a low fat diet would have an important role in maintaining a weight loss. There are reports that subjects who are successful in long-term weight maintenance eat a low fat diet (45), but there is a great need for more data in this area. It may be that there are important individual differences in the effectiveness of a low fat diet in producing and maintaining weight loss.

The decline in physical activity in the U.S. is an important contributor to the obesity epidemic. Despite recommendations to participate in 30 minutes of regular physical activity a day (46–48), 25% of U.S. adults are completely sedentary, according to a report issued by the Surgeon General (47). Physical inactivity is associated with a low energy requirement, and unless energy intake is decreased accordingly, weight gain will ensue. It is important to appreciate that a small daily imbalance between energy intake and expenditure can result significant change in body weight over a decade (49).

TREATMENT/ MANAGEMENT APPROACHES

Weight loss, even relatively moderate weight loss (i.e., 5 to 10% of body weight), has been demonstrated to reduce obesity-related comorbidities such as Type 2 diabetes, hypertension, and cardiovascular disease, and improve lipid profiles (1,11,17,19,50). However, differences of opinion have been expressed regarding the potential benefits and risks of weight loss (27). Questions regarding who and how to treat obesity/overweight recently led a federal government panel to critically review the published scientific literature and develop evidence-based clinical guidelines to identify, evaluate, and treat overweight/obese individuals (1).

The first step in the treatment of obesity is to determine who should be treated (1). Three key measures are recommended to determine the degree of overweight and overall risk: BMI which is highly correlated with total body fat content in adults; waist circumference which indicates abdomi-

> *Weight loss has been associated with bone loss. For this reason, adults following weight loss diets should consume an adequate intake of calcium-rich foods such as low fat dairy foods to maintain their bone strength and reduce risk of osteoporosis.*

nal fat accumulation; and the presence of comorbidities such as Type 2 diabetes, coronary heart disease, hypertension, gallstones, etc. (1). An individual's motivation or readiness to follow a weight loss regimen is another important consideration. The government panel concluded that treatment of overweight differs from that of obesity (1). Treatment of overweight is recommended only when an individual has two or more risk factors and should focus on changing dietary and physical activity patterns to produce moderate weight loss and avoid further weight gain (1). For obese individuals, treatment should focus on producing substantial weight loss for a prolonged period.

The general goals of treatment are threefold: to prevent further weight gain, reduce body weight, and maintain a prolonged lower body weight (1). A 10% reduction in body weight after the first six months of treatment with a weight loss of 1 to 2 pounds per week is recommended (1). This guideline is consistent with the Dietary Guidelines for Americans (15). Achieving this weight loss means an energy deficit of about 300 to 500 kcal/day for overweight individuals and 500 to 1000 kcal/day for more severely obese individuals (1). After six months, the rate of weight loss generally decreases and weight plateaus because of a decline in energy expenditure at a lower body weight. If necessary, further weight loss can be attempted. If not, a weight maintenance program should be followed indefinitely (1).

Numerous effective options are available to treat/manage overweight/obese individuals (1). These include dietary therapy, increasing physical activity, behavior therapy techniques, pharmacotherapy, surgery, and combinations of the above (1). This *Digest* discusses diet, physical activity, and behavior modification. Pharmacotherapy and surgery are generally reserved for select patients with clinically severe obesity and/or whom standard treatments have been unsuccessful. Information on these more aggressive approaches to weight control can be found in several references (1,28,51–53).

Diet Therapy. Diets ranging from modest energy restriction, to very low energy diets, to controlled fasting are available for weight loss (1,2,16). The government panel recommends an energy deficit of 500 to 1000 kcal/day which means a diet containing about 1000 to 1200 kcal/day for women and 1200 to 1500 kcal/day for men (1). Total fat intake should be 30% or less of total energy intake. Reducing fat as part of a calorie-reduced diet is a practical means to reduce calories. However, reducing fat alone will not lead to substantial weight loss unless total energy intake is also reduced (1).

Very low calorie diets (i.e., 400 to 800 kcal/day) can produce greater initial weight loss than moderate low calorie diets, but over the long term (>1 year) there is no difference in weight loss (1). Very low calorie diets may also lead to eating disorders in some individuals (16). Other risks associated with very low calorie diets include gout, gallstones, cardiac complications, and a sense of failure upon weight gain (54). Weight cycling may not be physiologically harmful (55), but it may have a psychological cost (54).

Regardless of the weight loss diet selected, it should be individually planned, meet nutritional needs, and not contribute to other health problems (1,3,16). For example, care should be taken to consume an adequate intake of calcium (56,57). According to a recent prospective study, a weight loss of 10% or more in men was linked to decreased bone density and increased risk of hip fractures (56). Increasing calcium intake reduced the risk of hip fracture (56). In another investigation, increasing calcium intake by 1000mg/day (i.e., a total of about 1500mg/day) in obese postmenopausal women consuming a moderate energy-restricted diet prevented the increase in bone turnover rate caused by a 10% loss in body weight (57).

Physical Activity. The U.S. is said to be facing not only an epidemic of obesity, but also of inactivity (58). Although increasing physical activity may produce only a modest weight loss, it is an important component of a comprehensive weight loss and weight maintenance program (1,3,53,58,59). Physical activity contributes to weight loss in overweight and obese adults; may favorably affect distribution of body fat; increases cardiorespiratory fitness; helps to maintain long-term weight loss; and confers a variety of health-related benefits even in the absence of weight loss (1,3,53,58). Also, physical activity offers psychological benefits (e.g., improved body image) which may help individuals overcome stressful situations that may sabotage their attempts to lose or maintain body weight (58,60). Physical activity is especially valuable in maintaining weight loss (1,3,53,58).

Walking (i.e., 30 minutes for 3 days/week, gradually building up to 45 minutes of more intense walking at least 5 days/week) or swimming at a low pace are convenient ways for adults to increase their physical activity (1,58). Exercise can be done at a single time or intermittently during the day. All adults are encouraged to set a goal of at least 30 minutes or more of moderate-intensity physical activity on most, and preferably, all

---

The challenge for health professionals is to reduce the prevalence of obesity. The solution lies in preventing obesity beginning in childhood and continuing throughout life.

---

days of the week (46–48). In addition, increasing "everyday" activities such as taking the stairs instead of the elevator is encouraged (1).

Behavioral Modification. Most people have difficulty losing weight and, in particular, maintaining weight loss. However, several behavior-change strategies can be used to help people alter their behavior to lose weight and maintain weight loss (61,62). These include self-monitoring (e.g., recording behaviors to increase awareness of obesity-related behaviors); stimulus control (i.e., identifying and learning how to control environmental cues associated with overeating and inactivity); cognitive restructuring (i.e., changing one's mindset); stress management; social support; and relapse prevention (i.e., training to prepare for setbacks) (61,62).

Combined Therapy. A combined intervention including a reduced energy diet, increased physical activity, and behavior modification is the most successful strategy for weight loss and weight maintenance (1). According to The American Dietetic Association (16), "successful weight management for adults requires a lifelong commitment to healthful lifestyle behaviors emphasizing eating practices and daily physical activity that are sustainable and enjoyable."

PREVENTION

Considering the magnitude of the obesity problem, its adverse consequences, and the disappointing outcome of many weight management approaches, primary prevention of overweight/obesity is a public health priority (1,11,12,28,29,34). Also important is prevention of weight regain following weight loss and further weight increases in individuals unable to lose weight (1).

Primary prevention of overweight/obesity beginning in childhood and continuing throughout life should focus on environmental and behavioral factors that contribute to overeating and physical inactivity (1,34,49). Education is needed to increase awareness of the dangers of moderate obesity, and to provide strategies to avoid gaining excess weight (e.g., attention to portion sizes of foods) (32,34). Clearly, weight management is an important challenge for the nation as well as the world (11).

REFERENCES

1. Expert Panel on the Identification, Evaluation, and Treatment of Overweight in Adults. *Am. J. Clin. Nutr.* 68: 899, 1998. The full report is available on the Internet at *www.nhlbi.nih.gov/nhlbi/*.
2. Rippe, J.M. *J. Am. Diet. Assoc.* 98(s): 5s, 1998.
3. Coulston, A.M. *J. Am. Diet. Assoc.* 98(s): 6s, 1998.

4 ❖ FAT AND WEIGHT CONTROL

4. Troiano, R.P., and F.M. Flegal. Pediatrics *101(s):* 497, 1998.
5. Freedman, D.S., S.R.Srinivasan, R.A. Valdez, et. al. Pediatrics *99:* 420, 1997.
6. Anonymous. JAMA *277:* 1111, 1997.
7. Whitaker, R.C., J.A. Wright, M.S. Pepe, et. al. N. Engl. J. Med. *337:* 869, 1997.
8. Dietz, W.H. J. Nutr. *128(s):* 411s, 1998.
9. Popkin, B.M., and C.M. Doak. Nutr. Rev. *56:* 106, 1998.
10. Flegal, K.M., M.D. Carrol, R.J. Kuczmarski, et. al. Int. J. Obes. Relat. Metab. Disord. *22:* 39, 1998.
11. Rippe, J.M., S. Crossley, and R. Ringer. J. Am. Diet. Assoc. *98(s):* 9s, 1998.
12. World Health Organization. *Obesity: Preventing and Managing the Global Epidemic.* Report of a WHO Consultation of Obesity. Geneva. June 3–5, 1997.
13. U.S. Department of Health and Human Services. *Healthy People 2000: National Health Promotion and Disease Prevention Objectives.* DHHS Publ. No. (PHS) 91-50213. Washington, DC: Public Health Service, 1991.
14. Food and Nutrition Board, Institute of Medicine. *Weighing the Options: Criteria for Evaluating Weight Management Programs.* P.R. Thomas (Ed.). Committee to Develop Criteria for Evaluating the Outcomes of Approaches to Prevent and Treat Obesity. Washington, DC: National Academy Press, 1995.
15. U.S. Department of Agriculture and Health and Human Services. *Nutrition and Your Health: Dietary Guidelines for Americans.* 4th ed. Home and Garden Bulletin. DHHS (PHS) Publication No. 88-50210. Washington, DC: U.S. Department of Agriculture and Health and Human Services, 1995.
16. The American Dietetic Association. J. Am. Diet. Assoc. *97:* 71, 1997.
17. Rippe, J.M. Nutr. Clin. Care *1(s):* 3, 1998.
18. Eckel, R. Circulation *96:* 3248, 1997.
19. Krauss, R.M., and M. Winston. Circulation *98:* 1472, 1998.
20. Heyka, R.J. Nutr. Clin. Care *1(s):* 30, 1998.
21. Kelley, D.E. Nutr. Clin. Care *1(s):* 38s, 1998.
22. World Cancer Research Fund in Association with American Institute for Cancer Research. *Food, Nutrition, and the Prevention of Cancer: a Global Perspective.* Washington, DC: American Institute for Cancer Research, 1997.
23. Siervogel, R.M., L. Wisemandle, L.M. Maynard, et. al. Arterioscler. Thromb. Vasc. Biol. *18:* 1759, 1998.
24. Rexrode, K.M., V.J. Carey, C.H. Hennekens, et. al. JAMA *280:* 1843, 1998.
25. Solomon, C.G., and J.E. Manson. Am. J. Clin. Nutr. *66(s):* 1044s, 1997.
26. Wolf, A.M., and G.A. Colditz. Obes. Res. *6:* 97, 1998.
27. Wickelgren, I. Science *280:* 1364, 1998.
28. Rosenbaum, M., R.L. Leibel, and J. Hirsch. N. Engl. J. Med. *337:* 396, 1997.
29. Grundy, S.M. Am. J. Clin. Nutr. *67(s):* 563s, 1998.
30. Wolff, G.L. J. Nutr. *127(s):* 1871s, 1997.
31. Comuzzie, A.G., and D.B. Allison. Science *280:* 1374, 1998.
32. Chagnon, Y.C., L. Perusse, and C. Bouchard. Obes. Res. *6:* 76, 1998.
33. Montague, C.T., I.S. Faroogi, J.P. Whitehead, et. al. Nature *387:* 903, 1997.
34. Hill, J.O., and J.C. Peters. Science *280:* 1371, 1998.
35. Jeffrey, R.W., and S.A. French. Am. J. Publ. Health *88:* 277, 1998.
36. Grundy, S.M. Am. J. Clin. Nutr. *67(s):* 497s, 1998.
37. Willett, W.C. Am. J. Clin. Nutr. *67(s):* 556s, 1998.
38. Willett, W.C. Am. J. Clin. Nutr. *68:* 1149, 1998.
39. Bray, G.A., and B.M. Popkin. Am. J. Clin. Nutr. *68:* 1157, 1998.
40. Bell, E.A., V.H. Castellanos, C.L. Pelkman, et. al. Am. J. Clin. Nutr. *67:* 412, 1998.
41. Seidell, J. Am. J. Clin. Nutr. *67(s):* 546s, 1998.
42. Saltzman, E., G.E. Dallal, and S.B. Roberts. Am. J. Clin. Nutr. *66:* 1332, 1997.
43. Roberts, S.B., F.X. Pi-Sunyer, M. Dreher, et. al. Nutr. Rev. *56(s):* 29s, 1998.
44. Astrup, A., S. Toubro, A. Raben, et. al. J. Am. Diet. Assoc. *97(s):* 82s, 1997.
45. Klem, M.L., R.R. Wing, M.T. McGuire, et. al. Am. J. Clin. Nutr. *66:* 239, 1997.
46. Pate, R.R., M. Pratt, S.N. Blair, et. al. JAMA *273,* 402, 1995.
47. U.S. Department of Health and Human Services, Centers for Disease Control and Prevention. *Physical Activity and Health: A Report of the Surgeon General.* Atlanta: USDHHS, National Center for Chronic Disease Prevention and Health Promotion, 1996.
48. American College of Sports Medicine. Med. Sci. Sports Exerc. *6:* 975, 1998.
49. St. Jeor, S.T. J. Am. Diet. Assoc. *97:* 1096, 1997.
50. Ditschuneit, H.H., M. Flechtner-Mors, T.D. Johnson, et. al. Am. J. Clin. Nutr. *69:* 198, 1999.
51. Aronne, L.J. J. Am. Diet. Assoc. *98(s):* 23s, 1998.
52. Cathelineau, G. Int. J. Obesity *22(s):* 1(s), 1998.
53. Atkinson, R.L. J. Nutr. Biochem. *9:* 546, 1998.
54. Foreyt, J.P., R.L. Brunner, G.K. Goodrick, et. al. Int. J. Eating Disord. *17:* 263, 1995.
55. National Task Force on the Prevention and Treatment of Obesity. JAMA *272:* 1196, 1994.
56. Mussolino, M.E., A.C. Looker, J.H. Madans, et. al. J. Bone Miner. Res. *13:* 918, 1998.
57. Ricci, T.A., H.A. Chowdhury, S.B. Heymsfield, et. al. J. Bone Miner. Res. *13:* 1045, 1998.
58. Rippe, J.M., and S. Hess. J. Am. Diet. Assoc. *98(s):* 31s, 1998.
59. Mattfeldt-Beman, M.K., S.A. Corrigan, V.J. Stevens, et. al. J. Am. Diet. Assoc. *99:* 66, 1999.
60. Foreyt, J.P., R.L. Brunner, G.K. Goodrick, et. al. Int. J. Obes. Relat. Metab. Disord. *19(s):* 69s, 1995.
61. Foreyt, J.P., and W.S.C. Poston, II. J. Am. Diet. Assoc. *98(s):* 27s, 1998.
62. Wing, R.R. In: *Handbook of Obesity.* G.A. Bray, C. Bouchard, and W.P.T. James (Eds). New York: Marcel Dekker, 1998, pp. 855–873.

ACKNOWLEDGMENTS

National Dairy Council® assumes the responsibility for this publication. However, we would like to acknowledge the help and suggestions of the following reviewers in its preparation:

- J.P. Foreyt, Ph.D.
  Director, Nutrition Research Clinic
  Baylor College of Medicine
  Houston, Texas
- J.O. Hill, Ph.D.
  Director, Center for Human Nutrition
  University of Colorado Health Services Center
  Denver, Colorado

The *Dairy Council Digest®* is written and edited by Lois D. McBean, M.S., R.D.

Childhood Obesity and Family SES Racial Differences

by Patricia B. Crawford, PhD, Allison Drury, and Sheila Stern, MA

It has been documented that childhood obesity is more common in families of lower socioeconomic status (SES). During the last 30 years going back to Huenemann and her colleagues at the University of California in Berkeley in 1969, studies have shown that childhood obesity is more common in families with low income and in families with parents of low educational level.[1-4]

Most of the studies that found SES inversely related to childhood obesity examined predominantly white populations, and it was not known if the findings could be generalized to African-American children. Recently, data from the longitudinal NHLBI Growth and Health Study allowed meaningful comparisons of 9- and 10-year-old white and African-American girls with regard to the relationship of SES to childhood obesity.

Racial differences

After careful analysis of data from the Growth and Health Study, it became evident that the association between childhood obesity and socioeconomic factors was different for girls depending on their race.[5] For the white girls, as expected, the prevalence of obesity dropped with higher parental education and higher household income. But, surprisingly, we found no significant correlation between these socioeconomic indicators and obesity in African-American girls.

The same dramatic racial difference was found when using parental employment versus unemployment as an indicator of SES. White girls with highly educated, employed parents were unlikely to be obese, while white girls with parents who were unemployed or not well-educated were more prone to obesity. No similar effects were found among the African-American girls, where the daughters of employed college graduates were as likely to be obese as the daughters of unemployed parents who had no formal education beyond high school.

Racial similarities

Similarities were found between the African-American and white girls when the focus was shifted from indicators of SES to other demographic factors more closely related to family structure. Other studies have shown that the risk of childhood obesity is higher for first-born children and decreases with an increasing number of siblings in the home.[6,7] This is the first study to find a similar relationship for both African-American and white girls. Similarly an association was observed between maternal age and obesity at 9 and 10 years in girls of both races. The older their mothers or female guardians, the more likely both African-American and white girls were to be obese. A similar relationship between child obesity and age of mother and number of siblings for girls of both races points to possible common patterns of family behavior. It is speculated that the age of the mother affects parenting practices and attitudes toward food. It is possible that with more siblings, there are more companions and opportunities for physically active play. Children with few siblings may be more likely to sit in front of a TV set or engage in other less active pursuits.

Research design

The NHLBI Growth and Health Study (NGHS), funded by the National Institutes of Health, National Heart, Lung, and Blood Institutes, is the largest study to compare obesity risk factors in African-American and white girls.[8] The study group provided a full spectrum of education and income levels for each race. The cohort of 2,379 9- and 10-year-old girls (1,213 African-American, 1,166 white) was identified in 1987 in three locations (Richmond, California; Cincinnati, Ohio; and Washington DC). Factors examined were dietary intakes, nutritional and physical activity patterns, lipid profiles, anthropometry, blood pressure, maturation, demographic data, health beliefs and attitudes, and other psychosocial parameters. Obesity was defined for the 9- and 10-year old girls using a body mass index (weight in kilograms/height in meters)^2 of greater than 19.6 and 20.9 respectively.

Income was categorized as 1) less than $20,000, 2) $20,000 to $39,999, or 3) $40,000 and above. Parental education was defined by the highest level of education attained by either parent/guardian, categorized as 1) high school or less, 2) some college, 3) 4 or more years of college. Parental employment status was assessed in two categories: neither parent/guardian employed, or at least one parent/guardian employed. All of the sociodemographic factors were analyzed in relation to obesity in the girls, while controlling for maturation stage.

Why these differences?

What is the significance of the widely divergent impact of SES on obesity in black and white girls? One can only speculate. Perhaps the impact of belonging to a particular racial group outweighs the impact of economic class more for African-American girls than for white girls. For example, it could be that African-American children with higher SES are more likely to socialize or attend school with their lower-income peers than are higher SES white girls. Previous studies have indicated that the societal pressures to be thin and cultural preferences for certain body shapes are not the same among African-American and white girls. African-American girls may be more insulated from the emphasis of popular cultures on the virtues of being thin. It could be that African-American families achieved their successes with higher income and education level more recently than white families, thus lessening the impact of SES on childhood weight. Future examination of the longitudinal data will review differences in the relationship between sociodemographic factors and childhood obesity in African-American and white girls of older ages. The authors' findings make it clear that sociodemographic factors are very important in the development of childhood obesity and must be taken into account when prevention strategies are being developed.

Patricia Crawford, DrPH, is Project Manager for the NHLBI Growth and Health Study, 140 Warren Hall, School of Public Health, University of California, Berkeley, CA 94720. E-mail: pbcraw@uclink4.berkeley.edu. Allison Drury is a graduate student at the School of Public Health, University of California, Berkeley. **Sheila Stern, MA,** is an Analyst with the Growth and Health Study.

The research was performed under contracts N01-HC-55023-26 of the National Heart, Lung, and Blood Institute (NHLBI), National Institutes of Health, Bethesda, MD. The authors wish to gratefully acknowledge the investigators, staff and participants of the NHLBI Growth and Health Study.

References

1. Sobal J, Stunkard AJ. Socioeconomic status and obesity: a review of the literature. Psychol Bull 1989; 105:260–275.
2. Huenemann RL. Factors associated with teenage obesity. In: Wilson NL, ed. Obesity. Philadelphia, PA: FA Davis Co, 1969:55–66.
3. Garn SM, Clark DC. Trends in fatness and the origins of obesity. Pediatrics 1976; 57:443–456.
4. Khoury PR, Morrison JA., Laskarzewski P, et al. Relationship of education and occupation to coronary heart disease risk factors in school children and adults: the Princeton School District Study. Am J Epidemiol 1981; 113:378–395.
5. Patterson ML, Stern S, Crawford PB, et al. Sociodemographic factors and obesity in preadolescent black and white girls: NHLBI's Growth and Health Study. J Natl Med Assoc 1997; 89:594–600.
6. Whitelaw GL. Association of social class and sibling number with skinfold thickness in London school boys. Human Biol 1971; 43:414–442.
7. Rona RN, Chinn S. National Study of Health and Growth: social and family factors and obesity in primary school children. Ann Hum Biol 1982; 9:131–145.
8. NHLBI Growth & Health Study Research Group. Obesity and cardiovascular disease risk factors in black and white girls: the NHLBI Growth and Health Study. Am J Public Health 1992; 82:1613–1620.

NIH Guidelines: An Evaluation

by Frances M. Berg, MS

The first National institutes of Health guidelines on the treatment of obesity were released on June 17, 1998, to a storm of controversy. The *Clinical Guidelines on the Identification, Evaluation, and Treatment of Overweight and Obesity in Adults,* developed by a 24-member panel of specialists convened by the National Heart, Lung, and Blood Institute in cooperation with the National Institute of Diabetes and Digestive and Kidney Diseases, bring together much valuable information, but at the same time raise numerous questions.[1]

Their purpose is to furnish health professionals with the best available information about who is at risk and what treatment is most appropriate. However, the guidelines are based on two assumptions which seem invalid to many experts in the field. These are, first, that a body mass index (BMI) of 25 constitutes a health risk and, second, that safe and effective weight loss therapy exists. The guidelines lower the level at which a person is defined as overweight and at health risk and includes 55 percent of American adults. (This lowers the previous level of a BMI of 27.3 for women and 27.8 for men set by the National Center for Health Statistics.) They also provide six weight loss methods said to be effective.

They focus on weight loss rather than improved health. They do not warn of potential harm from the recommendations given, or evaluate research on the risks of dieting and weight loss, dysfunctional eating, eating disorders, weight cycling, fraudulent weight loss promotions, or the difficulty in long-term weight loss maintenance. They barely mention obesity prevention, and then, oddly, mainly in connection with preventing weight regain after weight loss.

Validity of claim for risks at a body mass index of 25

"All overweight and obese adults with a BMI of 25 or more are considered at risk," the guidelines state.

What is the evidence that these people are at risk?

Slight increases in risk factors may occur at lower weights for some conditions, the report suggests, but it clearly regards most differences at this level, if any, as minimal. Nearly all research discussed by the guidelines on the risks of related conditions focus on risks at a BMI of 30 or more. Exceptions are its numerous references to the Nurses' Health Study, which finds higher risks above a BMI of 22 for several disease conditions. However, the NIH guidelines profess to be based on research from 236 randomized controlled trials, so it lessens credibility to extensively reference a self-reported, nonrandomized, noncontrolled study such as the Nurses' Study. It also raises the question: if stronger references were available, would they not have been cited instead?

The guidelines report that a BMI of close to 25 (24.8 for white men and 24.3 for white women) is the level of lowest morality. For ethnic and racial minorities they find this to be higher, about 27 for African-Americans, and much higher or no relationship at all for Pima Indian men and women. For older adults, age 55 to 74, the report says the lowest mortality occurs in the BMI range of 25 to 30, even after adjusting for smoking status and pre-existing illness.

This leaves two weak reasons for the cut-off level of a BMI of 25. In defense, its most vocal proponent, George Bray, MD, of the Pennington Biomedical Research Center, Baton Rouge, Louisiana, says that increments of 5 are a good way to divide categories, simple and easy to use; cutoff points of 20, 25, 30, 35, and 40 provide "simplicity and reasonableness."[2] Second, he says that using a BMI of 25 brings the NIH recommendations in line with what other groups advise. He fails to mention that others have adopted this standard through the efforts of like-minded people with whom he has networked for the past 20 years. Obesity experts worldwide are a small group who network extensively. Bray is listed as a backgrounding author for the 1998 World Health Organization report *Obesity: Preventing and Managing the Global Epidemic* which adopts the same standard.[3] Even in this latest defense by Bray, published in *Obesity Research,* he acknowledges that for men a BMI of 24 is associated with the lowest mortality, and for women it differs (rises) with age.

Thus, there appears to be no reasonable justification for setting a BMI of 25 as the level at which a person is defined as overweight and at health risk. The research cited in the report refutes the claim that this was an evidence-based decision.

Validity of efficacy claim

The guidelines claim, "A variety of effective options exist for the management of overweight and obese patients, including dietary therapy approaches such as low-calorie diets and lower-fat diets; altering physical activity patterns; behavior therapy techniques; pharmacotherapy; surgery; and combinations of these techniques." In support of this statement, the panel evaluated a great many short-term studies of 4 months or more and defined 1-year studies as being long term.

However, it is well known that both levels are far too short a time to be relevant.

Long-term weight loss is not 1 year, but keeping off lost weight for 2 years or more after the end of any maintenance program, according to the Federal Trade Commission. The American Heart Association guidelines call for 5 years: "If there are no data to demonstrate that program participants maintain their weight losses for 5 years or more, there is no scientific evidence of long-term results of the program."[4]

The NIH guidelines recommend losing 10 percent of baseline weight, or about 1 to 2 pounds per week for 6 months, with "subsequent strategy based on the amount of weight lost." They recommend that a weight maintenance program begin at 6 months, but are vague about its nature or how successful it might be.

Most studies suggest such a maintenance program has little likelihood of success.

"No plan has demonstrated significant success in weight maintenance beyond 6 to 12 months," writes Ann Coulston, MS, RD, senior research dietitian with the General Clinical Research Center at Stanford University Medical Center, in the lead article of the recent obesity supplement to the *Journal of the American Dietetic Association*.[5]

Thus, the standards for evaluating weight loss therapy in the NIH guidelines lack credibility, despite the many studies cited. No credible case has been made for the effectiveness of the six methods recommended.

Other evidence suggests that current methods are neither safe nor effective in the long term. Questioning the value of all methods of current obesity treatment in their January 1, 1998, editorial, Jerome P. Kassirer, MD, and Marcia Angell, MD, editors of the *New England Journal of Medicine*, made these four points:

- *Since many people cannot lose much weight no matter how hard they try, and promptly regain whatever they do lose, the vast amounts of money spent on diet clubs, special foods, and over-the-counter remedies, estimated to be on the order of $30 to $50 billion yearly, is wasted.*
- *The latest magical cures are neither magical nor harmless.... Until we have better data about the risks of being overweight and the benefits and risks of trying to lose weight, we should remember that the cure for obesity may be worse than the condition.*
- *The data linking overweight and death are limited, fragmentary, and often ambiguous.*
- *Even granting an association between increasing body weight and higher mortality, at least for younger people, it does not follow that losing weight will reduce the risk. We simply do not know.*[6,7]

The NIH guidelines reveal strong evidence that physical activity alone, without weight loss, reduces the risk for cardiovascular disease and other disease factors. Yet physical activity is emphasized primarily as a component of weight loss therapy. It is not advanced on its own as a safe and proven method of reducing risk factors associated with obesity.

In one about-face, the panel members do not recommend the very low calorie diet of 800 calories or less, even though it has been long endorsed by obesity specialists and National Institute of Diabetes and Digestive and Kidney Diseases official policy, and could be justified as readily as the six other methods on the basis of 4-month trials.

Why are these experts now willing to acknowledge that the very low calorie diet has been unsuccessful in achieving long-term weight loss, that it risks nutritional inadequacies, causes increased risk of gallstones, means more weight is usually regained, and does not allow for gradual eating behavior change? How will they admit this for other methods?

The panel members considered patient motivation a key factor, despite acknowledging that they could find no evidence that motivation makes any difference in successful weight loss. Yet they urge physicians to heighten patients' motivation, and recommend two strategies. First, the doctor is to explain the dangers of obesity and, second, how "the new treatment plan will be different."

This is astonishing advice that seems to encourage physicians to manipulate their patients with scare tactics and false promises. How the new plan will be different is not explained, since the six weight loss methods described have been in use for many decades and often have failed both patient and doctor. It seems inconceivable that many experienced physicians will follow this advice.

Whose needs do the guidelines serve?

Again, the professed purpose of the NIH guidelines is to advise health professionals in the best ways to treat their large patients by determining who is at risk and what treatment is most appropriate. But an objective evaluation can only conclude that they accomplish neither of these objectives.

Is there, then, perhaps a hidden agenda? And if so, could it be to get more people on weight loss programs, regardless of the consequences? Such question lead inevitably to another: Are the NIH guidelines aimed in part at serving the needs of the weight loss industry?

If true, this would explain one paradox contained in the guidelines. The NIH guidelines seem to advocate separating maintenance from weight loss, defining them as two separate therapies, as in this advice: "After 6 months, efforts to maintain weight loss should be put in place."

A sounder public health policy than is in place today would require weight loss therapy to prove long-term maintenance before any weight is lost, thus avoiding the risks of weight cycling

---

Weight loss maintenance then becomes a part of obesity prevention, as in this definition: "Prevention includes primary prevention of overweight or obesity itself, *secondary prevention or avoidance of weight regain following weight loss,* and prevention of further weight increases in obese individuals unable to lose weight."

This makes no apparent sense and confuses both issues. However, it can serve the needs of the weight loss industry. If this concept is accepted, the industry can continue to document success for short-term weight loss and avoid the need to show long-term maintenance.

However, logic suggests that weight loss and maintenance belong together, placing the responsibility for long-term results with the weight loss program itself. A sounder public health policy than is in place today would require weight loss therapy to prove long-term maintenance before any weight is lost, thus avoiding the risks of weight cycling. It would no longer be acceptable to urge people to lose weight, by any method, and then in 6 months—as advocated here—begin some vague kind of maintenance program that has no track record of success.

Similarly, a clearer definition of prevention would include as the primary goal preventing overweight, and as secondary goals preventing further weight increases and associated risks. This is a definition that can be implemented now and begin to move prevention efforts forward.

Vested interests may play a role

As timely as ever is the protest of Thaddeus Prout, MD, former chair of the Food and Drug Administration Committee on Anorectic Drugs, and of the Committee on Drugs for the American Board of Internal Medicine, when he testified before the 1990 Congressional hearings investigating the weight loss industry: "The same faces, the same people who have been doing industry-paid research for two decades are before us.... In July of 1983 we discussed this same question... We listened to their data, looked at their paltry studies. We are hearing all the exaggerated claims of success again.... The medical profession has learned that they need not waste the time or postage [with] an entrenched and persuasive pharmaceutical industry. What can we do? Shall we wait another decade and have a new generation of concerned physicians wringing their hands and bumping their heads against the stone wall of industry?"[8]

The issue of vested interests is complex, yet cannot be ignored. How many of the 24 NIH panel members have vested interests in the diet industry, or feel pressures to comply with its demands? These are respected scientists making health decisions in the national interest according to their highest ethics. Yet one may argue that many academics make accommodations almost daily to the issues of research funding, financial affiliations, consultancies, and the politics of power. Disclosure of financial affiliations was not requested from members of the panel, chaired by F. Xavier Pi-Sunyer, director of the federally-funded Obesity Research Center, St. Luke's/ Roosevelt Hospital Center in New York City.

It appears the NIH guidelines serve the weight loss industry better than health professionals or consumers

---

However, when disclosure was required of a related group for the *Journal of the American Medical Association,* it was revealed that eight of the nine members of the National Task Force on the Prevention and Treatment of Obesity were receiving funding from at least two and as many as eight commercial weight-loss companies.[9] At that time, Pi-Sunyer's financial affiliations included being on the advisory boards of Wyeth-Ayerst and Knoll pharmaceuticals, and being a consultant to Lilly Pharmaceuticals, Genentech, Hoffman-LaRoche, Knoll, Weight Watchers, and Neutrogen. Others on both the NIH panel and the Task Force are William H. Dietz, James O. Hill, and G. Terence Wilson, each listed as having at least two financial affiliations with these same companies.

It also may be suggested that the new guidelines appear designed to replace the industry-financed "Guidance for Treatment of Adult Obesity" distributed to physicians by Shape Up America and the American Obesity Association in 1996, and made obsolete when the drugs it advocated were withdrawn from the market.

In recent months, drug companies involved in producing diet drugs have distributed versions of the NIH guidelines to health professionals at medical conferences and financed special editions on obesity for subscribers of medical, health, and nutrition journals.

Conclusion

In summary, it appears the NIH guidelines serve the weight loss industry better than they serve health professionals or consumers. They overestimate the risks of obesity and the number of people at risk, assume that people can easily lose 10 percent of their weight and keep it off, promote weight loss treatments that have little chance of long-term success, encourage physicians to manipulate their patients with scare tactics and false promises, and appear likely to spread a sense of alarm, while doing nothing to further prevention efforts. Thus, the new NIH guidelines are unlikely to benefit the public, or to help health care providers deal in effective ways with the problems of obesity.

References

1. Clinical guidelines on the identification, evaluation, and treatment of overweight and obesity in adults: the evidence report. Bethesda, MD: National Institutes of Health, National Heart, Lung, and Blood Institute. Preprint June 1998.
2. Bray G. In defense of a body mass index of 25 as the cut-off point for defining overweight. Obes Res 1998; 6:461–462.
3. Obesity: Preventing and managing the global epidemic: report of a WHO consultation on obesity. WHO/NUT/NCD/98.1. Geneva, Switzerland: World Health Organization, 1998.
4. American Heart Association Guidelines. HWJ 1997; 11:108–110.
5. Coulston AM. Obesity as an epidemic: facing the challenge. J Am Diet Assoc 1998; 98:10(Suppl. 2):16–22.
6. Kassirer JP, Angell M. Losing weight—an ill-fated New Year's resolution. N Engl J Med 1998; 338:52–54.
7. Berg F. Medical journal questions obesity treatment. HWJ 1998; 12:36.
8. Berg F. Witnesses charge diet drug is hazardous. Obes Health 1991; 5:9–12. (Sept 24, 1990, Congressional hearings, U.S. House of Representatives Small Business Subcommittee on Regulation, Business Opportunities and Energy).
9. National Task Force on the Prevention and Treatment of Obesity. Drug therapy. JAMA. 1996; 276:1907–1915. (Berg F. Task Force advises against diet drugs. HWJ 1997; 11:27).

The great weight debate

A major medical journal says people should worry less about their weight. The government says worry more. Here's what we say.

Last January, The New England Journal of Medicine published an editorial with the blasphemous title "Losing Weight—An Ill-Fated New Year's Resolution." The editors suggested that "the cure of obesity may be worse than the condition." That triggered a flood of media coverage, including a U.S. News & World Report cover story called "The New Truth About Fat." The story elaborated on the suggestion that most people don't need to worry about their weight since the risks of fat are overblown, efforts to lose weight futile.

Five months later, the government flatly contradicted that message by issuing new guidelines that lowered the threshold for being overweight—and pushed 30 million Americans over the line from fit to fat. The guidelines classify as overweight anyone with

> **The percentage of people who are obese has risen, especially in the past decade.**

a body mass index (BMI) of 25 or more. Someone who's 5-feet 8-inches tall and weighs 165 pounds, for example, has a BMI of 25. The previous threshold for overweight, 27, allowed that person to hit 180 pounds or so before sounding an alarm. (To calculate your BMI, see the flowchart *Do you really need to lose weight?*)

The government took that step partly to underscore its concern about the fattening of America: The percentage of people who are obese, with a BMI of 30 or more, has risen considerably in the last 30 years, mainly in the past decade. More important, the government claims that excess weight can harm, and that shedding pounds can help.

Whom should you believe?

Teasing out the truth

The New England Journal editorial was right on several counts. It *is* hard to lose weight permanently. America does have an obsession with thinness, which drives millions of people, including many with no weight problem, to spend big bucks on dangerous or worthless drugs and fads. And certain people probably don't need to worry if they gain a few pounds.

But the editorial understated the risks of excess weight. The government guidelines, created by an expert panel after a comprehensive research review, provide solid evidence that weight matters. And the guidelines clarify *when* excess weight poses a significant threat by considering factors beyond just pounds: your health, the location of the fat, and, to a lesser extent, the proportion of fat versus muscle and bone.

Your health

As the Journal editorial acknowledged, the risk of hypertension, coronary heart disease, and diabetes rises as people get heavier, even if they're only moderately overweight, with a BMI of at least 25 but less than 30. Weaker evidence suggests that the risk of other disorders—breast cancer in postmenopausal women, colon cancer, infertility, thrombotic stroke (the kind caused by blood clots), gallstones, and osteoarthritis—also rises with BMI. Increasing weight may be similarly linked to increased mortality.

Dozens of clinical trials have shown that *losing* weight can reduce certain risk factors for disease, such as high blood pressure, high cholesterol levels, and a high blood-sugar level. There's not much direct evidence on how weight loss affects either the risk of disease itself or the overall death rate. However, some research suggests that slimming down

The skinny on how to lose weight

Losing weight and keeping it off is hard—but hardly impossible. And dropping even a few pounds can reduce certain major risk factors for major diseases (see story). Here's how to maximize the chance of success.

■ **Work it off.** To slim down permanently, you need to keep exercising. Strength training—using weights, machines, or elastic bands—builds muscle and bone; aerobic exercise, such as bicycling or brisk walking, can at least help preserve them. That's important, since muscle burns lots of calories, even when you're resting. And exercise, particularly aerobic exercise, burns calories during the workout and at a slightly elevated rate for a few hours afterwards.

Moderately paced activities may be better than intense workouts for losing weight, because the average overweight person can't do vigorous exercise long enough, at least at first, to burn enough calories. Aim for at least four weekly sessions of at least 45 to 60 minutes each. (Of course, building up to a faster pace will let you burn more calories.) Two or preferably three times a week, devote some of those minutes to strength training. That regimen may be all you need if you're only a little overweight.

Older people who need to lose should focus more on exercise—especially strength training and other weight-bearing exercises—than on diet. That's partly because they need to bolster their muscles and bones, partly because many of them are already eating an inadequate diet. Young and old alike should take a similar approach if their only body-fat problem is a chubby belly plus a weak physique.

Whatever your approach, try to make it fun. If you can't stand walking a treadmill or logging laps, choose workouts that don't seem like work, such as sports, hiking, or bird watching. At the very least, vary your regimen. (For more ways to make exercise enjoyable, see our April 1997 report.)

■ **Cut your calories.** To lose more than just a little weight, you'll almost surely have to eat less. A reasonable goal is to cut your daily intake by 300 to 500 calories. That step, combined with regular exercise, should help you lose about a pound a week. More drastic diets are less likely to yield long-lasting weight loss—and may be harmful.

Eating less fat is a simple, healthful way to cut calories. But it won't help if you compensate by consuming more calories overall, as many people do. (Note that "low-fat" foods often contain as many calories as regular versions, since manufacturers often adjust for the loss of tasty fat by adding extra sugar and other carbohydrates.) The most reliable way to reduce both calories and fat is to replace sugary or fatty foods with whole grains, beans, and produce. Of course, you could also eat smaller portions.

To stick with that leaner approach, keep looking for new foods, recipes, and restaurants that minimize the calories while maximizing the taste. Try to distinguish physical hunger from psychological appetite—and substitute interests and rewards that don't involve eating. Finally, set modest, reasonable goals, and don't obsess about your weight: Eating wisely and exercising regularly will improve your health whether or not it trims your waistline as much as you'd hoped. (For further tips on sticking with a healthful diet, see our May 1998 issue.)

■ **Think twice about fat pills.** Over-the-counter drugs and supplements that supposedly burn fat have little if any value. Prescription drugs may help some obese individuals, but the two most popular ones—dexfenfluramine (*Redux*) and fenfluramine (*Pondimin*)—were yanked off the market last year over concerns about possible heart-valve damage. That leaves only two drug options. One, the stimulant phentermine (*Fastin, Ionamin*), has only limited efficacy, and it often causes strong side effects, including agitation and insomnia. The other drug, sibutramine (*Meridia*), must be taken under close supervision, since it can cause potentially dangerous increases in heart rate and blood pressure.

The FDA may soon approve another medication, orlistat (*Xenical*), which inactivates certain intestinal enzymes needed to absorb fat from food. As a result, users may experience bloating, gas, and loose stools if they consume lots of fat. It may also block absorption of fat-soluble vitamins, including vitamins A, D, and E, so users should take a multivitamin supplement.

In addition to the short-term risks of those drugs, their long-term safety won't be known until they've been used extensively. You and your doctor shouldn't even consider such medication unless you're extremely obese and have truly tried and failed to lose weight without drugs.

---

may prolong life, both in obese people and in certain moderately overweight individuals. For example, a study of some 44,000 overweight women linked weight loss with a 20 percent lower death rate—but only in those who had at least one weight-related risk factor or disease. A similar study in overweight men suggested that shedding pounds may lengthen life only in those with diabetes.

Anyone whose BMI is 30 or more clearly needs to lose weight. The government advises people with a BMI of at least 25 but less than 30 to slim down if they have two or more risk factors—including some that have little to do with weight—or weight-related diseases (see flowchart for list). However, it's probably wise for moderately overweight people to shed pounds if they have even one of those factors or one weight-linked disease. Moderately heavy people who have *no* such factors or ailments—especially those with a BMI of 27 or more—may also want to lose weight, though the benefits are less clear. At the very least, anyone with a BMI of 25 or more should try to avoid gaining weight.

Where's the fat?

Fat on the belly is more metabolically active than fat on the hips or thighs. And when belly fat is metabolized, the byproducts can raise blood-cholesterol levels and reduce the

Do you really need to lose weight?

To answer that question, first determine your body-mass index (BMI), using this formula: Multiply your weight in pounds by 705. Divide the result by your height in inches. Then divide by your height in inches again to arrive at your BMI.

Next, assess how much abdominal fat you have. If your BMI is 25 or more, simply measure your waist. The threshold for concern is 35 inches in women, 40 inches in men. That method doesn't work if your BMI is less than 25. Instead, measure your waist at its narrowest point and your hips at their widest; then divide the waist measurement by the hip measurement. Men are at increased risk if their waist-to-hip ratio exceeds 0.95, women if it exceeds 0.80.

Now follow the flowchart to see if you should lose weight.

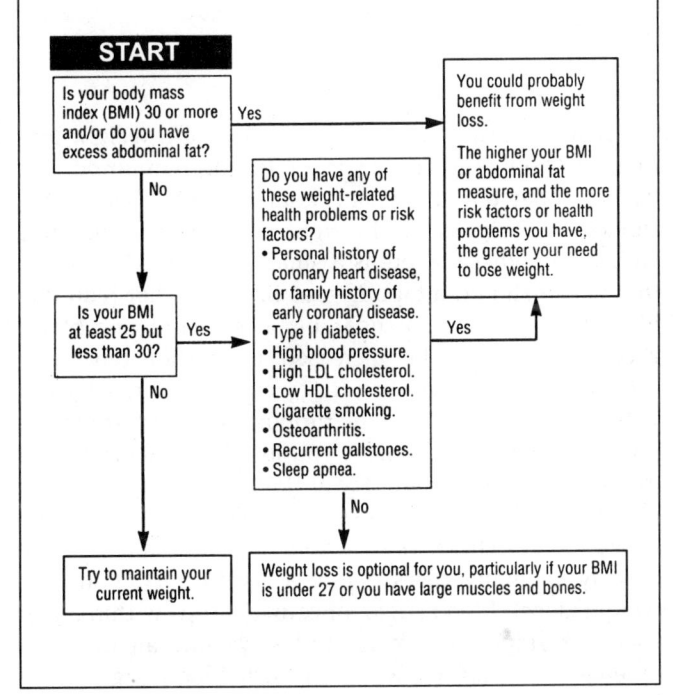

```
START
Is your body mass index (BMI) 30 or more and/or do you have excess abdominal fat?
  Yes → You could probably benefit from weight loss.
        The higher your BMI or abdominal fat measure, and the more risk factors or health problems you have, the greater your need to lose weight.
  No ↓
Is your BMI at least 25 but less than 30?
  Yes → Do you have any of these weight-related health problems or risk factors?
        • Personal history of coronary heart disease, or family history of early coronary disease.
        • Type II diabetes.
        • High blood pressure.
        • High LDL cholesterol.
        • Low HDL cholesterol.
        • Cigarette smoking.
        • Osteoarthritis.
        • Recurrent gallstones.
        • Sleep apnea.
          Yes → (benefit from weight loss)
          No ↓
          Weight loss is optional for you, particularly if your BMI is under 27 or you have large muscles and bones.
  No ↓
Try to maintain your current weight.
```

body's sensitivity to the hormone insulin. That reduced sensitivity causes blood-sugar levels to rise, which the body tries to control by churning out more insulin. Rising insulin levels may then increase blood pressure and, in theory, also trigger cancerous changes in colon cells. Moreover, abdominal fat produces more estrogen—which fuels the growth of breast cancer—than hip or thigh fat does.

All that may help explain why observational studies have linked big bellies with an increased risk of hypertension, coronary disease, diabetes, and, to a lesser extent, colon cancer and postmenopausal breast cancer. Many studies have found that a big tummy may pose greater risks than an elevated BMI does. In fact, a pot belly appears to threaten even people who aren't overweight at all. Note that the opposite case—being somewhat "overweight" due to big muscles and bones rather than a flabby belly—typically poses no threat to health. (To assess your abdominal fat, see flowchart.)

Does age matter?

That controversial New England Journal editorial was inspired by a study suggesting that the link between BMI and death rates grows progressively weaker as people grow older. In a subsequent study, moderately overweight people actually had the lowest mortality after age 55.

But those studies had several major weaknesses. First, some of the volunteers may have had a low BMI because they were wasting away from some serious disease, not because they were trim and fit. Further, older people tend to lose muscle and bone and to put on fat, particularly abdominal fat. But BMI doesn't distinguish fat from other tissue. So a substantial number of older people with a seemingly favorable BMI may actually have too little lean tissue and too much total and belly fat—a decidedly unhealthy combination. The loss of muscle and bone increases the risk of deadly falls and fractures. And excess abdominal fat, unlike BMI, remains strongly correlated with increased mortality in old age.

So the criteria for who needs to lose weight are probably still the same for young and old alike. But the best *approach* to slimming down does depend partly on age (see "The skinny on how to lose weight").

Summing up

Obese people, with a BMI of 30 or more, clearly need to lose weight. So do those with lots of belly fat, regardless of their BMI.

There's no definitive proof that losing weight helps people who are only moderately overweight, with a BMI of 25 to 30. But the risks clearly do rise as people get heavier. Slimming down improves key risk factors, and it seems to cut mortality, at least in susceptible people. So virtually all moderately heavy people should at least consider losing weight. Those at greatest risk—due to health, health habits, or family history—should start trying to slim down.

Article 35

Exploding the Myth: Weight Loss Makes You Healthier

by Paul Ernsberger, PhD

The advice to lose weight is the most common medical advice given today. The demand for weight reduction arises not only in the doctor's office, but also from nutritionists and dietitians, nurses and other health professionals, psychologists and other therapists and counselors, and all of the mass media. It is no wonder that the majority of North Americans want to lose weight and that health concerns are the number one stated reason for the pursuit of a slender figure.

Correlates between weight and health

Weight loss is put forth as treatment for a large array of disorders, but plays its most prominent role in the medical management of three diseases: diabetes type 2, hypertension or high blood pressure, and hypercholesterolemia or high cholesterol. All three are risk factors for atherosclerosis (hardening of the arteries) and heart attack. All three conditions are strongly related to body weight. In one study cited by the World Health Organization,[1] diabetes type 2 is 40 times more common in women with a body mass index (BMI) of 30 relative to lean women with a BMI of less than 22. Hypertension is two to three times more common in obese women and men. Hypercholesterolemia, on the other hand, is only weakly related to body weight. The correlation between BMI and cholesterol level in most studies is about 0.1 in women and 0.2 in men.[2] Blood pressure correlates better with BMI, usually around 0.4 in middle-age.[3] Put another way, if you know a woman's BMI, you can predict her cholesterol level with an accuracy only 1 percent better than pure chance. Blood pressure can be predicted a little better on the basis of BMI, with an accuracy of 16 percent better than chance.

What physical changes happen during a weight loss diet, and how long do they take? Timing is an important clue to understanding what is going on in the body. Consider the concept of ideal weight. According to the ideal weight hypothesis, there is a small range of BMI values that we all should attain. If your BMI is higher than this ideal, then your blood sugar, blood pressure, and blood cholesterol should be increased proportionately with each excess pound. As you lose weight, your risk factors will decline according to the proportion of excess weight you have removed. Thus, if you lose 10 percent of your excess weight, you should lose 10 percent of your excess blood pressure. Does this happen? The answer appears to be "no." These risk factors are normalized very quickly, in many cases before a significant amount of weight is lost. Blood sugar, of course, drops within a few hours or skipping a meal, and stays low all the time when you are on a low calorie diet. Blood sugar stays low even when you go off the diet, because your tissues readily take up nutrients after a period of deprivation. Blood pressure also drops quickly on a very low calorie diet, usually within a week, before there is much loss of body fat.[3] When calorie restriction is moderate, the drop in blood pressure is less and it takes longer to develop. A reduction in cholesterol level takes a few weeks to develop, but the full drop in cholesterol is achieved after only a fraction of excess weight is lost.[4] In fact, "bad" cholesterol (LDL) reaches its lowest level 8 weeks into a diet and actually rises with additional weight loss.[4] Improvements in cholesterol profile were related more directly to improved dietary habits such as reduced saturated fat intake than to the amount of weight loss. Therefore, the reductions in risk factors for heart attack that are seen with reduced calorie regimens are not solely the result of body fat loss. That being the case, we must reject the ideal weight hypothesis and come up with a new theory.

Short-term improvement, long-term deterioration

Why do risk factors drop so quickly compared to the slow and gradual loss of body fat? (Remember that much of the initial weight loss on low calorie diets is water, and fat is lost only at a rate of 1 kg per week or less). One explanation is that the fall in risk factors is a biologic response to mild starvation, rather than the result of reducing body fat stores. The author tested this idea a few years ago with a meta-analysis of trials of weight loss for the treatment of blood pressure.[3] There was no correlation between the amount of weight lost and decreases in blood pressure. On the other hand, if you looked at the rate of weight loss per week, there was a strong relationship. Gradual weight loss had little effect, whereas there were dramatic drops in blood pressure with rapid weight loss, especially with very low-calorie formulas. By the same token, diets providing very few calories (300–800 per day) led to large drops in blood pressure, whereas more moderate diets with 1200–1800 calories seldom lowered pressure. This means that the process of "going on a diet" and entering a state of deprivation results in a lowering of blood pressure. Part of the benefit may result from the consumption of healthier "diet" foods such as fruits and vegetables and the avoidance of high-fat and high-sodium "junk" foods. In the long run, however, this blood pressure lowering effect is not sustained after the diet ends.

How effective is weight loss as a medical treatment for disease? A great many studies have looked at the short-term benefits of weight loss programs, usually while the participants are still on the restrictive regimen. Many authors have reviewed the apparent risk factor improvements that take place during the initial phase of weight loss and in early maintenance.[1] Here, we will consider only those few studies that included at least a 6-month follow-up. For type 2 diabetics, the critical factor to monitor is glycosylated hemoglobin, which provides a picture of the prevailing glucose levels over several weeks. A review of all the controlled trials of weight loss in type 2 diabetes showed that there were initial improvements immediately after the weight loss program, but follow-up at 6 to 18 months showed a deterioration back to starting values, even when weight loss persisted.[5] In 21 experimental groups where there was follow-up, long-term benefit was found in only three, despite maintained weight losses of 3 to 9 kg. A 1-year follow up study of a behavior modification weight loss program showed that, for diabetics, weight loss was actually detrimental after 1 year. Overall, it appears that existing very low-calorie diets or strict behavior modification programs have no beneficial effect at 1 year of follow-up, even when weight loss is maintained. Despite these poor results, weight loss is still usually considered the cornerstone of diabetes treatment. As noted 12 years ago in the *New England Journal of Medicine*,[6] "Tradition, as opposed to scientific evidence, has had a remarkable influence on the prescription of dietary therapy for diabetes."

Weight loss is the most common nondrug treatment recommended for hypertension. However, as with diabetes, the long-term results are disappointing, even when massive amounts of weight are lost after gastric surgery.[3] Promising results have been obtained with trials of multifactorial interventions that have included exercise, sodium restriction, healthful overall diets, and stress management along with weight loss. For multifactorial programs, it is impossible to say how much of the blood pressure reduction is due to the small loss of body weight that accompanies these lifestyle modifications.

Most patients with high cholesterol are treated first with a weight loss regimen before any drug therapies are given. However, despite short-term changes, there is limited long-term effectiveness of weight loss as a cholesterol-lowering therapy.[4,7] In one study, obese patients were placed on a 1000 calorie diet until they reached their insurance table weight.[7] Importantly, their diet was controlled so that they consumed the same amount and type of dietary fat before and after losing weight. After a temporary dip during the weight loss process, levels of LDL cholesterol returned to the starting obese level. Thus, provided that dietary fat intake is not changed, weight loss does not improve cholesterol levels. One exception to this is weight loss by surgical methods such as gastric or biliopancreatic bypass. By interfering with the absorption of dietary fat, these operations can significantly lower cholesterol. Similarly, the new Hoffman-LaRoche drug orlistat (Xenical) can lower cholesterol by preventing the uptake of dietary fats from the digestive tract. The effectiveness of these surgical and pharmaceutical interventions does not arise from loss of body fat, but from direct intestinal action.

Undeniably, weight loss programs can benefit health. This is especially true when these programs emphasize permanent lifestyle changes and encourage exercise and healthier food choices. On the other hand, positive lifestyle changes can be encouraged without a primary focus on weight loss. Thus, exercise programs and low-fat diets can yield real and lasting improvements in risk factors while failing to correct obesity.[8] Importantly, improvements in cholesterol and other risk factors stemming from improved diet are maintained as long as the dietary guidelines are followed and do not dissipate with time.

Medication as a more effective treatment

The poor effectiveness of weight loss stands in marked contrast to the increasing effectiveness of medications.

New and highly potent treatments for type 2 diabetes, hypertension, and hypercholesterolemia have appeared in the last few years. Often new and old drugs can be combined for even greater effectiveness. A drawback of relying on weight loss as a first line of treatment is that chronically ill patients may be denied truly effective pharmaceutical therapy while pursuing the elusive goal of permanent weight loss. Weight reduction should be considered at most an adjunct to treatment rather than a primary goal.

Harmful effects of weight loss

Weight loss may not only be ineffective as a tool for managing chronic disease, but may even cause harm in the long run. Weight loss is not usually permanent, regardless of the intervention used. When lost weight is regained, all of the short-term benefits of weight loss are undone, and in many cases risk factors become worse than they were before the weight was regained.[9] Blood pressure increases significantly during the relapse to obesity in humans and in laboratory animals. Worsening of risk factors during regain probably accounts for the increased heart attack deaths seen in persons who lose and regain weight.

Another potentially harmful effect of weight loss regimens is that they can trigger binge eating. Bingeing is never healthy, but in persons with chronic disease it can be seriously harmful. People with diabetes need to maintain a steady level of food intake to keep their blood sugar levels tightly regulated. Alternately starving and bingeing can compromise blood sugar control. Similarly, chaotic eating patterns can hamper the therapy of high blood pressure and hypercholesterolemia.

Benefits are illusory, harm is real

The position of weight loss in medicine today can be compared to the role of bloodletting 150 years ago. Bloodletting became popular because doctors found that if a feverish patient was bled, their fever would break and their skin became cool and clammy. Thus, bloodletting improved the symptoms of sick patients. Of course, we now know that blood loss creates a state of shock that lowers body temperature but ultimately increases the risk of death. Similarly, weight loss produces short-term improvements in symptoms, but may not be ultimately beneficial. Before weight loss can be removed from its exalted status as a therapy, a revolution in medicine may be required, comparable to the one that brought an end to the practice of bloodletting.

To summarize, weight loss programs can produce many short-term benefits, which have been documented in literally thousands of medical studies. However, those few trials with follow-up beyond 6 months have failed to show lasting benefit. Weight loss programs can actually do harm by diverting the patient from more effective and reliable treatments with modern drugs or with sustainable lifestyle changes. Furthermore, when lost weight is regained, the patient may be worse off than when she started because of the harmful consequences of weight cycling. All of these limitations of weight loss programs compel the creation of a new paradigm, which incorporates the health-promoting aspects of permanent lifestyle changes without a focus on the correction of obesity.

References

1. Akram, D-S, Astrup A. V., Atinmo, T., et al. Obesity: Preventing and managing the global epidemic. Report of a WHO Consultation on Obesity. Geneva, Switzerland: World Health Organization, 1997.
2. Garn, S. M., Bailey, S. M., Block, W. D. Relationships between fatness and lipid level in adults. Am J Clin Nutr 1979; 32:733–735.
3. Ernsberger, P., Nelson, D. O. Effects of fasting and refeeding on blood pressure are determined by nutritional state, not by body weight change. Am J Hypertens 1988; 1(Suppl):153S–157S.
4. Andersen, R. E., Wadden, T. A., Bartlett, S. J., et al. Relation of weight loss to changes in serum lipids and lipoproteins in obese women. Am J Clin Nutr 1995; 62:350–357.
5. Ciliska, D., Kelly, C., Petrov, N., Chalmers, J. A review of weight loss interventions for obese people with noninsulin-dependent diabetes mellitus. Can J Diabet Care 1995; 19:10–15.
6. Wood, F. C., Bierman, E. L. Is diet the cornerstone in management of diabetes? N Engl J Med 1986; 315:1224–1227.
7. Wolf, R. N., Grundy, S. M. Influence of weight reduction on plasma lipoproteins in obese patients. Arteriosclerosis 1983; 3:160–169.
8. Dengel, J. L., Katzel, L. I., Goldberg, A. P. Effect of an American Heart Association diet, with or without weight loss, on lipids in obese middle-aged and older men. Am J Clin Nutr 1995; 62:715–721.
9. Ernsberger, P., Koletsky, R. J., Baskin, J. Z., Collins, L. A. Consequences of weight cycling in obese spontaneously hypertensive rats. Am J Physiol Regul Integr Comp Physiol 1996; 270:R864–R872.

Paul Ernsberger, PhD, is Associate Professor of Nutrition, Medicine (Hypertension), Pharmacology and Neuroscience, at Case Western Reserve University in Cleveland. Telephone: 216–368–4738, Fax: 216–368–4752, e-mail: *pre@po.cwru.edu*

Simplifying the Advice for Slimming Down

How to avoid the pitfalls of fad diets

IT'S KIND OF IRONIC. Weight Watchers, TOPS (Take Off Pounds Sensibly), Jenny Craig, and other weight-loss organizations that already promote sensible eating without too much hype have voluntarily adopted a code of stricter standards. That is, they have joined the Federal Trade Commission (FTC) Partnership for Healthy Weight Management, agreeing to disclose to consumers:

- any risks associated with their plans
- cost of the plans
- qualifications of the staff who administer the plans
- advice about the difficulty of maintaining weight loss once the pounds come off.

On the other hand, the creators of popular diets that need the *most* policing—because they promote unhealthful practices that promise much more than they can deliver—are free to ignore the guidelines' call. Among the plans rife with dietary imbalances and false promises: those espoused in *Sugar Busters!, Dr. Atkins' New Diet Revolution, Enter the Zone, The Five Day Miracle Diet, The New Beverly Hills Diet,* and *Protein Power.* Their sponsors are staying away even though the FTC's partnership is open to individuals as well as weight-loss companies (and has also been joined by health-promoting organizations such as The American Dietetic Association and the Centers for Disease Control and Prevention).

Though the lack of participation by the sponsors of the unsound plans is ironic, it's not surprising, because these diets do not live up to some of the major tenets of the Partnership for Healthy Weight Management. Among those tenets subscribed to by the Partnership:

- Products and programs that promise quick and easy results are misleading, since successful weight loss is a gradual process that requires focus on many fronts, including food choices, activity level, and how likely you are to eat in response to stress.

- Any ad that says you can lose weight without paying attention to calories "is selling fantasy and false hope."

- Any plan that eschews one or more food groups is setting people up for a lack of balance and potential nutrient deficiencies.

Just how far short do many of the popular plans fall? Tufts researchers Jeanne Goldberg, PhD, RD, and Julie Smith, MS, RD, have taken a systematic look at 10 of the popular diet books out there and found an alarming gap between the healthful eating promoted by the partnership guidelines and the food plans these books offer. For instance, the "induction phase" of *Dr. Atkins' New Diet Revolution* contains less than 60 percent of the fiber, copper, magnesium, manganese, and potassium that Americans should be consuming—no doubt because the diet is low in complex carbohydrates as well as fruits and vegetables.

Enter the Zone is lacking in fiber and vitamin D, while *The Five Day Miracle Diet* and *The New Beverly Hills Diet,* both low in dairy foods and starches, are deficient in calcium, carbohydrates, and zinc. *Sugar Busters!,* too, is low in calcium, in addition to fiber—and potentially high in unhealthful saturated fat.

All of this is to say nothing of the false promises made in the books espousing these plans. *Sugar Busters!* and *Enter the Zone,* for example, wrongly suggest that calories don't count. And all of the books tend to make weight loss sound much easier than it actually is.

Are the Diets Dangerous, or Just Useless?

Jane Kirby, RD, author of The American Dietetic Association's *Dieting for Dummies* (IDG Books Worldwide, Foster City, CA, 1998, $19.99), a sensible guide to weight loss that includes advice on spotting a fraud diet, says that for people in decent health, the biggest problem with going on fad diets is not nutrition status. Rather, it's "quality of life."

"Most unhealthful diets [that focus on just one food or eliminate whole food groups] are not going to harm you because they're so boring and impossible to stick with for too long," Ms. Kirby comments. "Just how much cabbage soup can you eat?" she asks rhetorically, referring to one of many diets that limits food choices.

It's the same with high-protein, low-carbohydrate diets that call for giving up everything from bread to bananas. You'll lose weight on such plans, Ms. Kirby says, because of the limited choices. But, she adds, "it can't work over the long term because we need flavor and texture diversity. We're hard-wired for it by nature. So you'll go off the diet. **You'll eventually realize that you really *do* want a bagel. This egg-white thing is not going to cut it."**

Tufts's Dr. Goldberg agrees with Ms. Kirby that people tend not to stick to any one of these diets for too long. But, she says, many people go from one poor diet to another, and that's where nutrient deficiencies become a concern.

For instance, she points out, the low-carbohydrate, high-protein diets that are currently popular—*Atkins, Sugar Busters!*—are "remarkably consistent with respect to their nutrient deficiencies." All have too little calcium. "Women take in too little calcium to begin with," she says. "On these diets, they get even less.

"And then there's very little vitamin D, so they don't adequately absorb the calcium they do take in. So what happens when they go from the *Zone* to *Sugar Busters!* to *Atkins*? I'm concerned that it magnifies the problem.

"You can always find a few people who went on a fad diet, lost weight, and kept it off because after they slimmed down, they told themselves they would start to eat reasonably," Dr. Goldberg says. "I'm sure they're out there. But that's very atypical. More often what you'll find is the chronic dieter who goes from one diet to the next to the next."

The funny thing about all these diets, Dr. Goldberg says, is that "the pitfalls have been pointed out." People know what they are.

They also know the choices they *really* have to make—more fruits and vegetables, few fatty and sugary treats, more exercise. As the Partnership for Healthy Weight Management says, "Be sure to include at least five servings a day of fruits and vegetables, along with whole grains, lean meat, and low fat dairy products. It may not produce headlines, but it can reduce waistlines."

Unfortunately, Dr. Goldberg points out, "I don't think people are paying attention. They want the quick fix. They are going to some tropical island in two weeks. They don't want someone telling them that the weight loss on a high-protein diet is going to be all water and that the minute they go off the diet, they're going to gain it all back and more."

Getting around the quick-fix mentality

For people who really want to get off the diet merry-go-round and lose a significant amount of weight once and for all, Dr. Goldberg suggests paying attention to some of the lessons coming out of the National Weight Control Registry. The Registry, maintained by researchers at the University of Pittsburgh School of Medicine and the University of Colorado Health Sciences Center, is a record of hundreds of people who have lost weight (at least 30 pounds) and kept it off (for at least one year).

"This is information for the real world," Dr. Goldberg says. "It's a compilation of techniques people really are living with" as opposed to advice being used to sell a diet program. She boils down the experience of the Weight Control Registry participants to five messages:

1 To lose weight, combine different methods. Some people start to lose weight using a structured plan such as Weight Watchers, Dr. Goldberg says. But then they might go off the plan and tailor a diet and exercise routine more to their own liking. The commercial plan may have just been what they needed to get started. As long as it works and doesn't exclude any foods or food groups, switching around or using a variety of methods at the same time is fine.

Likewise, Dr. Goldberg says, successful weight losers may have at different points paid more attention to total fat intake than to total calories. They weren't afraid to use what worked for them at a particular time.

What very few of them did, however, was follow a diet in which they restricted their intake to a very narrow group of foods, which Dr. Goldberg says was crucial to their loss of weight over the long term. Less than 5 percent of Registry participants succeeded that way.

2 Identify a weight-loss trigger. The Registry members were able to identify a particular aspect or point in their lives that was "overwhelmingly important" in getting started on the road to permanent weight loss, Dr. Goldberg says.

"You don't have to wait for the trigger to hit you over the head unexpectedly," she adds. "Hit *yourself* over the head. Make a proactive search. Don't wait to wake up one day and suddenly be inspired to diet."

For men, she points out, the trigger more often is about health. For

36. Simplifying the Advice for Slimming Down

women, it tends to involve an emotional consideration. Thus, a man may want to ask himself, "do I want to get rid of my blood pressure medication?" For a woman, the triggering question might be, "is there something about the way I carry myself that I really would feel more comfortable about if . . . ?"

3 Exercise. The members of the Weight Control Registry exercise a lot, Dr. Goldberg says. In fact, they walk an average of four miles a day, or 28 miles a week.

4 Forget all-or-nothing. People tend to say, "you've got to do it all or it isn't worth doing," Dr. Goldberg remarks. But that's not true. If you can't exercise the equivalent of walking 28 miles a week, it doesn't mean you shouldn't exercise at all. Make a start. Do what you *can* do. Something is always better than nothing. Nothing is exactly that—nothing.

It's the same with food restriction, Dr. Goldberg says. If you're eating 3,000 calories a day, maybe it's not realistic to try to cut back to 1,500 calories, or even 2,000 calories. **Maybe it makes more sense to acclimate yourself to weight loss by cutting out only 200 to 300 calories at first and going from there. By cutting out 200 calories daily, you'll lose about 20 pounds in the first year** (more if you walk a little, too).

5 Monitor yourself. "When you look at the histories that successful weight losers provide," Dr. Goldberg says, "it's clear that they get on the scale at least once a week, on average." And they count calories, or fat, or both. In other words, they use at least one kind of concrete system for making sure that they're adhering to the plan.

The history of dieting and its effectiveness

by Wayne C. Miller, PhD

How effective have diets and dieting programs been in producing weight loss?

Throughout the years, dietitians and nutritionists have advocated moderate consistent weight loss through a balanced, energy controlled diet in conjunction with lifestyle changes. Although this may be the healthiest way to lose weight, it is not necessarily the way the public attempts to lose weight.

In the late 1950s and early 1960s, total fasting was used to reduce weight in the massively obese. Weight loss through fasting amounted to 1.0 kg per day the first month followed by 0.5 kg a day thereafter.[1] Although the desired outcome, weight loss, was achieved through fasting, serious side effects such as loss of lean body mass, depleted electrolytes, and death caused fasting to quickly wane in popularity.[1,2,3]

Next on the scene came the high-protein, low-carbohydrate diets of the 1960s and early 1970s. The theory of this epic, which still lingers today, was that carbohydrates (particularly starch) make you fat. Popular diets of that time (e.g. Stillman, Atkins) provided 1,200 to 2,000+ calories per day, with only 5 to 10 percent coming from carbohydrates.[4] On the other hand, 50 to 70 percent of the energy intake on these diets came from fat. The justification of this diet composition was that the high protein content prevented the loss of lean tissue, while the high fat content produced ketosis with its associated appetite suppression. Weight loss on these diets was rapid because of depleted glycogen stores and diuresis, but side effects included nausea, hyperuricemia, fatigue, and refeeding edema.[5]

VLCD liquids

During the mid 1970s very low calorie liquid diets became commercially available. These diets were known as protein-sparing-modified fasts or liquid protein diets. Their extremely low caloric content (300–400 calories per day) caused rapid weight loss. However, in spite of medical supervision, high quality protein, and potassium supplementation, several deaths due to ventricular arrhythmia occurred with prolonged use. These liquid protein diets were subsequently banned until research studies could assure their safety.[6]

A second generation of very low calorie formula diets became popu-

---

'Long term weight loss following any type of intervention was limited to only a small minority of the obese people studied'
— NIH

lar in the 1980s. These commercial formula products, such as Optifast and Health Management Resources, became part of a medical approach including patient counseling and support. Diets of 400 to 500 calories per day were offered as well as the option of an 800-calorie plan. At the same time, franchises like Nutri-System and Jenny Craig offered clients pre-packaged foods along with exercise and nutrition counseling. This second generation of very low calorie formula diets and pre-packaged foods has evolved to where many of these commercial programs now offer individualized approaches that emphasize exercise and behavior change.[7] These programs can cost up to $3,000 and/or $70 to $90 per week for food products.[7] Another problem is that these programs have not been well researched for safety and may be as detrimental to health as any other rapid weight loss regimen.[8]

Lowfat diets

Research related to the health risks of dietary fat in the 1970s and 1980s has spawned a fat-phobic society. Thus, the newest trend in the dieting realm is non-fat or low-fat diets. Fat-free and low-fat versions of foods have become popular while the Pritikin diet, which was first used in the 1970s to combat the risks of degenerative diseases, has been resurrected as a weight-loss diet. Other low-fat programs, like the T-Factor diet, promote counting fat grams rather than calories for weight control. Average weight loss due to reducing dietary fat alone is only 0.1 to 0.2 kg per week.[9,10] Moreover, there is some concern that the abundance of low-fat fat-free calorie-rich snack foods on the market will encourage overconsumption by should-be dieters who concern themselves only with dietary fat.

Diets challenged

Obesity researchers have been fighting an uphill battle ever since Stunkard and McLaren-Hume concluded that dieting was ineffective for 95 percent of those in a hospital nutrition clinic.[11] Since that time, the use of diets for weight control has been challenged by the public, a growing number of health care professionals, as well as some obesity researchers themselves.[8]

Hence, the National Institutes of Health (NIH) recently convened a Technology Assessment Conference to evaluate the effectiveness of voluntary methods for weight loss and control.

The report for very low calorie diets (VLCDs) revealed that weight loss following a 12-week VLCD totaled 20 kg, with a 35 to 50 percent weight regain after one year.[12,13] Furthermore, dropout rates in some VLCD programs can reach 80 percent. The less restrictive low calorie diets (LCDs) are even less effective. Following a 20-week LCD program, average weight loss is 8.5 kg, with a 33 percent regain after one year, and a 100 percent regain after five years.[14,15]

Nutrition education and behavior modification programs have become popular because they are supposedly self-empowering. However, success on these programs isn't any better than on VLCDs or LCDs. An 18-week behavior modification program will bring about a 10 kg weight loss, with a 95 percent relapse after two years.[15] Similarly discouraging is the finding that community programs, worksite interventions, and home correspondence programs show negligible success after one to three years.[16]

Weak data advanced

Data to support the effectiveness claims of commercial weight-loss programs was requested by the NIH and FDA at the time of the Technology Assessment Conference. Material was received from only five companies, three representing non-physician-directed programs and two representing physician-directed programs. For the nonphysician-directed programs, one company submitted one research study and several abstracts. The study demonstrated reduced cardiovascular disease risk following short-term use of the program; the abstracts were judged scientifically inadequate. The second company representing nonphysician-directed programs submitted four research studies, but later withdrew the studies from the NIH review. The third company data was judged inadequate to evaluate.

For the physician-directed programs, one company submitted three research articles and several abstracts. Data from this company was evaluated as inconclusive. The other company representing a physician-directed program was the only company in the industry that submitted data that was scientifically sound. Although this company submitted 55 quality research reports, the NIH committee determined that long-term weight loss following this program was questionable.[17]

Odd conclusion

Surprisingly enough, even though only one commercial program in the whole industry provided data that could be seen as adequate, and that data provided no evidence for long-term success for weight control, the NIH assessment team concluded: *"Regardless of products used, successful weight loss and control is limited to and requires individualized programs consisting of restricted caloric intake, behavior modification and exercise.[17]"*

It is puzzling how the NIH could come to any effectiveness conclusion based on the paucity of data they received which they themselves judged to be inadequate, questionable, and inconclusive.[17] Only two conclusions seem possible to have been drawn, either 1) no conclusion can be made because there is no data upon which to base a conclusion, or 2) no commercial program is effective at producing long-term weight loss because no company could provide data to show otherwise.

It seems the NIH conclusion for commercial program effectiveness was based on an assumption or hope of what should be effective, not on the data evaluated.

The overall conclusion from NIH as to the effectiveness of any type of method for voluntary weight loss and control was more true to the facts than their conclusion for the commercial industry. The universal consensus of the conference was:

"Long term weight loss following any type of intervention was limited to only a small minority of the obese people studied.[18]*"*

Thus, it seems apparent that there is not enough data to support the claim that diet programs are effective in long-term weight control for a majority of the obese.

The question that is most relevant now is, *what intervention strategies should be used to promote health in the obese, if intervention is deemed appropriate at all?* This question will be addressed in the next issue of *Healthy Weight Journal.*

Wayne C. Miller, PhD, is Professor of Exercise Science and Nutrition at George Washington University Medical Center, Washington, DC.

REFERENCES

1. J Am Med Assoc 1964; 187: 100–106
2. J Am Diet Assoc 1990; 90: 722–726
3. J Nutr 1986; 116: 918–919
4. J Am Diet Assoc 1985; 85: 450–454
5. Clinical Nutrition and Dietetics. New York: Macmillan Publishing Co.; 1991.
6. Am J. Clin Nutr 1981; 34: 453–461
7. Environmental Nutr 1994; 17: 1, 3
8. Health Risks of Weight Loss. Hettinger, ND: Healthy Weight Journal; 1995
9. Am J Clin Nutr 1991; 53: 1124–1129
10. Am J Clin Nutr 1991; 54: 821–828
11. J Am Diet Assoc 1991; 91: 1248–1251
12. Ann Int Med 1993; 119: 688–693
13. Ann Int Med 1993; 119: 764–770
14. Behav Ther 1987; 18: 353–374
15. Int J Obesity 1989; 13: 123–136
16. Ann Int Med 1993; 119: 719–721
17. Ann Int Med 1993; 119: 681–687
18. Ann Int Med 1993; 119: 764–770

Dieting Disorder

THE STORY

Despite 15 years of media coverage of the physical and emotional ravages of eating disorders, an estimated 5 million Americans every year still battle anorexia, bulimia and related disorders. While awareness and treatment have improved, no one has yet defined what triggers the problem. In an attempt to understand more, Australian researchers recently followed nearly 2,000 teens for three years to look for common characteristics among those who eventually developed eating disorders. Though we still don't fully understand why eating disorders develop, the results confirm what many specialists already believed: Serious dieting is a powerful predictor that an eating disorder may emerge.

During any six-month period, girls who dieted severely were 18 times more likely to develop an eating disorder than nondieters; they had an almost one in five chance of developing an eating disorder within a year. Female moderate dieters (which included 60 percent of girls at the beginning of the study) were five times more likely to develop an eating disorder than nondieters and over 12 months had a 1 in 40 chance of developing a new eating disorder. Neither weight nor extent of exercise was associated strongly with developing an eating disorder, although psychiatric illness was. The findings, reported in the March 20 *British Medical Journal*, suggest that two-thirds of new cases of eating disorders arise in females who have dieted moderately.

All the new cases were bulimia nervosa, which involves binge eating followed by purging (self-induced vomiting or use of laxatives) or excessive exercise to prevent weight gain. This is more common than the more visible anorexia nervosa, in which weight drops to an unhealthy level.

Eating disorders are serious: They can lead to stomach problems and tooth decay, bone loss, blood and endocrine abnormalities, infertility—and ultimately death from starvation, suicide or heart problems. Treatment described in an April 8 summary in the *New England Journal of Medicine* involves education about nutrition, medical supervision, and a combination of individual, group or family therapy. Fluoxetine (Prozac) and other antidepressants have been helpful, especially in bulimia.

Is it possible to identify early signs of an eating disorder and find help before the problem becomes serious?—*The Editors*

THE PHYSICIAN'S PERSPECTIVE

David Rosen, M.D.
Associate Editor

Anorexia nervosa and bulimia nervosa—the more severe eating disorders—affect approximately 3 percent of young women. More than twice that number have other forms of disordered eating, a precursor that includes day-long preoccupation with food (counting calories and fat grams and planning or avoiding food), and weight loss or bingeing not severe enough to meet the official criteria for an eating disorder. Older adults, men and preadolescents are also susceptible.

Research over the last two decades has helped us recognize that disordered eating and the more severe eating disorders result from complex interactions among genetic predisposition, personal psychology, family dynamics and sociocultural influences. Several recent studies have added to the evidence that these disorders have some basis in brain chemistry and may be inherited. In one, women who had recovered from bulimia nervosa showed higher levels of by-products of the brain chemical serotonin. Three other studies confirm that the disorder occurs in some families at rates much higher than in the general population. Still, no one completely understands why or how disordered eating arises in certain people. This frustrates our efforts to predict who is at greatest risk for these conditions or to reliably prevent their occurrence.

The Australian study gives us an important clue. Whatever the underlying factors are, severe dieting seems to be an important gateway to the development of these conditions in teens. So identifying dieting teens becomes an extremely useful strategy in offering earlier intervention to those at high risk. We know that early intervention improves the prognosis for disordered eating. And it is at least

POSSIBLE SIGNS OF AN EATING DISORDER

- Arrested growth
- Marked weight change
- Inability to gain weight
- Fatigue
- Constipation or diarrhea
- Susceptibility to fractures
- Disrupted menstruation
- Change in eating habits
- Difficulty eating in social settings
- Reluctance to be weighed
- Depression or social withdrawal
- Absence from school or work
- Deceptive or secretive behavior
- Excessive exercise

Source: Adapted from the New England Journal of Medicine, April 8, 1999.

plausible (though not proven) that by preventing dieting behavior altogether, we might be able to interrupt the pathway by which these conditions develop.

Sadly, we know that dieting behavior sometimes begins as young as 6 or 7 years of age. By middle school, most girls say they've dieted at least once. So what can be done?

• Emphasize "healthy" bodies. The goal should be fitness, not thinness.

• Praise kids for the things they do, rather than for the way they look.

• Don't diet yourself. Commit to lifelong healthy eating, rather than quick-fix diets.

• If a child insists on dieting, insist that the diet be medically supervised.

• Get rid of the scale.

• Prepare kids, especially girls, for the changes of puberty, which may be interpreted as "getting fat."

• Forbid teasing about appearance. Even playful teasing has powerful negative effects.

• Encourage an active lifestyle. This needn't involve organized athletics, but rather any movement—walking, dancing, biking—that is pleasurable enough to do every day.

It is time to seek help when a teen— or adult—can't give up dieting. That person is at risk for an eating disorder and should be helped to see a health-care professional as soon as possible.

FOR MORE INFORMATION

▼ *Eating Disorders Awareness and Prevention, 800-931-2237, members.aol.com/edapinc*

The Effects of Starvation on Behavior: Implications for Dieting and Eating Disorders

by David M. Garner, PhD

One of the most important advances in the understanding of eating disorders is the recognition that severe and prolonged dietary restriction can lead to serious physical and psychological complications.[1] Many of the symptoms once thought to be primary features of anorexia nervosa are actually symptoms of starvation. Given what we know about the biology of weight regulation, what is the impact of weight suppression on the individual? This question is particularly relevant for health professionals who treat eating disorders, but is also important in obesity treatment, for dieters, and for others who have lost significant amounts of body weight.

Perhaps the most powerful illustration of the effects of restrictive dieting and weight loss on behavior is an experimental study conducted over 50 years ago and published in 1950 by Ancel Keys and his colleagues at the University of Minnesota.[2] The experiment involved carefully studying 36 young, healthy, psychologically normal men while restricting their caloric intake for 6 months. More than 100 men volunteered for the study as an alternative to military service; the 36 selected had the highest levels of physical and psychological health, as well as the most commitment to the objectives of the experiment. What makes the "starvation study," as it is commonly known, so important is that many of the experiences observed in the volunteers are the same as those experienced by patients with eating disorders as well as some people who have undergone weight loss programs.

During the first 3 months of the semistarvation experiment, the volunteers ate normally while their behavior, personality, and eating patterns were studied in detail. During the next 6 months, the men were restricted to approximately half of their former food intake and lost, on average, approximately 25 percent of their former weight. Although this was described as a study of "semistarvation," it is important to keep in mind that cutting the men's rations to half of their former intake (to an average of 1,570 calories) is precisely the level of caloric deficit used to define "conservative" treatments for obesity.[3] The 6 months of weight loss were followed by 3 months of rehabilitation, during which the men were gradually refed. A subgroup was followed for almost 9 months after the refeeding began. Most of the results were reported for only 32 men, because four men were withdrawn either during or at the end of the semistarvation phase. Although the individual responses to weight loss varied considerably, the men experienced dramatic physical, psychological, and social changes. In most cases, these changes persisted during the rehabilitation or renourishment phase.

Attitudes and behavior related to food and eating

One of the most striking changes that occurred in the volunteers was a dramatic increase in food preoccupation. The men found concentration on their usual activities increasingly difficult, because they became plagued by incessant thoughts of food and eating. During the semistarvation phase of the experiment, food became a principal topic of conversation, reading, and daydreams. Rating scales revealed that the men experienced increase in thoughts about food, as well as corresponding decreases in interest in sex and activity during semistarvation. The actual words used in the original report are particularly

Many of the symptoms that might have been thought to be specific to anorexia nervosa and bulimia nervosa are actually the result of starvation.

revealing and the following quotations followed by page numbers in parentheses are from Keys et al. with permission from the University of Minnesota Press.

"As starvation progressed, the number of men who toyed with their food increased. They made what under normal conditions would be weird and distasteful concoctions, (p. 832)... Those who ate in the common dining room smuggled out bits of food and consumed them on their bunks in a long-drawn-out ritual, (p. 833)... Toward the end of starvation some of the men would dawdle for almost 2 hours after a meal which previously they would have consumed in a matter of minutes, (p. 833)... Cookbooks, menus, and information bulletins on food production became intensely interesting to many of the men who previously had little or no interest in dietetics or agriculture, (p. 833)... [The volunteers] often reported that they got a vivid vicarious pleasure from watching other persons eat or from just smelling food (p. 834)..."

In addition to reading cookbooks and collecting recipes, some of the men even began collecting coffeepots, hot plates, and other kitchen utensils. According to the original report, hoarding even extended to non-food-related items such as "old books, unnecessary second-hand clothes, knick knacks, and other 'junk.' Often after making such purchases, which could be afforded only with sacrifice, the men would be puzzled as to why they had bought such more or less useless articles" (p. 837). One man even began rummaging through garbage cans. This general tendency to hoard has been observed in starved anorexic patients and even in rats deprived of food.[4,5] Despite little interest in culinary matters prior to the experiment, almost 40 percent of the men mentioned cooking as one of their postexperiment plans. For some, the fascination was so great *that they actually changed occupations after the experiment;* three became chefs!

The Minnesota subjects often were caught between conflicting desires to gulp their food down ravenously and consume it slowly so that the taste and odor of each morsel would be fully appreciated.

They did much planning as to how they would handle their day's allotment of food (p. 833). The men demanded that their food be served hot, and they made unusual concoctions by mixing foods together, as noted above. There also was a marked increase in the use of salt and spices. The consumption of coffee and tea increased so dramatically that the men had to be limited to nine cups per day; similarly, gum chewing became excessive and had to be limited after it was discovered that one man was chewing as many as 40 packages of gum a day and "developed a sore mouth from such continuous exercise" (p. 835).

During the 12-week refeeding phase of the experiment, most of the abnormal attitudes and behaviors related to food persisted.

Binge eating

During the restrictive dieting phase of the experiment, all of the volunteers reported increased hunger. Some appeared able to tolerate the experience fairly well, but for others it created intense concern and led to a complete breakdown in control. Several men were unable to adhere to their diets and reported episodes of binge eating followed by self-reproach. During the eighth week of starvation, one volunteer flagrantly broke the dietary rules, eating several sundaes and malted milks; he even stole some penny candies. He promptly confessed the whole episode, [and] became self-deprecatory (p. 884). While working in a grocery store, another man suffered a complete loss of will power and ate several cookies, a sack of popcorn, and two overripe bananas before he could regain control of himself. He immediately suffered a severe emotional upset, with nausea, and upon returning to the laboratory he vomited... He was self-deprecatory, expressing disgust and self-criticism (p. 887).

One man was released from the experiment at the end of the semistarvation period because of suspicions that he was unable to adhere to the diet. He experienced serious difficulties when confronted with unlimited access to food: "He repeatedly went through the cycle of eating tremendous quantities of food, becoming sick, and then starting all over again" (p. 890). During the refeeding phase of the experiment, many of the men lost control of their appetites and "ate more or less continuously" (p. 843). Even after 12 weeks of refeeding, the men frequently complained of increased hunger immediately following a large meal.

"[One of the volunteers] ate immense meals (a daily estimate of 5,000 to 6,000 calories) and yet started snacking an hour after he finished a meal. [Another] ate as much as he could hold during the three regular meals and ate snacks in the morning, afternoon, and evening, (p. 846)... Several men had spells of nausea and vomiting. One man required aspiration and hospitalization for several days, (p. 843)..."

During the weekends in particular, some of the men found it difficult to stop eating. Their daily intake commonly ranged between 8,000 and 10,000 calories, and their eating patterns were described as follows:

Subject No. 20 stuffs himself and he is bursting at the seams, to the point of being nearly sick and still feels hungry; No. 120 reported that he had to discipline himself to keep from eating so much as to become ill; No. 1 ate until he was uncomfortably full; and subject No. 30 had so little control over the mechanics of "piling it in" that he simply had to stay away from food because he could not find a point of satiation even when he was "full to the gills...," "I ate practically all weekend," reported subject No. 26... Subject No. 26 would just as soon have eaten six meals instead of three. (p. 847)

After about 5 months of refeeding, the majority of the men reported some normalization of their eating patterns, but for some the extreme overconsumption persisted "No. 108 would eat and eat until he could hardly swallow any more and then he felt like eating half an hour later" (p. 847). More than 8 months after renourishment began, most men had returned to normal eating patterns; however, a few were still eating abnormal amounts. "No. 9 ate about 25 percent more than his prestarvation amount; once he started to reduce but got so hungry he could not stand it" (p. 847).

Factors distinguishing men who rapidly normalized their eating from those who continued to eat prodigious amounts were not identified. Nevertheless, the main findings here are as follows: *Serious binge eating developed in a subgroup of men, and this tendency persisted in some cases for months after free access to food was reintroduced; however, the majority of men reported gradually returning to eating normal amounts of food after about 5 months of refeeding.* Thus, the fact that binge eating was experimentally produced in some of these normal young men should temper speculations about primary psychological disturbances as the cause of binge eating in patients with eating disorders.

These findings are supported by a large body of research indicating that habitual dieters display marked overcompensation in eating behavior that is similar to the binge eating observed in eating disorders.[6-8] Polivy et al. compared a group of former World War II prisoners of war and noninterned veterans and found that the former prisoners who had lost an average of 10.5 kg while prisoners of war, reported a significantly higher frequency of binge eating than noninterned veterans according to a self-report questionnaire sent by mail.

Emotional and personality changes

The experimental procedures involved selecting volunteers who were the most physically and psychologically robust. "The psychobiologic 'stamina' of the subjects was unquestionably superior to that likely to be found in any random or more generally representative sample of the population" (pp. 915–916).

Although the subjects were psychologically healthy prior to the experiment, most experienced significant emotional deterioration as a result of semistarvation. Most subjects experienced periods during which their emotional distress was quite severe; almost 20 percent had extreme emotional deterioration that markedly interfered with their functioning. **Depression** became more severe during the course of the experiment. Mood swings were extreme for some of the volunteers:

> [One subject] experienced a number of periods in which his spirits were definitely high... These elated periods alternated with times in which he suffered "a deep dark depression." (p. 903)

Irritability and frequent outbursts of **anger** were common, although the men had fairly tolerant dispositions prior to starvation. For most subjects, **anxiety** became more evident. As the experiment progressed, many of the formerly even-tempered men began biting their nails or smoking because they felt nervous. **Apathy** also became common, and some men who had been moderately fastidious neglected various aspects of personal hygiene. During semistarvation, two subjects developed disturbances of **psychotic** proportions. During the refeeding period, emotional disturbance did not vanish immediately but persisted for several weeks, with some men actually becoming more depressed, irritable, argumentative, and negativistic than they had been during semistarvation. After 2 weeks of refeeding, one man reported his extreme reaction in his diary:

> *I have been more depressed than ever in my life... I thought that there was only one thing that would pull me out of the doldrums, that is release from C.P.S. [the experiment] I decided to get rid of some fingers. Ten days ago, I jacked up my car and let the car fall on these fingers... It was premeditated.* (pp. 894–895)

Several days later, this man actually did *chop off three fingers of one hand* in response to the stress.

Standardized personality testing with the Minnesota Multiphasic Personality Inventory (MMPI) revealed that semistarvation resulted in significant increases on the Depression, Hysteria, and Hypochondriasis scales. The MMPI profiles for a small minority of subjects confirmed the clinical impression of incredible deterioration as a result of semistarvation. One man scored well within normal limits at initial testing, but after 10 weeks of semistarvation and a weight loss of only about 4.5 kg (10 pounds, or approximately 7 percent of his original body weight), gross personality disturbances were evident on the MMPI.

Social and sexual changes

The extraordinary impact of semistarvation was reflected in the social changes experienced by most of the volunteers. Although originally quite gregarious, the men became progressively more withdrawn and isolated. Humor and the sense of comradeship diminished amidst growing feelings of social inadequacy. The volunteers' social contacts with women also declined sharply during semistarvation. Those who continued to see women socially found that the relationships became strained. These changes are illustrated in the account from one man's diary:

> *I am one of about three or four who still go out with girls. I fell in love with a girl during the control period but I see her only occasionally now. It's almost too much trouble to see her even when she visits me in the lab. It requires effort to hold her hand. Entertainment must be tame. If we see a*

show, the most interesting part of it is contained in scenes where people are eating. (p. 853)

Sexual interests were likewise drastically reduced. Masturbation, sexual fantasies, and sexual impulses either ceased or became much less common. One subject graphically stated that he had "no more sexual feeling than a sick oyster." (Even this peculiar metaphor made reference to food.) Keys et al. observed that "many of the men welcomed the freedom from sexual tensions and frustrations normally present in young adult men" (p. 840). The fact that starvation perceptibly altered sexual urges and associated conflicts is of particular interest, since it has been hypothesized that this process is the driving force behind the dieting of many anorexia nervosa patients. According to Crisp, anorexia nervosa is an adaptive disorder in the sense that it curtails sexual concerns for which the adolescent feels unprepared.[10] During rehabilitation, sexual interest was slow to return. Even after 3 months, the men judged themselves to be far from normal in this area. However, after 8 months of renourishment, virtually all of the men had recovered their interest in sex.

Cognitive and physical changes

The volunteers reported impaired concentration, alertness, comprehension, and judgment during semistarvation; however, formal intellectual testing revealed no signs of diminished intellectual abilities. As the 6 months of semistarvation progressed, the volunteers exhibited many physical changes, including gastrointestinal discomfort; decreased need for sleep; dizziness; headaches; hypersensitivity to noise and light; reduced strength; poor motor control; edema (an excess of fluid causing swelling); hair loss; decreased tolerance for cold temperatures (cold hands and feet); visual disturbances (i.e., inability to focus, eye aches, "spots" in the visual fields); auditory disturbances (i.e., ringing noise in the ears); and paresthesias (i.e., abnormal tingling or prickling sensations, especially in the hands or feet).

Various changes reflected an overall slowing of the body's physiologic processes. There were decreases in body temperature, heart rate, and respiration, as well as in basal metabolic rate (BMR), the amount of energy (in calories) that the body requires at rest (i.e., no physical activity) to carry out normal physiologic processes. It accounts for about two thirds of the body's total energy needs, with the remainder being used during physical activity. At the end of semistarvation, the men's BMRs had dropped by about 40 percent from normal levels. This drop, as well as other physical changes, reflect the body's extraordinary ability to adapt to low caloric intake by reducing its need for energy. More recent research has shown that metabolic rate is markedly reduced even among dieters who do not have a history of dramatic weight loss.[11] During refeeding, Keys et al. found that metabolism speeded up, with those consuming the greatest number of calories experiencing the greatest rise in BMR. The group of volunteers who received a relatively small increment in calories during refeeding (400 calories more than during semistarvation) had no rise in BMR for the first 3 weeks. Consuming larger amounts of food caused a sharp increase in the energy burned through metabolic processes.

Significance of the "Starvation Study"

As is readily apparent from the preceding description of the Minnesota experiment, many of the symptoms that might have been thought to be specific to anorexia nervosa and bulimia nervosa are actually the result of starvation.[12] These are not limited to food and weight, but extend to virtually all areas of psychological and social functioning. Since many of the symptoms postulated to cause these disorders may actually result from undernutrition, it is absolutely essential that weight be returned to "normal" levels so that psychological functioning can be accurately assessed.

The profound effects of starvation also illustrate the tremendous adaptive capacity of the human body and the intense biologic pressure on the organism to maintain a relatively consistent body weight. This makes complete evolutionary sense. Over hundreds of thousands of years of human evolution, a major threat to the survival of the organism was starvation. If weight had not been carefully modulated and controlled internally, early humans most certainly would simply have died when food was scarce or when their interest was captured by countless other aspects of living. The "starvation study" by Keys et al. illustrates how the human being becomes more oriented toward food when starved and how other pursuits important to the survival of the species (e.g., social and sexual functioning) become subordinate to the primary drive toward food.

Some researchers have indicated publicly that this study could not be conducted today because of the stringent ethical guidelines for research using human subjects. However, rarely have ethical concerns been raised regarding the use of very low calorie diets that involve a level of calorie restriction that is approximately one half of that used in the "starvation study." In light of the profound changes observed in the "starvation study," it would seem mandatory to warn participants of these potentially untoward effects as well as to carefully study the psychological and physical impact of these programs.

Providing patients with eating disorders with the above account of the semistarvation study can be very useful in giving them an explanation for many of the emotional, cognitive, and behavioral symptoms that they experience. Recommendations to use the findings of this study, as well as other educational materials,[1] are based on the assumption that patients with eating disorder often suffer from misconceptions about the factors that cause and then maintain symptoms. It is further assumed that patients may be less likely to persist in self-defeating symptoms if they are made truly aware of the scientific evidence regarding factors that perpetuate eating disorders.

One of the most notable implications of the Minnesota experiment is that it challenges the popular notion that body weight is easily altered if one simply exercises a bit of "willpower." It also demonstrates that the body is not simply "reprogrammed" at a lower set point once weight loss has been achieved. The volunteers' experimental diet was unsuccessful in overriding their bodies' strong propensity to defend a particular weight level. Again, it is important to emphasize that following the months of refeeding, the Minnesota volunteers did not skyrocket into obesity. On average, they gained back their original weight plus about 10 percent; then, over the next 6 months, their weight gradually declined. By the end of the follow up period, they were approaching their pre-experiment weight levels.

References

1. Garner DM. Psychoeducational principles in the treatment of eating disorders. In: Garner DM, Garfinkel PE, eds. Handbook for treatment of eating disorders. New York: Guilford Press, 1997:145–177.
2. Keys A, Brozek J, Henschel A, et al. The biology of human starvation. Vols 1 and 2. Minneapolis: University of Minnesota Press, 1950.
3. Stunkard AJ. Introduction and overview. In: Stunkard AJ, Wadden TA, eds. Obesity: theory and therapy. 2nd Ed. New York: Raven Press, 1993:1–10.
4. Crisp AH, Hsu LKG, Harding B. The starving hoarder and voracious spender: stealing in anorexia nervosa. J Psychosom Res 1980; 24:225–231.
5. Fantino M, Cabanac M. Body weight regulation with a proportional hoarding response in the rat. Physiol Behav 1980; 24:939–942.
6. Polivy J, Herman CP. Dieting and bingeing: a causal analysis. Am Psychol 1985; 40:193–201.
7. Polivy J, Herman CP. Diagnosis and treatment of normal eating. J. Consult Clin Psychol 1987; 55:635–644.
8. Wardle J, Beinart H. Binge eating: a theoretical review. Br J Clin Psychol 1981; 19,20:97–109.
9. Polivy J, Zeitlin SB, Herman CP, Beal AL. Food restriction and binge eating: a study of former prisoners of war. J Abnorm Psychol 1994; 103:409–411.
10. Crisp AJ. Anorexia nervosa: let me be. London: Academic Press, 1980.
11. Platte P, Wurmser H, Wade SE, et al. Resting metabolic rate and diet-induced thermogenesis in restrained and unrestrained eaters. Int J Eat Disord 1996; 20:33–41.
12. Pirke KM, Ploog D. Biology of human starvation. In: Beaumont PJV, Burrows GD, Casper RC, eds. Handbook of eating disorders: Part I. Anorexia and bulimia nervosa. New York: Elsevier, 1987:79–102.

Adapted by the author from Garner and Garfinkel (ref. 1). David M. Garner, PhD, is the director of the Toledo Center for Eating Disorders and an adjunct professor of psychology at Bowling Green State University and of women's studies at the University of Toledo, Ohio. He is co-editor of the *Handbook of Treatment of Eating Disorders*. He can be reached at 419–843–2000 or by e-mail at garnerdm@aol.com.

Unit 5

Unit Selections

40. **Food Safety: Don't Get Burned,** Consumer Reports on Health
41. **Audits International's Home Food Safety Survey** Audits International
42. **Avoiding Cross-Contamination in the Home,** Institute of Food Science & Technology
43. **Why You Need a Kitchen Thermometer,** Tufts University Health & Nutrition Letter
44. **Campylobacter: Low-Profile Bug Is Food Poisoning Leader,** Audrey Hingley
45. **E. Coli 0157:H7—How Dangerous Has It Become?** Nutrition & the M.D.
46. **A Crackdown on Bad Eggs,** Amanda Spake
47. **Irradiation: A Safe Measure for Safer Food,** John Henkel
48. **Questions Keep Sprouting about Sprouts,** Paula Kurtzweil

Key Points to Consider

❖ Rank order three issues of food safety that you think are the most important and justify your selection.

❖ Observe yourself when you handle food. In what ways might you be the vector of food-borne illness?

❖ What measures would you suggest to counteract misinformation about food safety and the tactics used by activist organizations?

❖ Find articles in newspapers and magazines that will chronicle the events of the trade wars with Europe over the use of hormones with dairy cows and beef cattle. Why do we view the issues differently? How should this be resolved? Do the same for the acceptance of genetically altered foods.

❖ Read Upton Sinclair's muckraking novel *The Jungle.* Compare conditions and problems described in this book with today's procedures for ensuring a safe food supply.

DUSHKIN ONLINE Links   www.dushkin.com/online/

27. **Centers for Disease Control and Prevention**
    http://www.cdc.gov
28. **FDA Center for Food Safety and Applied Nutrition**
    http://vm.cfsan.fda.gov
29. **Food Safety Information from North Carolina**
    http://www.ces.ncsu.edu/depts/foodsci/agentinfo/
30. **Food Safety Project**
    http://www.exnet.iastate.edu/Pages/families/fs/
31. **USDA Food Safety and Inspection Service**
    http://www.fsis.usda.gov

These sites are annotated on pages 4 and 5.

Food Safety

It is important for consumers to understand that absolutely risk-free food cannot exist.
—*Professor Dean O. Cliver, Ph.D., University of California, Davis*

During the Spanish-American War of 1898, more U.S. troops died from food poisoning than died from battle wounds. In 1906, with the passage of the first Food and Drug Act, the federal government assumed some responsibility for food safety. Increased governmental involvement has been an inevitable trend ever since. With the 1950s came a fear that chemicals in the food supply, especially additives, might be carcinogenic. Congress responded with tighter control on the use and testing of additives. In 1958, the Delaney Clause prevented the use of any additive found to induce cancer in man or experimental animals, and the GRAS (Generally Recognized as Safe) list identified those believed by scientists to be safe for human consumption. This list is periodically revised, and the testing and retesting of additives continues. The Food and Drug Administration (FDA) governs all of these procedures, and books of regulations cover all aspects of food production and service.

Given the complexity of biological interactions, the uniqueness of each human organism, and the multitude of chemicals that potentially could interact, few knowledgeable people would contend that the absolute safety of anything can be ensured. Yet activist groups demand just that and have become experts at escalating a minor or nonexistent issue into a major catastrophe. It has been argued that if it takes programs like *60 Minutes*, or a partisan political group such as the National Resources Defense Council, or a self-appointed watchdog group such as Food and Water, Inc., to create a public issue, then it probably isn't a safety issue at all. Alar—a growth regulator used in apple orchards—is a good example. The scare over Alar's safety appears to have been media hype, but it seriously hurt the apple industry and shook parents' confidence in apple juice for their children.

The United States' food supply is among the world's safest; yet food safety has become a major national issue. This is hardly surprising, given the media coverage of food-borne illness outbreaks due to cyclospora on raspberries from Guatemala, salmonella at church suppers, and *E. coli* from a variety of products. Although the incidence of some types of food-borne illness has dropped in recent years, it cannot be denied that significant numbers of people become ill. The Council for Agricultural Science and Technology recently reported 33 million cases and 9 thousand deaths for a single year. Other sources suggest that the figures may be much higher. Annual costs of these illnesses are estimated by the USDA at $7–35 billion.

Some of today's most prevalent food-borne organisms were not public health issues 20 years ago, a sign that conditions and lifestyles have changed. One of these is *E. coli* 0157:H7, which is infamous for causing a 1991 outbreak of food poisoning in Washington State from undercooked hamburger. After repeated outbreaks involving a variety of foods, it has become clear that this type of contamination is truly serious, sometimes resulting in hemolytic uremic syndrome, kidney failure, and death. This organism must be aggressively controlled both in the processing industry and in the kitchen. Pasteurization and irradiation are two powerful measures currently used commercially, and new technology suggests that feeding calves a nonpathogenic form of bacteria may work prophylactically.

Many people blame the food industry or the government's food inspection procedures for the presence of illness-producing organisms in the food supply. And, indeed, government agencies are responding to the challenge. A state-of-the-art surveillance system now permits scientists to determine the cause of an illness outbreak within 24 hours by entering the DNA fingerprinting of a pathogen into a national data base. This speeds up intervention strategies to stop outbreaks with only a few illnesses. The FDA has adopted HACCP (Hazard Analysis and Critical Control Points) rules to improve safety control and monitoring in the food production of meat, poultry, and seafood. Microwave pasteurization, high-voltage pulses of electricity, and chemical dehairing of carcasses *before* cutting are among the new methods for controlling bacterial growth in the food supply.

People often assume that food-borne illness is contracted primarily in restaurants, and some statistics support this supposition. A few states, most recently California, have enacted laws that require food-service workers to be specially trained in safe food handling. But it is revealing to discover that in our own kitchens, we are our own worst enemies. A survey has shown that people do not follow proper sanitation techniques over 95 percent of the time, even when they know better and have agreed to be observed.

Food irradiation, addressed in an article by John Henkel, has been both a food safety issue and a political issue. For years activist groups effectively used aggressive scare tactics to delay irradiation in this country. Although it was approved previously in the United States for poultry, fresh produce, and spices, only at the end of 1997 was irradiation finally approved for use with red meat. The World Health Organization (WHO), however, has recommended radiation for years and nearly 30 countries use it effectively to destroy pathogenic bacteria and to maintain high quality produce over a prolonged shelf life.

A number of current issues related to safety have international implications. One of these, and a highly controversial one, is the use of hormones to increase milk production and to add leaner weight more efficiently to cattle prior to market. Europeans have very little tolerance for this practice, which is fairly common in the U.S. Nor are Europeans willing to accept our genetically altered crops, a matter of considerable concern to our farmers and an issue included in unit 1. In Europe, a concern of major significance is the new variant of Creutzfeldt-Jakob Disease (CJD). First discovered in the 1920s, CJD is a rare neurological disease that affects about a million people per year worldwide.

Consumers are often misinformed concerning the terms "natural" and organic." While the common belief is that both terms connote healthier, safer products, neither may be true. Snake venom and amanita mushrooms are both quite natural and very dangerous. Furthermore, the safety of organic produce is questioned by many—although supported by others—because the use of animal manure and, sometimes, unchlorinated water make the presence and growth of harmful bacteria more likely. Problems arising over the safety of food supplies can be documented throughout history. As consumers, we must accept personal responsibility for safe food handling.

Article 40

Food safety: Don't get burned

Common misconceptions can spoil your barbecue—or your health

Summertime: Time to fire up the grill, cook some burgers, and let the good times roll. But to safeguard the fun, you need to take some sensible precautions. Meat sometimes harbors harmful bacteria, which may flourish during barbecue season. Unfortunately, some of the conventional wisdom on the safety of meat and other foods isn't very useful—and a few supposedly helpful preventive measures might actually *increase* your risk of contracting foodborne illness. Here's the lowdown on several misconceptions about what will—and won't—keep what you eat from making you sick.

❶ Myth: You can tell whether a burger is safe to eat by checking whether it's brown in the middle.

Truth: Brownness and pinkness do not accurately reflect doneness. Government researchers have found that more than one-fourth of fresh burger patties and up to two-thirds of frozen patties turn brown before they've been cooked to a safe temperature. Some hamburgers may be predisposed to early browning because they've been exposed excessively to air, kept for too long before they're cooked, or not chilled sufficiently during storage. On the flip side, some burgers still look pink in the middle even when they're well cooked.

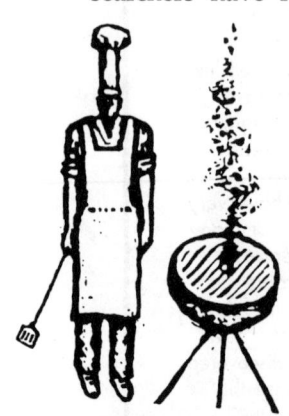

The chance of getting a truly dangerous illness from eating a hamburger—mainly due to contamination with a virulent strain called *E. coli 0157:H7*—is very small. So you may decide it's not worth spending much effort to avoid that risk. But if you want to be completely safe—which is particularly important if you're cooking for children, older people, or sick or immunocompromised individuals—you should consider using a meat thermometer. Lift the meat off the grill and, for thin burgers, insert the thermometer into the side of the patty. (If you don't want to bother checking every single piece of meat, you might do a *rough* check by spot-testing a few pieces on different parts of the grill.) Using a thermometer can help ensure that you've cooked the meat to the following minimum temperatures for killing potentially harmful bacteria:

- Ground beef, 160° F; ground turkey, 165° F.
- Unground beef, veal, or lamb, 145° F.
- Pork, 160° F.
- Chicken breasts, 170° F; other parts, 180° F.
- Whole turkey, 180° F (in the inner thigh); stuffing, 165° F.
- Fish, 145° F—and then continue to cook it for another five minutes.
- Leftovers, 165° F.

❷ Myth: Raw meat and poultry should always be rinsed thoroughly before cooking to wash away the bacteria on the surface.

Truth: Sustained cooking almost always kills all of the *Salmonella, E. coli,* and other bacteria that may be lurking on meat and poultry, since the surface is almost always heated to lethal temperatures.

But if you do rinse those foods, be sure to clean up carefully afterward. That's because the water washes the germs into the sink—a prime breeding ground for bacteria and the very area where you may be handling fresh produce. If you wipe the sink with a damp dishcloth or sponge, you're likely to spread the organisms everywhere. Indeed, a study of 15 households in Tucson, Ariz., showed that the most germ-infested spots in the house are the kitchen sponge or dishcloth and the sink.

> Brownness may not reflect doneness.

40. Food Safety: Don't Get Burned

To keep bacteria at bay, pack each piece of raw meat in a plastic bag at the store and keep the meat in the bag when you get home so the juices won't contaminate other foods. Try to handle raw meat and poultry in just one part of the kitchen—say, on a particular cutting board. Mop up spilled juices with paper towels. Then wash with hot soapy water any faucets, sink handles, counters, and utensils that you touched while handling the food. (And wash your hands, too.) Don't put the cooked meat or poultry back on the same plate that held it raw, and don't pour leftover marinade over cooked food unless you've first heated it to a boil.

For extra protection, periodically add bleach—a particularly effective bacteria buster—to your cleanup routine. Douse the sink, cutting board, and surrounding area with a solution of 2 teaspoons of bleach per quart of water; after a few minutes, rinse and air-dry. Disinfect the kitchen sponge daily, if possible, in one of these ways: Pop it in the basket of the dishwasher or in the washing machine, heat it in the microwave till it's steaming hot, or soak it in a bleach solution.

Myth: Plastic or glass cutting boards are safer than wooden ones, which harbor bacteria.

Truth: Some research has suggested that bacteria can get trapped in wood, lie dormant, and possibly resurface the next time a board is used. But other research suggests that some types of wood have antimicrobial properties that render most micro-organisms harmless. So no one really knows whether wood, plastic, or glass is inherently safer. But if you handle the boards properly, *all* types can be equally safe.

Regardless of what they're made of, cutting boards should be washed with either a bleach solution or hot soapy water after each use, rinsed thoroughly, and either air-dried or patted dry with paper towels. Boards riddled with hard-to-clean grooves should be replaced. For further protection, reserve one cutting board for produce, another for meat and poultry. That reduces the risk that bacteria left behind after cutting, say, raw chicken might contaminate a tomato cut on the same board later.

Myth: You can generally spot contaminated food because it looks, smells, or tastes bad.

Truth: Any potentially dangerous bacteria lurking in a food are more likely to have multiplied if the food is old or spoiled; that increases the risk of food poisoning in some cases. So you can indeed reduce your odds of getting sick by choosing foods that look or smell fresh. For meat, that means creamy-white to yellow chicken, bright-red beef, grayish-pink veal or pork, and pink lamb. For fish, it means a mild odor, moist and firm flesh, shiny skin, pink or red gills, clear, protruding eyes, and fillets without brown edges.

But you can't rely only on those signs. Many contaminated foods actually look, smell, and taste perfectly normal. That's because the bacteria that cause food poisoning are often different from those that cause spoilage. While freshness may lower the risk, it certainly doesn't guarantee safety.

To further reduce the odds of buying significantly contaminated food, try to avoid:

- Foods that have passed their "sell by" date.
- Frozen foods that don't feel solid or that have large ice crystals, a sign that they may have thawed and later become frozen again.
- Refrigerated foods that don't feel cold or that have rips or openings in the packaging.

Myth: Freezing effectively destroys bacteria.

Truth: Freezing to 0° F stalls the growth and activity of bacteria, but it kills only some of them. If a food is defrosted at a warm temperature, the surviving organisms resume multiplying even faster than before. That's because freezing breaks down some of the cells in food, giving the bacteria easier access to nutrients that fuel their growth. And it's the strongest organisms that survive.

To minimize that problem, make frozen foods your last purchase, then get them home from the store and into your freezer as soon as possible. And don't defrost foods on the kitchen counter. Long before the interior has thawed, the outside portions can rise to temperatures that let the bacteria start to thrive. Instead, defrost foods in the refrigerator to minimize bacterial growth. If that's too slow, use a microwave oven—but then cook the food right away, since microwaving may warm some portions to ideal temperatures for bacteria to proliferate.

In addition, take the following steps to freeze foods as quickly as possible. If your freezer has shelves, use them to spread the items in single layers. Don't stack the items until they're completely frozen. Divide large portions into smaller amounts and store them in shallow containers. Cut meat into portions no more than 2 inches thick. It takes about two hours for such portions to freeze solid. But it may take hours before the center of larger items drop even to 40° F and far longer to hit 0° F. And many people keep their refrigerator and freezer too warm in the first place. So buy a thermometer for each compartment and check it periodically, particularly if the temperature in your home changes substantially from season to season.

⑥ Myth: Food shouldn't be refrozen.

Truth: Performed at room temperature or in a microwave, the second *thawing* may give bacteria a second chance to overrun the food. But refreezing is safe if you defrost in the refrigerator (though the second freezing may hurt the food's taste or texture). It's also safe if you've cooked the food to the recommended temperature and returned it to the freezer within an hour or two—or to the refrigerator temporarily and then to the freezer.

Summing up

To reduce your risk of foodborne illness, follow these guidelines:

- Choose foods that seem to be fresh, appropriately frozen or cold, undamaged, and unopened.

- At home, chill foods immediately in a refrigerator set below 40° F or freeze them at 0° F or lower, as described above. Thaw frozen foods in the refrigerator or microwave, not on the countertop.

- Don't think you need to rinse raw meat (or fish or poultry); if you do rinse, clean the sink carefully afterward. Prepare meat and produce on separate cutting boards and in separate places. And cook meat to the recommended temperature.

- Regularly disinfect the sink, countertop, cutting boards, sponges, and dishcloths, particularly after you've handled raw meat.

Audits International's Home Food Safety Survey

Introduction

In 1997, Audits International conducted the initial Home Food Safety Survey because previous studies had been based on consumer knowledge without actually measuring performance. Due to the fact that Audits International has expert food safety auditors across North America, evaluating actual performance seemed like a natural fit. An overall deficiency in safe food handling practices was observed when just one of 106 participants met the standards Audits International had used in over 20,000 foodservice safety evaluations to date. Critical violations (those which in and of themselves may cause foodborne illness, and deem an establishment unacceptable) were found in 96% of the households evaluated. Whether or not deficient food safety practices were being used was no longer the question; the question became why.

Are people lacking the education to be aware of potential food safety issues? Or is the motivation behind avoiding the issues not strong enough? The estimated number of cases of foodborne illness in the U.S. ranges upward from 6 million annually including more than 9,000 deaths. These figures have lead to an increased media attention, which has both educated and motivated the public. The desire to gauge the reasons behind the general population's deficient food safety practices prompted Audits International to conduct the second home food safety survey.

The 1997 study was strictly designed to determine how often proper food safety practices were employed as part of home food preparation. The 1999 study also attempted to determine whether key food safety deficiencies are caused by a lack of knowledge or the lack of sufficient desire to follow proper food safety practices (motivation). These results can be used not only to raise public awareness and personalize the inadequacies of current practices, but also to guide the government, industry, and the media further in promoting proper food safety.

Methodology

Households selected in 1997 were not included in this study. Household selection was not random. Auditors asked acquaintances if they were willing to have their meal preparation practices evaluated as part of this survey. Those who participated knew they were being evaluated, probably believed they would perform well, and were better educated than the average U.S. population (71% college degree, 1% did not complete high school). It is our belief that each of these design biases suggest that the selected households were likely to perform better than if we had used an unannounced, stratified random sampling.

Auditors observed meal preparation, service, post-meal cleanup and leftover storage. The inspection process required 45–60 minutes of evaluation time but the evaluation was spread out over as much as seven hours from preparation to final handling of leftovers. Each auditor utilized a consistent and objec-

5 ❖ FOOD SAFETY

Critical Violations	Households Observed (n=121)
	Frequency (%)
Cross contamination observed	31
Improper cooling of leftovers	29
Neglected handwashing	29
Improper food preparation techniques	21
Cleaning supplies or chemicals improperly stored/labeled	20
Finished internal cooking temperatures too low	19
Refrigerated ingredient temperatures too high	9
Disposable plastic gloves not properly used	4
Dented, rusted, or swelling cans present	2
Sick/symptomatic foodhandler preparing food	2

Most Frequently Observed Critical Violations

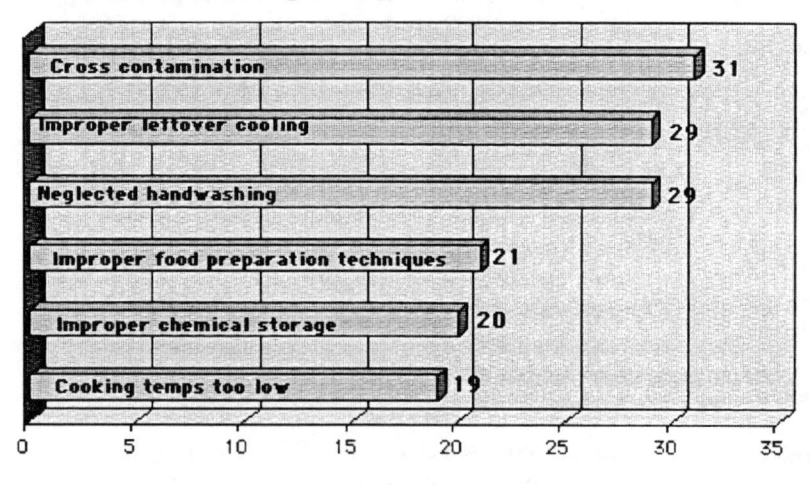

Violation	Value
Cross contamination	31
Improper leftover cooling	29
Neglected handwashing	29
Improper food preparation techniques	21
Improper chemical storage	20
Cooking temps too low	19

tive critical control point approach for home evaluation in a similar fashion to the Audits International Food Safety Inspection conducted in restaurants. Performance was compared to standards from the 1997 U.S. Food Code.

The following issues were evaluated:

- temperature taking practices
- storage and rotation practices (time, temperature, etc.)
- hot and cold ingredient preparation and holding (time, temperature, and product handling)
- sanitation and chemical storage
- personal practices (cross-contamination, handwashing, safety-related habits)
- general kitchen condition (infestation, maintenance, plumbing, etc.)

Violations were categorized as major or critical. A critical violation is defined as one that, by itself, can potentially lead to a foodborne illness or injury. Major violations, on their own, are unlikely to cause foodborne illness but are frequently cited as contributing factors. *To be classified as acceptable, a home was allowed zero critical violations and no more than four major violations.* This Audits International classification method has been used in foodservice institutions which have demonstrated the ability to consistently meet and exceed these criteria.

When auditors observed a critical violation in any of six areas of high concern (ingredient cooking, handwashing, cross contamination, chemical storage, handling of leftovers, and cold ingredient holding), the auditor would try to determine why the violation was committed through a series of questions. The goal of this exercise was to determine whether the violations were due to either a lack of education or motivation.

All participants were given a short quiz (4–6 questions) in each of the high concern categories listed above. The purpose of this exercise was to determine the correlation between testing what consumers know versus testing what they do.

Revisions to the 1997 Study

The 1997 study originally found that of 106 households, less than 1% met the minimal Audits International criteria for acceptable performance. Households averaged 2.8 critical violations and 5.8 major violations. In order to gauge any improvement in the 18 months since that study, 1997 results had to be reviewed against the current food safety standards employed by Audits International. Changes were made based on conversations with leading regulators and industry experts. These include:

Refrigerated product selection-

Auditors recorded the temperature of products based on whether the product was hazardous, rather than the location in the refrigerator. The 1997 study required one product temperature from the interior of the refrigerator and one from the door.

Although this change biased the temperature results favorably, it is reasonable because of its orientation to potentially hazardous foods.

Cutting board procedures-
Households were not to be required to wash and sanitize a cutting board between uses. While washing is still a necessary step, not sanitizing a cutting board in the home would no longer merit a critical violation.

Leftover labeling-
Leftover items were no longer required to be dated and timed (a major violation). Instead, refrigerators would be evaluated by how long leftovers had been present. Leftovers older than four days would result in a major violation.

After modifying the results of the 1997 study to reflect these changes, the percent of households deemed acceptable in the initial study increased from less than 1% to 4% (see Discussion section for further analysis). 1997 results refer to the revised results when referenced throughout the rest of the report.

Results

Overall Summary

Of the 121 households evaluated, 26% met the minimal Audits International criteria for acceptable performance. Households averaged 1.7 critical violatoins with a range from 0 to 5. At least one critical violation was observed in 69% of the households. Households averaged 3.2 major violations with a range from 0 to 8.

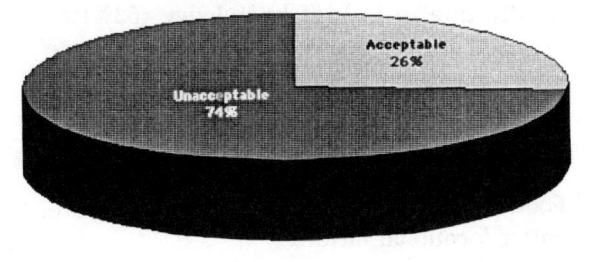

41. Audits International's Home Food Safety Survey

Major Violations

Education Versus Motivation

When auditors observed one of six chosen critical violations (cross contamination, handling of leftovers, handwashing, chemical storage, ingredient cooking, and cold ingredient holding) the auditor would point out the violation to the participant, then ask why the violation was committed. Responses were categorized either as lack of education (ex. "I was not aware I was doing it.") or lack of motivation (ex. "I don't think using proper practices is very important."). The responses offered by participants are as follows:

Major Violations	Households Observed (n=121)
	Frequency (%)
Improper thermometer use	79
Food handler smoking/eating/drinking/gum chewing	55
Common cloth/sponge/towel misused	49
Product present past "Use-by" date	46
Refrigerated ingredient temperatures too high	23
Clean dishes and pans not drying properly	17
Improper food preparation procedures	12
Cross contamination issues	12
Improper leftover procedures	11
Hand drying towels unavailable	5
Frozen ingredient temperatures too high	4
Pest activity evident in household	4

Most Frequently Observed Major Violations

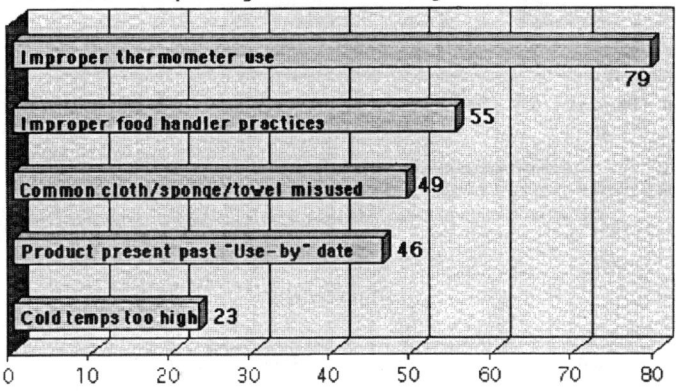

- Improper thermometer use: 79
- Improper food handler practices: 55
- Common cloth/sponge/towel misused: 49
- Product present past "Use-by" date: 46
- Cold temps too high: 23

5 ❖ FOOD SAFETY

Violation*	OA	CC	HL	HW	CS	IC	CH
	\multicolumn{7}{c}{Frequency (%)}
Educational Responses**	62	65	61	59	67	65	70
Motivational Responses	38	35	39	41	33	43	30
I don't think it is very important	11	16	6	19	5	0	20
I am willing to take the risk and ignore the guideline	7	10	6	9	10	0	0
It takes too much time to do it right	5	0	12	6	5	5	0
I have always done it this way and see no reason to change	5	3	3	6	0	19	0
I am confused by the multiple standards I have heard or read about	5	0	12	0	5	10	10
I don't agree with the safety principle	4	6	0	0	10	10	0

*OA = overall (combined); CC = cross contamination observed; HL = Improper cooling of leftovers; HW = Neglected handwashing; CS = cleaning supplies or chemicals improperly stored/labeled; IC = Finished internal cooking temperatures too low; CH = Refrigerated ingredient temperatures too high

Testing Knowledge Versus Testing Performance

Upon completion of the observational portion of the evaluation, auditors quizzed participants in each of six areas of high concern. The following table lists how often participants were able to answer all quiz questions for a category correctly and how often the participant met all criteria during observation (i.e. didn't receive a critical violation).

Violation*	OA	CC	HL	HW	CS	IC	C
	\multicolumn{7}{c}{Frequency (%)}
All questions in quiz answered correctly**	37	55	23	79	60	7	0.8
All criteria met during observation	77	69	71	71	80	81	91

**OA = overall (combined average of other six columns); CC = cross contamination observed; HL = Improper cooling of leftovers; HW = Neglected handwashing; CS = cleaning supplies or chemicals improperly stored/labeled; IC = Finished internal cooking temperatures too low; CH = Refrigerated ingredient temperatures too high

Discussion

Overall Improvement

Over six times as many households met criteria in this study compared to the 1997 results (4% vs. 26%). The frequency of households receiving at least one critical violation decreased from 96% to 69%. The number of critical violations observed per household also decreased between studies, from an adjusted average of 2.3 to 1.7 critical violations per household.

Results	1977	1999
	\multicolumn{2}{c}{Frequency (%)}
Household achieving acceptable standards	4	26
Number of critical violations per household	2.3	1.7
Number of critical violations per household	4.0	3.2

Although the increase in acceptable households is encouraging, nearly three-quarters of all households failed to meet criteria. The increase in acceptable households indicates that food safety awareness is reaching a higher level of consciousness, but further steps to motivate and educate the public are necessary.

Factors Causing Critical Violations

When a violation was observed, the follow-up questions identified that the violations were mostly due to lack of knowledge (62%) as opposed to a perceived lack of importance (38%). Based on this observation, attempting to change the population's food safety practices should continue to focus on education. One of the primary goals of the 2000 Home Food Safety Study will be to further investigate educational factors.

Media Driven Improvement

The increase in the frequency of acceptable households could be partially attributed to the recent attention the media is paying to food safety. While this study did not evaluate the *reasons* people change their practices, a non-published Audits International study conducted in 1998 investigated what was responsible for increasing awareness in food safety. Those participants not included in Audits International's 1997 study listed television (73%) and print media (63%) as the most significant reasons for raising their awareness of food safety, which could directly influence behavior. The responses given as what increased food safety awareness are listed below:

	Frequency(%)
Television	73
Newspapers	53
Magazines	41
Family and friends	35
Government	10
Advice from doctors	6
Schooling	4

Knowledge Is a Poor Indicator

When it comes to food safety, it is difficult to measure what the general population does by what they know. The ability to demonstrate knowledge did not correlate to proper performance. As an example, 79% of all participants could correctly identify each of five instances when handwashing was necessary. However, 20% of the respondents that did correctly identify all instances still received a critical violation for neglected handwashing.

Conversely, lack of knowledge did not mean a violation was imminent. Very few participants demonstrated knowledge in cooking ingredient to proper temperature (7%). Even without this knowledge, 81% of all households still cooked their foods to proper temperatures.

Children Are a Motivating Factor

Households with young children were over three times as likely to achieve acceptable standards as those without children. Children in households where the head of the kitchen was under 50 years old were considered young. Of thirty-two households with children and a head of kitchen under 50 years old, 28% were deemed acceptable. Just one of 13 households without children and a head of kitchen under 50 years old was acceptable (8%).

Advancing Awareness in Food Safety Is Everyone's Business

The 1997 study demonstrated that food safety must become everyone's concern. The improvement in overall results found in 1999 implies that the general population is becoming more aware of food safety issues. The kitchen is often the last chance we have to limit the risks of foodborne illness. It is imperative that those who prepare meals in their homes understand the importance of proper food safety practices. It is because of this that Audits International plans to conduct a home food safety survey each year to help increase public awareness.

Conclusions

The results of the 1999 home food safety survey demonstrate six key issues:

- the situation is improving with regards to home food safety but we still have a long way to go;
- knowledge tests do not necessarily indicate performance - it is important to observe what people are doing;
- the majority of errors (critical violations) are based on is education (knowledge or conscious awareness) rather than motivation;
- families with small children are more motivated than those without;
- media appear to be the driving force behind the change;
- it is in all of our interests to keep the ball rolling.

Questions to be answered in the Audits International 2000 home food safety study include:

- Where does the population as a whole stand in their food safety practices? It is our belief that the sample chosen here would do better that the general population. In order to answer the question, it is necessary to incorporate a more random stratified sample.
- What do people really know about food safety? Are the violations attributed to education caused by not knowing the standards, or a lack of conscious awareness of what they are doing?

Home Food Safety Survey Definition of Terms

Clean dishes and pans not air drying properly The process of stacking dishes or pans that are not completely dry in a fashion that could result in moisture trapped between two. This moisture provides an environment beneficial to some types of bacterial growth.

Common cloth/sponge/ towel misused Separate cloths, sponges, and towels should be used for washing dishes, wiping counters and tables, wiping hands, and drying clean dishes. *Using a common towel for more than one of these purposes could allow cross-contamination.*

Cross contamination A practice causing the potential transfer of harmful substances or disease-causing micro-organisms from one food or food ingredient to another. Other than neglected handwashing, the most frequently observed forms of cross-contamination were (1) failure to wash cutting board between uses. (2) storage of raw materials above ready-to-eat foods, (3) failure to wash whole produce, (4) cloth, sponge, or towel used in a manner resulting in a direct threat of cross-contamination, (5) utensils not washed with soap before use.

Dented, rusted, or swelling cans present Observation of any can which is swollen, or has flawed seals, seams, rust, dents or leaks.

Disposable plastic gloves not properly used Failure to cover bandages with gloves may permit the introduction of pathogenic bacteria to food

Finished internal cooking temperatures too low Cooking to less than the minimum safe internal temperature required to destroy pathogens (critical violation: Fruits and Vegetables < 140°F for 15 seconds; Commercially Pre-cooked Foods < 140°F for 15 seconds; Fish and Seafood < 145°F for 15 seconds; Beef <145°F for three minutes; Ground Beef < 155°F for 15 seconds; Pork < 155°F for 15 seconds; Poultry < 165°F for 15 seconds; Casserole < 165°F for 15 seconds; Reheated Leftovers < 165°F for 15 seconds).

Food handlers smoking/ eating/drinking/gum chewing These habits encourage mouth-to-hand-to-food contamination and can lead to the introduction of a foreign substance to food which may cause a foodborne illness.

Frozen ingredient temperatures too high Frozen product and ingredient temperatures which could permit rapid bacterial growth (critical violation: > 45°F; major violation: 29–45°F).

Hand drying towels unavailable To prevent the use of aprons or clothing for drying hands, each handwashing sink should have towels available.

Hot and cold water available at all sinks Each faucet should allow hot and cold water to mix to a temperature of at least 110°F.

Hot ingredient holding too cool Maintaining hot foods temperatures which permit rapid bacteria growth (critical violation: < 140°F; major violation: 140–144°F).

Improper chemical labeling Failure to keep household chemicals in labeled containers.

Improper chemical storage Chemicals stored in such a way that they may contaminate food, food contact surfaces, or equipment.

Improper cooling of leftovers Any food that is not cooled after cooking or hot holding from 140°F to 70°F in two hours and to 41°F in an additional four hours for a total of less than six hours cooling time.

41. Audits International's Home Food Safety Survey

Improper food preparation techniques and procedures	Conducting food preparation using any of the below described procedures can be the direct cause of or serve as a contributing factor in foodborne illness: 1. Use of non-pasteurized eggs for uncooked egg-based products (critical) 2. Leaving hazardous items unattended at room temperature (critical) 3. Incorrect thawing practices (definition listed-major) 4. Use of non-chilled ingredients to make sandwiches or salads (major) Use of non pre-chilled ingredients to make sandwiches or salads (ex. tuna salad). Ingredients that are not pre-chilled increase the temperature of the final product and increase the risk of the product being inside the temperature danger zone (40–140°F).
Improper leftover procedures	The presence of leftovers older than 4 days present or leftovers cooled to 42–45°F after six total hours of cooling.
Improper thermometer use	Failure to regularly measure temperatures of held or prepared foods
Incorrect thawing practices	Reducing food temperatures incorrectly from frozen to temperatures suitable for cooking rather than by using one of four proper techniques: 1. In a refrigerator 2. Under running drinkable water at 70°F or lower within two hours 3. As part of the cooking process 4. In a microwave (this method should always be followed by immediate cooking)
Neglected handwashing	Failing to wash hands (1) when first starting to handle food, (2) after using the phone, (3) after touching face, hair, body or other people, (4) after handling garbage, dirty dishes or cleaning, (5) after using the restroom.
Pest activity evident in household	Any indication that a foodservice area is inhabited by pests (insects/rodents).
Product past "Use-by" date	Expiration times are meant to maintain product quality and safety. Any ingredient past manufacturer's "use-by" date should be discarded.
Refrigerated ingredient temperatures too high	Refrigerated product and ingredient temperatures which permit rapid bacterial growth (critical violation: > 45°F; major violation: 42–45°F).
Sick/symptomatic food handler preparing food	Food handlers with cold or flu-like symptoms that may cause food to be contaminated.

Note: Definitions were adapted from the *ServSafe® Serving Safe Food Certification Coursebook*, Copyright 1995, by The Educational Foundation of the National Restaurant Association.

Article 42

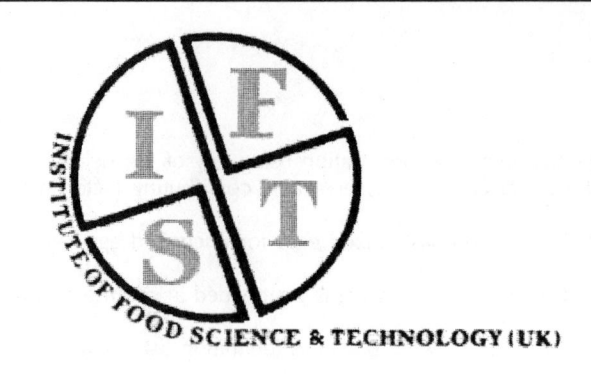

Avoiding cross-contamination in the home

The Institute of Food Science & Technology, through its Public Affairs and Technical & Legislative Committees, has authorised this paper, dated 25 May 1999, and prepared by its Professional Food Microbiology Group, as an IFST contribution to the 7th Foodlink National Food Safety Week which runs from 7–13 June 1999.

SUMMARY

Cross-contamination is a major cause of food poisoning. Food poisoning is preventable—avoiding cross-contamination is simple. Here we offer ten pointers for avoiding cross contamination in the home.

Where can germs be found?

Germs (food-poisoning organisms) exist harmlessly in many natural environments, for example farmyards and farm animals, poultry and wild birds and on fields that are fertilised with 'organic' manure. People and animals suffering from food-poisoning can also shed large numbers of germs, either through sickness or diarrhoea.

Insects, rodents and other pests ('vermin') as well as domestic pets can also harbour germs and transfer them from one place to another.

Germs may therefore be found in foods that are to be cooked. If the cooking is thorough, many types of germs (though not all) are killed, so their presence in raw foods such as meat, poultry, fish, eggs and vegetables may not be important provided these foods are cooked properly. However, these raw foods may spread contamination to other, unpackaged, ready-to-eat foods such as cheese, sandwiches, salad vegetables, cooked meats, pies and desserts.

What is cross-contamination and why must it be avoided?

Cross-contamination is the transfer of germs from their natural habitat to uncontaminated, ready to eat food.

Germs do not always cause food-poisoning, although for some people even low numbers may constitute a risk. The risk of food-poisoning increases greatly if germs are allowed to multiply ('breed'), either in the food itself or in a dirty place that can contaminate the food with large numbers of germs. Foods that not eaten immediately after thorough cooking should be stored in the 'fridge.

How does cross-contamination occur?

Cross-contamination, is its simplest form, occurs, for example, if blood from raw meat drips directly onto a ready-to-eat dessert placed at the bottom of the

42. Avoiding Cross-Contamination in the Home

'fridge, or in the shopping bag if the food is not properly wrapped.

Almost anything that is dirty can also transfer germs indirectly from a source of contamination to uncontaminated foods. Here are a few examples of common routes of cross-contamination:-

- hands
- dishcloths, teatowels, handtowels, aprons and floor cloths (especially if allowed to become dirty or remain wet)
- work surfaces
- packaging used for raw foods
- pets (especially if allowed to walk on the worktop)
- pets' bowls
- vermin
- dirty rinse water and washing up bowls
- waste bins and dustbins
- children's toys that have been in the garden
- dirty utensils or utensils that have been in contact with raw egg, meat or vegetables, for example chopping boards, knives, bowls and food processors.

Ten points for avoiding cross-contamination in the home

1. Remember that raw foods come from farms. Germs exist naturally even on the most hygienic farms so we must assume that raw food might be contaminated and keep it separate from ready-to-eat-food. This applies to **all** raw foods, even if 'free-range' or 'organic' and whether you have bought them in the village store or from the supermarket. Therefore **choose foods that have been processed for safety.** The World Health Organisation recommends that consumers should, for example:
   - always buy pasteurised milk
   - thoroughly wash certain foods eaten raw, such as lettuce, other salad vegetables and fruit.

2. **Keep raw and cooked foods apart during storage,** either in the refrigerator, the freezer or the larder. Store ready-to-eat food above raw meat and poultry. Commodities such as salad vegetables may be placed in the middle. Cover all food and place on a plate any food that is likely to drip.

3. **Use different utensils for preparing raw and cooked foods.** Don't, for example, prepare a raw chicken and then use the same unwashed cutting board and knife to carve the cooked bird. After preparing raw foods in a food processor, clean the parts thoroughly using hot water with detergent or in the dishwasher. Remember that using separate utensils is just as important when cooking on the barbeque!

4. **Wash hands, including finger-tips,** thoroughly with soap and water for at least 20 seconds and dry them thoroughly before you start preparing food. Do this **repeatedly** during food preparation—after every interruption and **always** if you have had to change the baby's nappy or have been to the toilet. After preparing raw foods such as fish, meat, or poultry, wash again before you start handling other foods. Rings can harbour germs—remove them before preparing food!

5. **Keep all kitchen surfaces meticulously clean** because every food scrap, crumb or spot is a potential reservoir of germs. The most important aspect of cleaning is physical removal of germs using hot water, a detergent and 'elbow grease' to remove food residues, especially fat. Disinfectants only work at their best on a surface that is already clean!

6. Frequently change cloths that come into contact with plates and utensils and wash in very hot water before re-use. **After use, dry dishcloths, teatowels, handtowels and aprons rapidly to stop any germs from breeding.** Don't use floorcloths for cleaning plates and utensils. Wash and dry floorcloths after use on floors!

7. **Dry the washing by allowing the items to drain naturally and rapidly or by using a dishwasher!** These are the most hygienic methods.

8. **Protect foods from domestic pets, insects and rodents. Do not allow domestic pets to walk on kitchen worktops!** Remember, too, that smaller pets such as birds and especially turtles often harbour germs.

9. **Always use clean, drinkable water for food preparation and for washing up.** After washing foods that are to be cooked, change the water before washing ready-to-eat foods.

10. **Do not prepare food for others if you are sick or have a severe skin infection.** Cover cuts with waterproof plasters.

Additional precautions

If you suspect cooked, or ready-to-eat/food might be contaminated, don't eat it!

Take the same precautions with cutting boards, utensils and other items that contain an antibacterial as with ordinary ones. Germs breed less quickly on those with built-in antimicrobial, but if they become contaminated they are just as liable to transmit contamination.

Remember:

Food-poisoning is preventable—avoiding cross-contamination is simple!

Also visit Foodlink at
http://www.curryhouse.co.uk/cw/foodlink.htm

The Institute of Food Science & Technology (IFST) is the independent professional qualifying body for food scientists and technologists. It is totally independent of government, of industry, and of any lobbying groups or special interest groups. Its professional members are elected by virtue of their academic qualifications and their relevant experience, and their signed undertaking to comply with the Institute's ethical Code of Professional Conduct. They are elected solely in their personal capacities and in no way representing organisations where they may be employed. They work in a variety of areas, including universities and other centres of higher education, research institutions, food and related industries, consultancy, food law enforcement authorities, and in government departments and agencies. The nature of the Institute and the mixture of these backgrounds on the working groups drafting IFST Position Statements, and on the two Committees responsible for finalising and approving them, ensure that the contents are entirely objective.

IFST recognises that research is constantly bringing new knowledge. However, collectively the profession is the repository of existing knowledge in its field. It includes researchers expanding the boundaries of knowledge and experts seeking to apply it for the public benefit.

Why You Need A Kitchen Thermometer

YOU'VE GRILLED YOUR hamburger until it looks brown in the middle, so it's safe to eat, right? Wrong, says the U.S. Department of Agriculture's Food Safety and Inspection Service. The government bacteria busters warn that you can't use visual cues like color or texture to judge whether ground meat has been cooked thoroughly enough to kill potentially harmful microbes.

The only way to know for sure whether ground beef—or any meat, poultry, or casserole—has been safely cooked is to use a kitchen thermometer. Unfortunately, in a survey conducted by the USDA, only about half of those questioned said they do. Considering that dangerous pathogens like *E. coli* 0157:H7 can be killed only at high temperatures, that's a lot of people who are putting themselves at unnecessary risk of foodborne illness.

The reason that using your eye to judge a burger's "doneness" won't cut it is that the natural pigment of raw red meat (which can range from purple to red to brown depending on the age of the animal and whether the meat was exposed to air) could change to brown before the meat is fully cooked, according to Bessie Berry, manager of the USDA's Meat and Poultry Hotline. Using marinades can also make a burger appear brown before it has reached a safe internal temperature.

Testing a burger to see whether the juices run clear is an equally faulty method. "What does 'clear' really mean?" challenges Ms. Berry. "Should the juice have no color at all? Or just no evidence of pink? The color you see could change according to the background lighting, the plate you use, and how much juice you squeeze out of the burger."

The meat thermometers that everyone should depend on (instead of their eyes) come in several models, and safe temperatures will differ according to what type of meat, poultry, or casserole you're cooking. (See charts at right.) When checking a meat's temperature, make sure to put the thermometer in the deepest, thickest part of the roast or patty. You may have to turn chops, chicken breasts, or burgers sideways to get an accurate reading. Make sure your thermometer is properly calibrated (you can do this by taking the temperature of boiling water, which should read 212 degrees Fahrenheit), and always wash it in hot, soapy water after each use.

Note: While checking temperatures at the grill or stove may sound cumbersome, some types of thermometers take only 10 seconds or so to get a reading.

Know When Your Dinner Is *Really* Done

Here are the minimum internal temperatures that different foods must reach to be safe to eat, according to the USDA. These temperatures apply whether the foods are roasted, broiled, grilled, baked, or fried.

	degrees Fahrenheit
Ground beef, veal, lamb, pork	160
Beef, veal, lamb (steaks, roasts, chops)	145
Pork (roasts, chops)	160
Ham	
uncooked	160
precooked	140
Poultry	
ground chicken, turkey	165
whole chicken, turkey	180
breasts	170
thighs, wings	180
Stuffing (cooked alone or in bird)	165
Egg dishes, casseroles	160
Leftovers*	165

* Reheated soups and gravies should be brought to a rolling boil. All other leftovers should be hot and steaming.

5 ❖ FOOD SAFETY

Finding a Food Thermometer

Type of Thermometer	What It's Best For*
Liquid-Filled	Roasts, casseroles, and soups. Thermometer can remain in food while it's cooking. Must be placed at least 2 inches deep; it can't measure temperature in thin foods. Takes 1 or 2 minutes to get a reading.
Bimetal [oven-safe]	Roasts, turkeys, or other large items. This is the traditional "meat thermometer" that remains in food throughout cooking; it can be read at a glance, but the long probe makes it a poor choice for foods less than 3 inches thick. Also, since the metal stem conducts heat, readings must be taken in two or three different places to avoid getting a false high reading. Takes 1 or 2 minutes to get a reading.
Bimetal [instant-read]	Roasts, casseroles, and soups. Since it reads temperature in 15 to 20 seconds, it can be used to check foods at the end of cooking time. However, it can't be used in the oven while food is cooking, and it must be inserted sideways into thin goods.
Thermistor [digital]	Any foods; especially good for thin foods like burgers because it needs to be inserted only ½ inch deep. Reads temperature in 10 seconds; digital face is easy to see. However, it can't be used in the oven while food is cooking.

* Based on technical information from the USDA Food Safety and Inspection Service

Campylobacter

Low-Profile Bug Is Food Poisoning Leader

by Audrey Hingley

When it comes to food poisoning, big outbreaks make headlines. E. coli in apple juice and alfalfa sprouts. *Listeria* in cheese and hot dogs. *Salmonella* in eggs and on poultry. But the most frequently diagnosed food-borne bacterium rarely makes the news. The name of the unsung bug? *Campylobacter.*

"Most *Campylobacter* infections are sporadic and not associated with an outbreak, but we know it causes up to 4 million human infections a year," says Frederick J. Angulo, D.V.M., an epidemiologist with the national Centers for Disease Control and Prevention.

Federal and state health experts have long recognized that *Campylobacter* causes disease in animals. Conclusive proof that the bacteria also causes human disease emerged in the 1970s, and by 1996, *Campylobacter* was sitting atop the bacterial heap as the number one cause of all domestic food-borne illness.

In addition, with the emergence of antibiotic-resistant *Campylobacter,* "the true magnitude of the problem is becoming clearer," says Angulo, who also heads the CDC arm of the National Antimicrobial Resistance Monitoring System.

Campylobacter is commonly found in the intestinal tracts of people or animals without causing any symptoms of illness. But eating contaminated or undercooked poultry or meat, or drinking raw milk or contaminated water, may cause *Campylobacter* infection, or campylobacteriosis.

Symptoms of campylobacteriosis usually occur within two to 10 days of ingesting the bacteria. Children, the elderly, and people with weakened immune systems are particularly at risk. The most common symptoms include mild to severe diarrhea, fever, nausea, vomiting, and abdominal pain.

Most people infected with *Campylobacter* can get well on their own without treatment, though antibiotics may be prescribed for severe cases. But complications can occur, such as urinary tract infections or meningitis. The bacteria also is now recognized as a major contributing factor to Guillain-Barré syndrome, the most common cause of acute paralysis in both children and adults.

Concerns About Chicken

Although found in many farm animals, *Campylobacter* in poultry is causing experts the most concern. There have been several studies pointing to high levels of *Campylobacter* present on poultry at the retail level, including a recent two-year Minnesota Department of Health study that found that 88 percent of poultry sampled from local supermarkets tested positive for the bacteria.

"The retail study was in collaboration with the Minnesota Department of Agriculture; their inspectors went to supermarkets throughout the St. Paul/Minneapolis Twin Cities area to cover a variety of supermarket types, from big chains to mom-and-pop stores," says Kirk E. Smith, D.V.M., a Minnesota state epidemiologist who participated in the study.

Many prior surveys have found *Campylobacter* contamination rates of between 40 and 60 percent, he says. "But 88 percent—this degree [of contamination] surprised even me," he admits.

In studies conducted by the U.S. Department of Agriculture's poultry microbiological safety research unit, more than 90 percent of poultry tested positive for *Campylobacter*, in levels ranging from one cell to over a million cells per bird.

Norman J. Stern, Ph.D., research leader for the unit, says the infection of poultry broiler flocks typically occurs at week three in the six-week growing cycle. It's not unusual, he says, for *Campylobacter* to infect the entire flock.

Things only get worse by the time the chickens reach the processing plant, he says. USDA studies have found a hundredfold increase in bacteria amounts on the birds' exterior from that detected on the farm. "The exterior contamination represents consumer exposure," he explains.

To help reduce that exposure, Stern says the poultry industry is currently participating in a USDA-led study that will cover "every element of production where chickens can become infected, from . . . shells to farmers' boots to wild bird droppings. When we're done . . . we will be able to genetically fingerprint the organism so we can ascribe a relationship between various environmental sources and the spread of pathogens." The study was slated to end in September.

Resistance to Antibiotics

According to the Minnesota Department of Health study, the number of *Campylobacter* infections that are resistant to a class of antibiotics called fluoroquinolones has been on the increase since 1992. While most Americans acquired the resistant infections while on foreign travel, Kirk explains, "we have been seeing a significant increase in domestically acquired resistant cases as well." The Food and Drug Administration approved the use of fluoroquinolones in food animals in 1995. The study concluded that antibiotic use in U.S. poultry is contributing to antibiotic resistance.

Resistance to fluoroquinolones, not only by *Campylobacter* but by other bacteria as well, is a concern, explains Jesse Goodman, M.D., chief of the division of infectious diseases at the University of Minnesota, "because fluoroquinolones are commonly used to treat severe infectious diarrhea, often before the specific cause has been identified. Fluoroquinolones are very important drugs for treating a variety of serious human infectious diseases."

CDC studies also show an increase in resistance to fluoroquinolones and this can be correlated to fluoroquinolone use in poultry, according to Angulo. In addition, "We did a case control study in 1997, comparing people with [nonresistant] *Campylobacter* infections with fluoroquinolone-resistant infections, and found that those with resistant infections [were] more likely to have severe infections, bloody diarrhea, and be hospitalized."

Because of the concern over antibiotic resistance, FDA is considering whether, before it reviews a new animal drug for approval, manufacturers must assess the likelihood that use of a certain drug in food animals will transfer resistance and create a public health problem. In addition, new procedures for monitoring antibiotic use and resistance after approval also are being considered.

"FDA believes a new regulatory framework is needed to address resistance concerns raised by the food animal use of antibiotics," says Goodman, who also serves as a deputy medical director for FDA.

The Animal Health Institute, a national trade association representing manufacturers of animal health products, says it also is concerned about the possibility of antibiotic use in food animals causing resistant bacteria to develop. But the organization believes that the requirements FDA is proposing may have "unintended negative consequences on animal health . . . and risk sending unhealthy animals into the food chain."

Hollinger says, "At this time we are not taking action toward withdrawal of these products from the market. We have asked the sponsors of poultry fluoroquinolone products to provide data that would describe the prevalence of resistance in poultry flocks and identify possible actions to prevent the emergence of disease in treated flocks."

Calling it a "farm to plate" approach, Hollinger says that the *Campylobacter* problem can be addressed "at any number of points" along the food chain. "They all need to be reviewed and evaluated for new methods to deal with the problems."

USDA's Stern says he believes the poultry industry is "trying very hard" to move toward enhanced food safety for economic as well as safety benefits. For example, he explains, a company could use extensive microbiological criteria to ensure safety as a marketing tool. Just as consumers are willing to pay more for "gourmet" coffees or specialty food items, an increasingly health-conscious consumer could be wooed by a health emphasis when it comes to safer poultry products, he says.

Vaccine on the Horizon

A team of Navy, Army, and drug industry researchers is also moving ahead in the development of a prototype vaccine for *Campylobacter*. The vaccine has shown promise in animal models and currently is undergoing clinical trials.

Capt. Louis A. Bourgeois, director of the enteric diseases program at the Naval Medical Research Center in Bethesda, Md., says the Navy has been involved in *Campylobacter* research since the early 1980s.

"Historically, the military has had longstanding diarrheal problems with troops deploying overseas," he explains. "*Campylobacter* was an emerging pathogen in the early '80s, and by the mid-1980s, we began doing more directed studies towards a vaccine development."

Bourgeois and his fellow researchers say an approved vaccine is likely "several years away" but they remain optimistic. Bourgeois says private companies are interested in a vaccine due to its possible application in "traveler's diarrhea," a common ailment.

"We know from animal model work that we can protect animals against *Campylobacter* colonization," says colleague Daniel Scott, M.D., deputy director of the Navy's enteric diseases program. "We have also gained an increasing amount of knowledge in the clinical and preclinical development of this product, especially in terms of what happens with the actual infection. We are already seeing some evidence that term protection can occur, which allows for a lot of optimism."

The Consumer's Role

While researchers, regulatory agencies, and scientists grapple with *Campylobacter*, what can you do to protect yourself?

"Consumers go to the supermarket thinking everything [there] is clean, and that is just not true," says Donald H. Burr, Ph.D., a research microbiologist in FDA's Center for Food Safety and Applied Nutrition. "People can't assume that anymore. Consumers have a responsibility in food safety."

Those responsibilities include prompt refrigeration, thorough cooking, avoiding cross-contamination, and washing hands and surfaces often. In addition:

- Don't let raw foods such as uncooked poultry touch other food, since bacteria can spread.
- Thaw raw poultry on a bottom shelf in the refrigerator so that blood or juices don't drip onto other foods.
- Do not reuse marinades from raw meat or poultry.
- Never put cooked poultry or meat back on the plate that held the raw product.
- Wash your hands frequently, especially after handling raw meat and poultry.
- Wash kitchen surfaces and cutting boards often, especially after they have come in contact with raw meat or poultry.

Audrey Hingley is a writer in Mechanicsville, Va.

Tracking Down Trouble

Bacteria That Cause Food-Borne Illness

Bacteria	Cases of Food-Borne Illness
Listeria	77
Vibrio	51
Yersinia	139
E. coli O157:H7	340
Shigella	1,263
Salmonella	2,207
Campylobacter	3,974
Total	8,051

Campylobacter was the culprit in an overwhelming number of cases detected by the FoodNet system in 1997. FoodNet, a joint project of FDA, the national Centers for Disease Control, and USDA's Food Safety and Inspection Service, tracks cases of food-borne infections at early-warning sites in several states. The numbers are combined totals from California, Connecticut, Georgia, Minnesota, and Oregon.

E. Coli 0157:H7—How Dangerous Has It Become?

Escherichia coli 0157:H7 is now recognized as an important cause of bloody diarrhea; it causes hemorrhagic colitis, which begins with watery diarrhea and severe abdominal pain and rapidly progresses to passage of bloody stools. It is the leading cause of postdiarrheal hemolytic-uremic syndrome (HUS), characterized by acute kidney failure, among children in the U.S. and Canada. Infection with *E. coli* 0157:H7 results in a disturbingly high frequency of serious complications. Data from outbreak investigations in the U.S. suggest 5%–10% of infected children develop HUS. Approximately 25,000 cases of food-borne illness can be attributed to *E. coli* 0157:H7 each year, resulting in as many as 100 deaths.

Among the identified dietary risk factors, foods of bovine origin, particularly undercooked ground beef, have been the most frequently implicated source. Other foods, such as apple cider and mayonnaise-containing sauces, have also been implicated in outbreaks. However, the original source of contamination in these cases was suspected of being of bovine or other animal origin. Nondietary risk factors include person-to-person transmission in daycare settings or swimming in contaminated water.

L. Slutsker et al. reported on a two-year case-control study in the U.S. in which 118 cases of *E. coli* 0157:H7 were found in 30,463 persons examined. Case questionnaires were completed by 93 patients. Eighty-six did not develop HUS, but 100% had diarrhea, 92% had abdominal cramps, 90% had bloody diarrhea, 45% had nausea, 45% had subjective fever, and 37% had vomiting. The seven patients with HUS ranged in age from one to 82 years. Vomiting within three days of diarrhea onset was the only symptom significantly associated with HUS. Those patients younger than 13 years old who developed HUS were more likely to have received an antimicrobial agent within three days after onset of their diarrhea. Other than hamburgers and hot dogs, no other foods were positively associated with illness, including other beef, poultry, or dairy products. (See *J Infect Dis*, 1998; 177:962.)

Consumption of visibly undercooked ground beef was the only dietary factor independently associated with *E. coli* 0157:H7-related diarrhea. The findings of the current study are supported by two Canadian studies that linked sporadic *E. coli* 0157:H7 infection with consumption of undercooked meat and undercooked ground beef at picnics or special events. The fact that undercooked ground beef rather than ground beef *per se* was a risk factor for infection underscores the importance of proper cooking for prevention of *E. coli* 0157:H7 infection.

Recently, outbreaks of *E. coli* 0157:H7 have been linked to fresh produce, specifically leaf and iceberg lettuce and unpasteurized apple cider and juice. Local unchlorinated water sources such as rural wells are also potential sources. Prevention of sporadic infection requires recognition and modification of risk factors. In addition, since the infectious dose for this pathogen is low and person-to-person spread not uncommon, it is important to identify cases to prevent secondary transmission in households and in the community.

The Source of *E. Coli* 0157:H7

How did the relatively innocuous bacterium *Escherichia coli* found in human and animal intestines become the deadly strain of *E. coli* 0157:H7? It is theorized that this deadly strain was created from a dysentery epidemic in Central America. Scientists believe that a virus, which invades cells like bacteria to reproduce, carried a toxin-producing gene from *Shigella*, the bacteria that were causing the epidemic, over to *E. coli*.

The resultant *E. coli* 0157:H7 is surprisingly tough and virulent. Most bacteria do not produce disease unless a person is exposed to millions of them, but as few as 10 *E. coli* 0157:H7 can produce illness—far too few to see or smell. While most bacteria, including those which cause botulism, cannot live in acidic environments, *E. coli* 0157:H7 is able to grow in foods like unpasteurized apple cider and commercial mayonnaise. This acid tolerance may also signal the pathogen's resistance to other protective measures such as heat, radiation, and antimicrobials. Successful prevention strategies must focus on eliminating the presence of the microorganism, rather than on preventing pathogen growth as is traditionally done.

Dairy cows and other cattle seem to be the "Typhoid Marys" of the epidemics, carrying the bacteria harmlessly in their feces. From there, the bacteria enter the food supply. A single contaminated carcass can be ground up with scores of other cows to produce hamburgers. *E. coli* 0157:H7 has gotten into apple cider possibly because farmers fertilized their crops with cow manure or cows grazed in the orchard. The same may be said for the lettuce and alfalfa sprouts. Washing prepackaged salad mixes and vegetables, even if the label says they are prewashed, would help prevent this source of contamination.

Preventive Measures

To kill any disease-causing bacteria, the following procedures are recommended. For whole cuts of meat, sear the entire surface; the interior of a whole cut is generally safe. Cook ground beef, veal, lamb, and pork to an internal temperature of 160° F; 165° F for ground poultry; and 180° F for whole poultry. Washing hands with soap and hot running water while rubbing hands together for 20 seconds is an effective preventive recommendation for all food handlers.

The FDA wants the food industry to take more responsibility. It is working on voluntary guidelines to encourage safer handling of fruits and vegetables, similar to the HACCP guidelines in place for fish, meats, poultry, dairy, and eggs.

Article 46

A crackdown on bad eggs

Egg-carton warnings sought to fight salmonella outbreaks

By Amanda Spake

The first call to the Henrico County, Va., Health Department on June 1 came from a concerned mother. Her teenager had ended up in the hospital emergency room with salmonella poisoning after a trip to the local International House of Pancakes, outside Richmond.

On June 2, the department's staff ordered the IHOP closed. Within days, hundreds of people called the health department complaining of diarrhea, vomiting, fever, and cramps. "We had 121 people confirmed with *Salmonella enteritidis*," says Elizabeth Barrett, assistant state epidemiologist. Many more people probably were sick; nationwide, only about 1 in 39 *Salmonella enteritidis* infections is reported to health departments. Barrett is certain of one thing: "Eggs appear to be the likely source of the outbreak."

The Virginia outbreak is just the latest of many problems with the safety of eggs. Last week, Congress's General Accounting Office released a report highly critical of the federal government's response to an estimated 661,633 food poisonings yearly from eggs contaminated with *Salmonella enteritidis* bacteria, and 331 deaths. In a congressional hearing last Thursday, Sen. Dick Durbin of Illinois took the U.S. Food and Drug Administration and the Department of Agriculture's Food Safety and Inspection Service to task for failing to set egg refrigeration rules mandated by Congress in 1991. "It took *eight years* just to come up with a temperature standard?" an incredulous Durbin asked. "Eight years?"

The long-awaited temperature standard, which takes effect next month, requires eggs be refrigerated to an air temperature of 45 degrees or below while in storage or shipment to retail outlets, since refrigeration retards bacterial growth. By week's end, the FDA had come up with a similar standard for supermarkets, restaurants, and other institutions. But the rule may not stop salmonella infections, according to the GAO, since FSIS studies show it is the *internal* temperature of the egg, not air temperature, that should remain at 45 degrees. So the FDA proposed what amounts to a warning label for egg cartons, saying that

---

PLAYING IT SAFE
Just say no to over easy

The egg-carton warning label proposed by the FDA would go a long way toward describing the safest way for consumers to handle fresh eggs. The labeling would read: "Eggs may contain harmful bacteria known to cause serious illness, especially in children, the elderly, and persons with weakened immune systems. For your protection: Keep eggs refrigerated; cook eggs until yolks are firm; and cook food containing eggs thoroughly."

Infections from *Salmonella enteritidis* result when raw or undercooked eggs contaminated with the bacteria are consumed. Even a small amount of the bacteria can cause illness. Specific steps for protection include:

■ Use eggs within 30 days of purchase and keep them in the refrigerator.
■ Don't use cracked or broken eggs.
■ Use pasteurized eggs in recipes that call for raw eggs, such as Caesar salad dressing or homemade ice cream.
■ Don't eat raw cake or cookie batter.
■ Make sure dishes containing eggs, such as lasagna or french toast, reach 160 degrees in the center.
■ Think twice about eating scrambled eggs on brunch buffets. Restaurants commonly "pool" eggs. One bad egg can infect a whole batch.
■ Don't eat eggs sunny-side up or with runny yolks.

"bacteria known to cause serious illness" may be present.

The proposed regulations may simply add more confusion to the crazy quilt of federal, state, and industry standards on egg safety. Some states require egg dating on cartons, for example. Yet there is no federal standard for how long eggs can be sold, even though scientists know that after about 28 days, the membrane around the yolk breaks down, allowing bacteria to multiply. Critics including Michael Jacobson, executive director of the Center for Science in the Public Interest, say the lack of a federal egg-safety plan has allowed salmonella to become "a national public-health epidemic."

Chicken or egg? In 1980, only about 6 percent of all salmonella infections were caused by *Salmonella enteritidis*. It was believed that eggs became contaminated when bacteria from fecal matter were drawn through the shell's pores into the egg. But in 1988, an experiment confirmed that when the ovaries of laying hens were infected with salmonella, their eggs, in turn, were tainted with the same strain. By 1994, *Salmonella enteritidis* had become the most frequently reported salmonella infection. Between 1985 and 1998, the CDC traced 794 outbreaks, resulting in 79 deaths.

But in the past two years, the infection rate has dropped 44 percent, according to FoodNet, a federal food-safety surveillance network. "I think we're seeing results from the egg quality assurance programs," says Morris Potter, the FDA's Director of Food Safety Initiatives. The programs, instituted by the egg industry in the mid-1990s, set standards for farming practices, refrigeration and dating of eggs, and diversion of contaminated eggs to plants where they are pasteurized, which kills the bacteria. According to the Egg Nutrition Center, 93 percent of the nation's largest egg producers adhere to these voluntary programs. Yet the USDA estimates that 1 in 20,000 eggs is still contaminated, about 3.4 billion eggs in 1998.

The major stumbling block to safer eggs, according to the GAO, Congress, and many scientists, is the absence of a plan to reduce transmission of bacteria from farm to table. This enormous task, according to the FDA's Potter, will be undertaken by members of the President's Council on Food Safety, which meets next week. A national plan for egg safety is expected by Nov. 1.

At the Richmond IHOP, they've decided not to wait. They now use pasteurized eggs.

Article 47

IRRADIATION

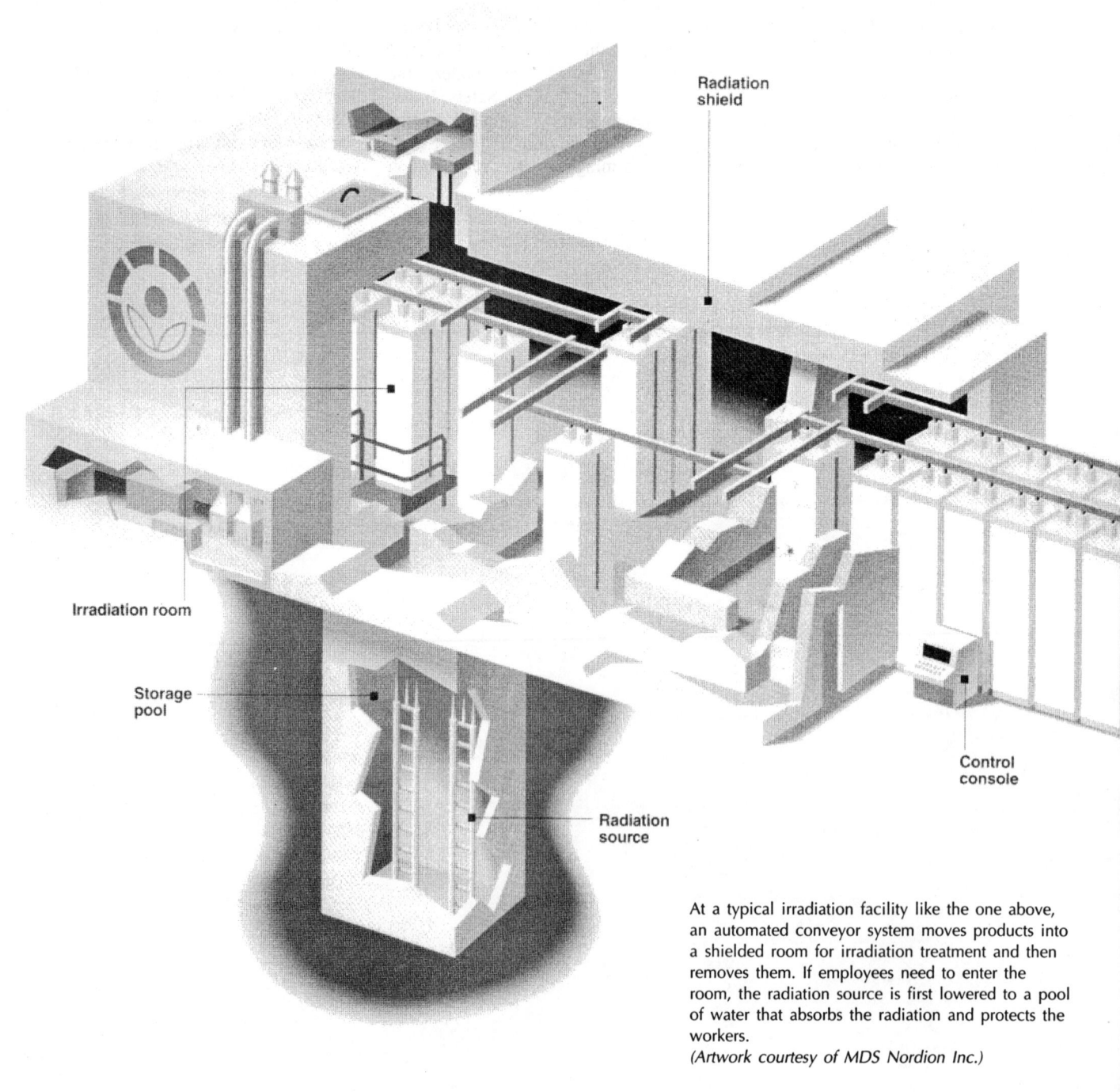

At a typical irradiation facility like the one above, an automated conveyor system moves products into a shielded room for irradiation treatment and then removes them. If employees need to enter the room, the radiation source is first lowered to a pool of water that absorbs the radiation and protects the workers.
(Artwork courtesy of MDS Nordion Inc.)

INFOGRAPHIC BY SAM WARD

47. Irradiation

A Safe Measure For Safer Food

BEEF is one of the U.S. food industry's hottest sellers—
to the tune of 8 billion pounds a year, according to trade figures.
Whether at a fast-food meal, a dinner on the town,
or a backyard barbecue, beef is often front and center
on America's tables.

by John Henkel

But in recent years, beef, especially ground beef, has shown a dark side: It can harbor the bacterium *E. coli* O157:H7, a pathogen that threatens the safety of the domestic food supply. If not properly prepared, beef tainted with *E. coli* O157:H7 can make people ill, and in rare instances, kill them. In 1993, *E. coli* O157:H7-contaminated hamburgers sold by a fast-food chain were linked to the deaths of four children and hundreds of illnesses in the Pacific Northwest.

In 1997, the potential extent of *E. coli* O157:H7 contamination came to light when Arkansas-based Hudson Foods Inc. voluntarily recalled 25 million pounds of hamburger suspected of containing *E. coli* O157:H7. It was the largest recall of meat products in U.S. history.

Nationally, *E. coli* O157:H7 causes about 20,000 illnesses and 500 deaths a year, according to the federal Centers for Disease Control and Prevention. Scientists have only known since 1982 that this form of *E. coli* causes human illness.

To help combat this public health problem, the Food and Drug Administration last December approved treating red meat products with a measured dose of radiation. This process, commonly called irradiation, has drawn praise from many food industry and health organizations because it can control *E. coli* O157:H7 and several other disease-causing microorganisms. As with other regulations governing meat and poultry products, irradiation will be authorized when the U.S. Department of Agriculture completes its implementing regulations.

Though irradiation is the latest step toward curbing food-borne illness, the federal government also is implementing other measures, which include developing new technologies and expanding the use of current technologies.

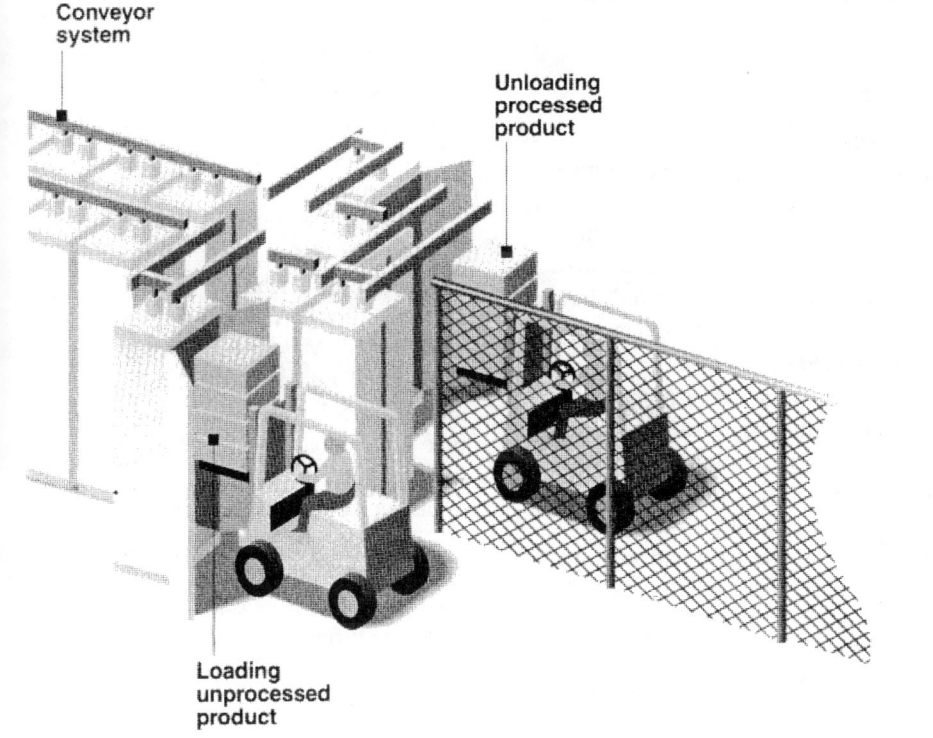

A Long Safety Record

FDA's red meat approval added another product category to the already lengthy list of foods the agency has approved for irradiation since 1963. These include poultry, fresh fruits and vegetables, dry spices, seasonings, and enzymes.

As part of its approval, FDA requires that irradiated foods include labeling with either the statement "treated with radiation" or "treated by irradiation" and the international symbol for irradiation, the radura (pictured

163

5 ❖ FOOD SAFETY

FDA'S approval of red meat irradiation adds to a lengthy list of foods approved for this process, including poultry, fresh fruits and vegetables, and dry spices.

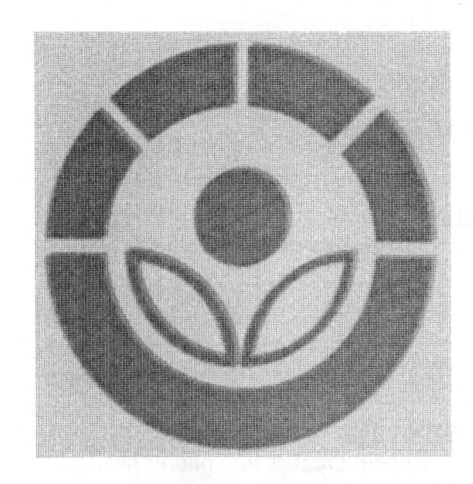

above). Irradiation labeling requirements apply only to foods sold in stores. For example, irradiated spices or fresh strawberries should be labeled. When used as ingredients in other foods, however, the label of the other food does not need to describe these ingredients as irradiated. Irradiation labeling also does not apply to restaurant foods.

FDA has evaluated irradiation safety for 40 years and found the process safe and effective for many foods. Before approving red meat irradiation, the agency reviewed numerous scientific studies conducted worldwide. These included research on the chemical effects of radiation on meat, the impact the process has on nutrient content, and potential toxicity concerns.

In this most recent review and in previous reviews of the irradiation process, FDA scientists concluded that irradiation reduces or eliminates pathogenic bacteria, insects and parasites. It reduces spoilage, and in certain fruits and vegetables, it inhibits sprouting and delays the ripening process. Also, it does not make food radioactive, compromise nutritional quality, or noticeably change food taste, texture or appearance as long as it's applied properly to a suitable product.

Health experts say that in addition to reducing *E. coli* O157:H7 contamination, irradiation can help control the potentially harmful bacteria *Salmonella* and *Campylobacter*, two chief causes of food-borne illness. The Centers for Disease Control and Prevention estimates that Salmonella—commonly found in poultry, eggs, meat, and milk—sickens as many as 4 million and kills 1,000 per year nationwide. *Campylobacter*, found mostly in poultry, is responsible for 6 million illnesses and 75 deaths per year in the United States. A May 1997 presidential report, "Food Safety from Farm to Table," estimates that "millions" of Americans are stricken by food-borne illness each year and some 9,000, mostly the very young and elderly, die as a result.

FDA officials emphasize that though irradiation is a useful tool for reducing food-borne disease risk, it complements, but doesn't replace, proper food handling practices by producers, processors and consumers.

Limited Success So Far

Though irradiation would appear to have much going for it, retail outlets have been slow to carry irradiated foods. This, experts say, is partially because many store owners and food producers fear consumers won't buy the products based on misgivings about radiation in general.

But some stores have plunged in anyway—with limited success. Carrot Top, a Chicago-area grocery market, was one of the first to carry irradiated fruits (see "Berry Successful Irradiation"). Owner Jim Corrigan says the products have been selling steadily since 1992. Other stores—mostly small, independent markets—have followed suit, offering irradiated vegetables, fruits and poultry to a modest, but loyal, group of irradiation-savvy customers.

Because irradiated red meat is not yet on the market, it remains to be seen if consumers will buy products such as irradiated ground beef—or if large food processors will even offer it. Irradiated products sold to date have cost slightly more than their untreated counterparts because of the extra step irradiation adds to food processing. But in the future, these costs could be offset by improved shelf life and increased consumer demand, according to food trade groups.

Major food companies such as poultry processors, meat packers, and grocery chains have yet to embrace irradiation, not only because of perceived consumer attitudes, but also due to logistics. Food Technology Service Inc., in Mulberry, Fla., is the only irradiating facility dedicated solely to treating agricultural products. More than 40 other facilities nationwide primarily handle sterilization of medical supplies, though these plants also can irradiate food products. In fact, it was a New Jersey-based medical irradiation company, Isomedix Inc., that petitioned FDA to approve red meat irradiation.

Beyond physical distances and lack of facilities, sheer product volume makes it unlikely that irradiation will be widespread anytime soon. The domestic poultry trade, for instance, processes about 25 billion pounds per year, according to industry figures. Says Kenneth May, spokesman for the National Broiler Council, which represents poultry producers: "We think [irradiation is] a process that will work. But for practical purposes, we just don't see anything happening with it in the near future." He adds, however, that if the public really wants an irradiated product, the poultry industry will find a way to deliver it.

Will Consumers Accept It?

Before irradiation can really take off, the public must "warm up" to a method associated with nuclear en-

Many spices are irradiated, which eliminates the need for chemical fumigation to control pests.

ergy, a source that carries its share of negative perceptions. George Pauli, Ph.D., FDA's food irradiation safety coordinator, compares irradiation to milk pasteurization, another decontaminating process that dramatically curbed disease but took decades before achieving public acceptance. "When the public finally sees a need for irradiation and realizes its value, I think people will accept it, maybe even demand it," Pauli says. "But you have to give them time."

A Louis Harris poll released in 1986 found that 76 percent of Americans considered irradiated food a hazard. But later studies have shown that consumer attitudes can be changed through education.

In 1995, researchers at the University of Georgia reported that 87.5 percent of consumers had heard of irradiation but knew little about it. So the university set up a "simulated supermarket setting" and labeled irradiated products, put posters at the point of sale, and developed a slide show explaining irradiation. "Our goal was to see which one of those techniques was most effective in changing people's attitudes," says Kay McWatters, agricultural research scientist and one of the study authors.

The study found that any kind of education helps convey the benefits of irradiation, McWatters says. "But the one that turned out most effective was the slide show, because visual images and [narration] are much more attention-getting than just a static label or poster."

After the study's education strategy, about 84 percent of participating consumers said irradiation is "somewhat necessary" or "very necessary." Fifty-eight percent said they would always buy irradiated chicken if available, and 27 percent said they would buy it sometimes.

Another study in 1997 by the Food Marketing Institute had similar results. After receiving education about the process, 60 percent of those in the study said they would buy irradiated foods.

Carrot Top owner Corrigan also discovered this on a small scale after sending his regular customers information about irradiation in periodic newsletters.

Luggage and Milk

Other studies, however, show that many consumers still question if irradiation is safe. They wonder if the process transfers radiation to the product or if it causes chemical changes in the food that might be hazardous. Even the word "irradiation" is scary to some, carrying images of atomic explosions or nuclear reactor accidents.

But as long as radiation is applied to foods in approved doses, it's safe, says FDA's Pauli. Similar to sending luggage through an airport scanner, the process passes food quickly through a radiation field—typically gamma rays produced from radioactive cobalt-60. That amount of energy is not strong enough to add any radioactive material to the food. The same irradiation process is used to sterilize medical products such as bandages, contact lens solutions, and hospital supplies such as gloves, sutures and gowns. Many spices sold in this country also are irradiated, which eliminates the need for chemical fumigation to control pests. American astronauts have eaten irradiated foods since 1972.

Irradiation is a "cold" process that gives off little heat, so foods can be irradiated within their packaging and remain protected against contamination until opened by users. Because a few bacteria can survive the process in poultry and meats, it's important, Pauli says, to keep products refrigerated and to cook them properly.

Berry Successful Irradiation

The huge sign hanging over the rows of boxed strawberries left little doubt for Chicago-area grocery shoppers that the produce before them was something new and unusual.

Not that the berries looked any different. But the massive poster above them bore a message in mammoth letters that might as well have been neon: "Treated by irradiation for freshness and health." To the store owner's surprise, patrons flocked to the new product, buying nine times more of it than of standard strawberries.

That scene took place in 1992 at Carrot Top, one of the first retail stores to venture into the then-uncharted realm of irradiated foods. The decision to stock radiation-treated berries in the store, however, came slowly. Owner Jim Corrigan spent about a year reading up on the irradiation process and passing details to his regular customers through periodic newsletters. He says informing customers before the store actually stocked the new products helped allay possible fears.

When the Florida-grown strawberries finally arrived, along with irradiated oranges and grapefruits, shoppers were well acquainted with the process and responded with sales.

Today, Corrigan remains enthusiastic. He says irradiation ensures that strawberries will be free of insects and will keep longer—in some cases, up to three weeks, versus three to five days for conventional berries.

"One of our ways of rating the freshness of strawberries is to examine the small hairs that grow by the seed," he says. "If they are standing up and plentiful, the strawberries are still fresh. [With irradiated strawberries] we see a lot of that after three weeks."

The products remain steady sellers, and Corrigan has since added irradiated onions and papayas to his stock.

—J.H.

5 ❖ FOOD SAFETY

Irradiating food is similar to passing luggage through an airport scanner.

Irradiation interferes with bacterial genetics, so the contaminating organism can no longer survive or multiply. Although chemicals called radiolytic products are created when food is irradiated, FDA has found them to pose no health hazard. In fact, the same kinds of products are formed when food is cooked.

Praises and Protests

Though irradiation has its share of detractors, many prestigious organizations endorse it, including the World Health Organization, the International Atomic Energy Agency, the American Medical Association, and the American Dietetic Association. Trade groups such as the National Meat Association, the Grocery Manufacturers of America, and the National Food Processors Association also support irradiation.

However, some groups have given irradiation a thumbs down. Consumer activist Jeremy Rifkin, president of the Pure Food Campaign, says more attention should be placed on raising healthier livestock, which he says would reduce pathogens and make irradiation unnecessary. The Center for Science in the Public Interest calls irradiation "expensive" and "an end-of-the-line solution to contamination problems that can and should be addressed earlier."

But with so many influential organizations backing irradiation, along with concerns about rising numbers of disease cases, the stage is set for the process to pick up momentum, despite negative sentiments, supporters say. First, however, says FDA's Pauli, the food industry needs to get more irradiated products into the marketplace. "Most people in this country haven't even seen an irradiated food," he says. "When products start appearing, then the public can make up its mind."

John Henkel is a staff writer for FDA Consumer.

Approved Uses of Irradiation

FDA approved the first use of irradiation on a food product in 1963 when it allowed radiation-treated wheat and wheat flour to be marketed. In approving a use of radiation, FDA sets the maximum radiation dose the product can be exposed to, measured in units called kiloGray (kGy). The following is a list of all approved uses of radiation on foods to date, the purpose for irradiating them, and the radiation dose allowed.

Food	Approved Use	Dose
Spices and dry vegetable seasoning	decontaminates and controls insects and microorganisms	30 kGy
Dry or dehydrated enzyme preparations	controls insects and microorgamisms	10 kGy
All foods	controls insects	1 kGY
Fresh foods	delays maturation	1 kGy
Poultry	controls disease-causing microorganisms	3 kGy
Red meat (such as beef, lamb and pork)	controls spoilage and disease-causing microorganisms	4.5 kGy (fresh) 7 kGy (frozen)

Radiation's Positive Side

Scientists first studied radiation as a way to improve food products in the 1930s, but research didn't begin in earnest until just after World War II. At that time, the U.S. Army was seeking a means to lessen dependence on refrigeration and replace K rations and other preserved products that troops used in the field.

In the early 1950s, the Atomic Energy Commission (now part of the U.S. Department of Energy) explored food irradiation as part of President Eisenhower's "Atoms for Peace" program. This research differed from the Army's in that it examined the effects smaller radiation doses had on certain fruits and vegetables. The end result was not a sterile product but one where insects would be killed or sterilized. Because this produce still could spoil, refrigeration was needed. But at least potentially harmful insects would not cross state or national borders.

Such research, augmented by studies from other countries, established that the most important benefit from irradiation could be the control of disease-causing pathogens and that the maximum practical and effective dose depended on the food and the purpose for irradiating. •

—J.H.

Radiolytic products, formed when food is irradiated, are similar to those formed by cooking food. FDA has found them to be safe.

QUESTIONS KEEP SPROUTING ABOUT SPROUTS

by Paula Kurtzweil

Sprouts—those crunchy, healthy newborn plants often associated with the hippie days of the 1960s—have in this decade become regulars in salad bars and produce departments across the country. But along with their increasing presence has come an increasing frequency of sprout-related food-borne illness.

The federal government has linked the most common kind—alfalfa sprouts—to a number of food-borne disease outbreaks, most occurring since 1995. The disease culprits included the bacteria *Salmonella* and *Escherichia coli* O157:H7, a particularly dangerous pathogen.

These outbreaks led the Food and Drug Administration in August 1998 to issue a health advisory for high-risk groups warning them not to eat raw alfalfa sprouts and, in September, to conduct a public hearing to determine what further steps, if any, are needed to ensure the safety of sprouts.

"There are some interesting questions raised about sprouts," says Karen Hulebak, a science policy analyst in FDA's Office of Policy. "What do we know about the source of sprout contamination? What should consumers do? . . . There are a lot of uncertainties."

What Are Sprouts?

Sprouts, which are the germinating form of seeds and beans, are easy to produce. They require no soil, only water and cool temperatures. They emerge in two to seven days, depending on the type of seed or bean. In addition to raw alfalfa sprouts, other varieties include clover, sunflower, broccoli, mustard, radish, garlic, dill, and pumpkin, as well as various beans, such as mung, kidney, pinto, navy and soy, and wheat berries. Many are sold individually, some in mixtures.

Potomac Glen Farms in Potomac, Md., sells a wide array. Each offers a distinct flavor, suggesting, as sprout growers like to point out, that sprouts indeed work well in a variety of dishes, such as soups, salads, sandwiches, and stir fries. Nancy Snider, owner of Potomac Glen Farms and president of the International Sprout Growers Association, says one of her favorite foods is sprouts with peanut butter and crackers.

While versatile, sprouts also are favored for their nutritional value. Like other fresh produce, sprouts are low in calories and fat and provide substantial amounts of key nutrients, such as vitamin C, folate and fiber. A 1997 Johns Hopkins University study suggested raw broccoli sprouts may be particularly rich in sulforaphane, a compound that may mobilize the body's natural cancer-fighting resources and reduce the risk of developing cancer.

Though popular in this country in only the past few decades, sprouts have actually been around for thousands of years. Mung beans have been used in Chinese foods for years—though usually in cooked dishes.

Today, sprouts in the United States are a $250-million market. Some 475 U.S. sprout growers produce 300,000 tons of sprouts every year, according to the International Sprout Growers Association. As many as 10 percent of Americans eat sprouts regularly.

Food-Borne Illnesses

Sprouts have only recently emerged as a recognized source of food-borne illness. Since 1995, health officials have attributed 13 food-borne disease outbreaks worldwide to sprouts. Ten of these outbreaks occurred in the United States, resulting in illnesses in at least 956 Americans and at least one death.

Four of the outbreaks were caused by *E. coli* bacteria, and three of those involved the most dangerous strain, *E. coli* O157:H7. The biggest outbreak occurred in Japan in 1996;

5 ❖ FOOD SAFETY

> ### How to Eat Sprouts Safely
>
> If you belong to one of the groups at high risk for food-borne disease—children, the elderly, and people with compromised immune systems—avoid raw alfalfa sprouts.
>
> If you are a healthy adult, follow these tips:
>
> 1. Buy only sprouts kept at refrigerator temperature. Select crisp-looking sprouts with the buds attached. Avoid musty-smelling, dark, or slimy-looking sprouts.
> 2. Refrigerate sprouts at home. The refrigerator should be set at no higher than 40 degrees Fahrenheit (4 degrees Celsius).
> 3. Wash hands with warm water and soap for at least 20 seconds before and after handling raw foods.
> 4. Rinse sprouts thoroughly with water before use. Rinsing can help remove surface dirt. Do not use soap or other detergents.
>
> —P.K.

9,000 people were sickened and 17 died after eating radish sprouts contaminated with *E. coli* O157:H7.

The O157:H7 strain produces toxin in the human gut that damages cells of the intestinal lining. This allows blood to pass into the stool. Other symptoms of O157:H7 infection are stomachache, nausea and vomiting. Infection can lead to hemolytic uremic syndrome (HUS), a major cause of acute kidney failure in children in this country. HUS is fatal in about 3 to 5 percent of cases.

Many of the outbreaks have involved raw alfalfa sprouts or mixed sprouts containing raw alfalfa sprouts contaminated with *Salmonella*.

In people, *Salmonella* can cause salmonellosis, an illness characterized by fever, stomach cramps, and diarrhea. The illness can last as long as seven days, and severe cases may require hospitalization. In some people, it can cause death. A small number of illnesses may develop into recurring joint pain and arthritis.

Where do these bacteria come from? It's believed that the seeds from which sprouts are derived are often the source. Some of the seeds may become contaminated by animals in the field or during post-harvest storage, for example. Also, the use of animal manure in fields of alfalfa intended for nonhuman use may be a problem if seed is used for sprouting.

The ideal conditions provided by germinating seeds and beans—namely abundant nutrients in this phase of plant growth, high levels of moisture needed to produce sprouts, and heat generated from the sprouting process—help ensure the survival and growth of bacteria. "In the sprouting environment, bacteria can grow quickly," says Robert Wick, Ph.D., a plant pathologist with the University of Massachusetts and one of the presenters at FDA's September 1998 public hearing on sprouts.

So far, mishandling of sprouts during production, packing or distribution has not been implicated as the source of sprout contamination. However, bacteria already present in the sprouting seed can continue to thrive in conditions in which poor food handling techniques are practiced—for example, lack of refrigeration, infected workers, and dirty and unsanitary sprouting facilities.

Preventive Measures

Following three 1998 food-borne disease outbreaks involving raw alfalfa sprouts, FDA in August reaffirmed a warning that had been issued by the national Centers for Disease Control and Prevention in 1997. The advisory urged people at high risk for severe food-borne disease—children, the elderly, and people with compromised immune systems—to avoid raw alfalfa sprouts until methods to improve the safety of sprouts can be identified and put in place.

In September, the agency held a two-day public meeting on sprout safety to learn, among other things, possible preventive measures to

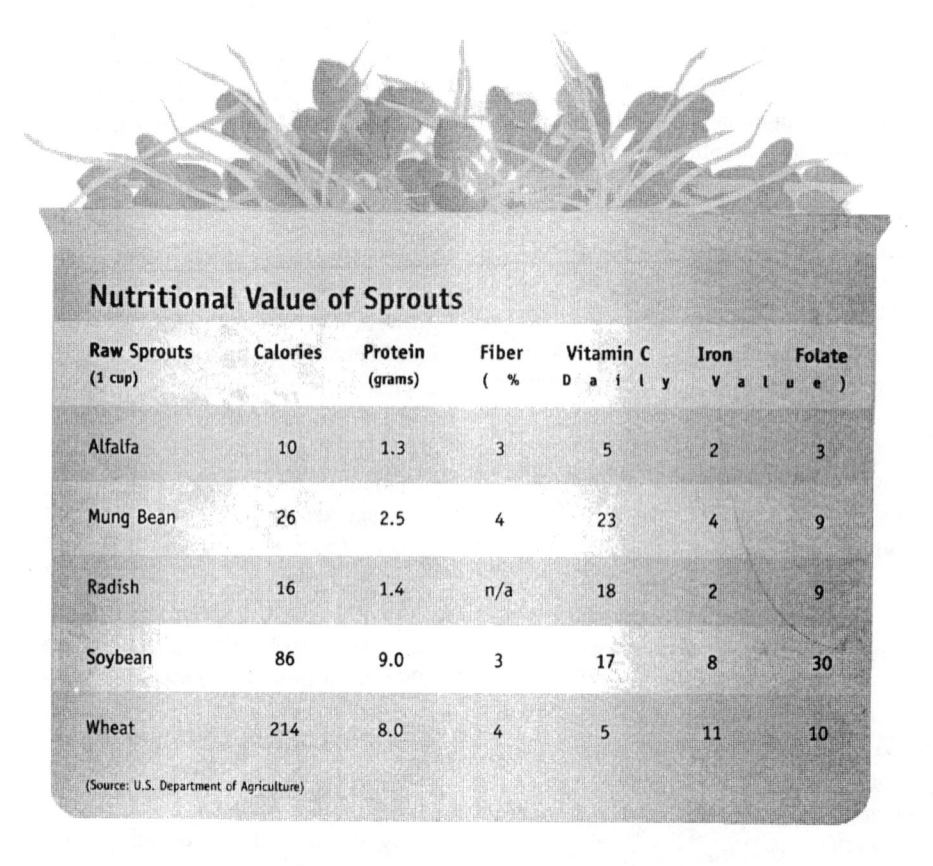

Nutritional Value of Sprouts

Raw Sprouts (1 cup)	Calories	Protein (grams)	Fiber (%	Vitamin C D a i l y	Iron V a l u	Folate e)
Alfalfa	10	1.3	3	5	2	3
Mung Bean	26	2.5	4	23	4	9
Radish	16	1.4	n/a	18	2	9
Soybean	86	9.0	3	17	8	30
Wheat	214	8.0	4	5	11	10

(Source: U.S. Department of Agriculture)

ensure safe sprouts. Representatives from the sprout industry and consumer groups, as well as scientists and regulators, presented information to the Fresh Produce Subcommittee of the National Advisory Committee on Microbiological Criteria for Food.

High on the list of possible strategies was decontamination of sprout seeds. The most promising method is chemical treatment with calcium hypochlorite. It already is in use in California on an emergency basis, as approved by the state's environmental protection agency. FDA is working with the U.S. Department of Agriculture to get the treatment approved by the U.S. Environmental Protection Agency, which oversees use of chemicals on raw agricultural products, such as sprout seeds.

Irradiation, in which a measured dose of ionizing radiation is applied to a food product, appears to work well in decontaminating sprout seeds, especially when used in conjunction with calcium hypochlorite. Irradiation of sprout seeds would require FDA approval. (See "Irradiation: A Safe Measure for Safer Food" in the May-June 1998 *FDA Consumer.*)

Heat treatment (the same as pasteurization) has limited appeal because there is such a fine threshold at which bacteria can be killed and germination not destroyed.

Other preventive measures would focus on production and distribution of sprouts. Possibilities include mandatory Hazard Analysis and Critical Control Point (HACCP) programs for sprout growers. HACCP focuses on identifying and preventing hazards, such as bacterial contamination, rather than relying on spot-checks of production processes and random sampling of finished products. Emphasis on good agricultural and manufacturing practices of sprouts also may help reduce the incidence of sprout-related food-borne disease outbreaks. Another option might be to include a list of safe handling practices or a mandatory warning on labels of sprout packages. The warning would echo FDA and CDC recommendations for high-risk groups.

According to LeAnne Jackson, Ph.D., a science policy analyst in FDA's Center for Food Safety and Applied Nutrition, the National Advisory Committee on Microbiological Criteria for Food was awaiting the subcommittee's recommendations at press time. If endorsed, the recommendations will be forwarded to FDA for consideration.

In the meantime, the International Sprout Growers Association planned to begin in November 1998 a voluntary quality assurance program in which sprout growers agree to follow ISGA-established sanitation guidelines based on good manufacturing practices. According to ISGA president Snider, sprout growers that participate could label their products as ISGA-certified as long as their facilities pass inspection by a third-party auditor.

The sprout industry also is working with the National Center for Food Safety and Technology—a consortium of government, industry and academia devoted to food safety research—in Summit-Argo, Ill., to study sprout safety. The center is conducting a six-month research project to verify the effects of chemical, heat and irradiation treatment of seeds on sprout safety.

Snider says the industry is involved because it wants to reduce any hazards associated with sprouts. "This is a difficult time for us," she acknowledges. "But out of difficulties, something good can come. We expect [these concerns over sprout safety] to turn out to be our best friend. We want our products to carry zero risk."

Paula Kurtzweil is a member of FDA's public affairs staff.

Unit 6

Unit Selections

49. **Twenty-Five Ways to Spot Quacks and Vitamin Pushers,** Stephen Barrett and Victor Herbert
50. **Yet Another Study—Should You Pay Attention?** Tufts University Health & Nutrition Letter
51. **Alternative Medicine—The Risks of Untested and Unregulated Remedies,** Marcia Angell and Jerome P. Kassirer
52. **The Mouse That Roared: Health Scares on the Internet,** Food Insight
53. **Uprooting Herbal Myths,** Consumer Reports on Health
54. **Herbal Weight Loss Tea: Beware the Unknown Brew,** Healthy Weight Journal
55. **5 Nutrition Topics That Are Not All They're Cracked Up to Be,** Tufts University Health & Nutrition Letter
56. **Pyruvate: Just the Facts,** Joseph P. Cannon
57. **Are Health Food Stores Better Bets than Traditional Supermarkets?** Tufts University Health & Nutrition Letter
58. **The Unethical Behavior of Pharmacists,** Stephen Barrett

Key Points to Consider

❖ Why do you think people are so vulnerable to quackery? When have you been a victim?

❖ Identify three current fallacies that you believe are the most dangerous to nutritional health. Why are they fallacies?

❖ Make a list of characteristics you would look for in a reliable information source. Use them to evaluate nutrition articles in your local newspaper or a nutrition-oriented talk show.

❖ Decide if there are any herbals you could safely use right now and which ones should wait for scientific testing and judgment. What criteria did you use? Where did you get your information?

❖ Explore a variety of Web sites for nutrition information and decide if they offer reliable information.

❖ How do you feel about pharmacies promoting supplements, herbals, and homeopathic remedies? What are the issues to consider?

DUSHKIN ONLINE Links
www.dushkin.com/online/

32. **Diet, Health & Fitness**
    http://www.ftc.gov/bcp/menu-health.htm
33. **National Council against Health Fraud**
    http://www.ncahf.org
34. **QuackWatch**
    http://www.quackwatch.com

These sites are annotated on pages 4 and 5.

Health Claims

Does it contain any experimental reasoning, concerning matter of fact and existence? No. Commit it then to the flames; for it can contain nothing but sophistry and illusion.
—David Hume in *An Enquiry Concerning Human Understanding*, 1748

In ancient Rome, Cato the elder prescribed cabbages to cure "everything that ails you" and continued to do so even though his wife died from the "fevers." London pharmacists, in 1632, believed that bananas were so important to health that only trained druggists should administer them. In the early years of this country, Elisha Perkins promoted vinegar as the cure for yellow fever, yet he died of this disease. All were sincere but wrong.

Quackery is misinformation about health, according to the Food and Drug Administration (FDA). Certain fallacious statements have been made repeatedly by promoters for years, among them: "The American food supply is worthless because it is grown on depleted soil," "Everybody needs vitamin supplements for insurance," "Sugar from honey is healthier than table sugar," and "Natural is better." Such misinformation may be easier to find than facts. For example, popular talk show hosts provide a good promotional forum for misinformation, since their need to capture a large audience draws sensationalism. Nutritionists often have despaired of counteracting the exaggeration and blatantly false information frequently distributed through the popular information media. This unit begins with 25 indicators that should cause the consumer to suspect quackery. Typically, those who misrepresent the truth warn that today's food supply is deficient, that processing techniques are harmful, and that dire consequences will result if one doesn't use supplements—their supplements.

Since surveys repeatedly have shown the media to be the primary source of nutrition and food-safety information, the accuracy of what is reported is an important issue. Hardly a newspaper or periodical is published without mention of a new study that has produced "important" information about a health issue. Often these reports predict dreadful consequences from something we commonly do or consume. "Yet Another Study—Should You Pay Attention?" suggests a set of guidelines to assist the consumer in deciding what to ignore and when to take a study seriously.

Many of us rely more and more on the Internet for answers to our questions. Here, too, we must be watchful—perhaps even more so, for Web sites and e-mail capabilities allow the easy and rapid promotion of virtually anything. Guidelines for recognizing and avoiding unreliable sites are suggested in the article entitled "The Mouse that Roared." Some Web sites make a point of exposing fraudulent information. One such site that may benefit the reader is www.quackwatch.com.

An editorial from *The New England Journal of Medicine* on alternative medicine offers a dissertation on the risks of untested and unregulated remedies, which often take the form of herbals and other dietary supplements. This is also the subject of two articles on herbals. Increasingly popular herbals are classified as food supplements under the Dietary Supplement Health and Education Act (DSHEA) of 1994, and currently account for about $1 billion in annual sales. Given that herbals have medicinal qualities, questions of safety and efficacy must be raised. Some argue that, because herbs are natural, safety is a nonissue, although this can be refuted easily by pointing out that the amanita mushroom and hurricanes are also quite natural but potentially deadly. To be sure, nearly one-third of modern drugs are derived from herbs and other plants, and undoubtedly more will be found to advance the modern medical arsenal against disease. But there is a clear distinction between pharmaceuticals, which must stand up to rigorous testing and have carefully controlled active ingredients, and herbals, which are not subject to strict controls and where the amounts of active ingredients depend more on how they are grown, harvested, and stored. Most herbal literature is still grounded in folklore and tradition, not in scientific research. There are no guarantees of safety, and serious side effects have included life-threatening allergic reactions, kidney failure, liver damage, and heart rhythm abnormalities. Some, such as sassafras and comfrey, are known to contain carcinogens.

Some progress regarding herbals can be found. The herbal industry has made some attempts to police itself, even suggesting manufacturing standards, although they have yet to go into effect. These recommendations, however, would ensure the identity and quality of products but would not address their effectiveness. A physician's desk reference for herbal medicines has been published, and courses on botanicals are being offered in a few schools of medicine and pharmacology. Also the FTC (Federal Trade Commission) has been able to take action against a few manufacturers who did not conform to the requirement for truthful and verifiable advertising. However, the Food and Drug Administration can restrict herbal sales only if well-documented reports of health problems are received. It took the FDA 4 years, more than 100 reports of life-threatening symptoms, and nearly 40 deaths to take action against ma huang (ephedra). Another concern of many professionals is the phenomenal growth of food products called functional foods that are claimed to provide a specific health benefit and that, it can be argued, truly resemble medicinals. We have become accustomed to milk being fortified, cereals enriched, and calcium being added to orange juice. Now herbals are added to foods as well. Soft drinks and soups to which echinaciea, St. John's wort, or other substances have been added are readily available. The FDA does not yet have a definition for functional foods or a policy in place to regulate the industry.

Quackery in the new century also includes other compounds that are touted to have special healthful effects. An article on pyruvate is an example. Another such compound of current interest is vitamin O, which is claimed to provide the body with more oxygen, thereby increasing energy levels, curing many serious diseases, improving memory, and eliminating fatigue. Selling at $10 per ounce, it was found to contain nothing but salt water.

Finally, you will discover that buying from a health food store is not a guarantee of healthful products. And, if you have wondered why most pharmacies appear to promote supplements and dubious alternative products, while nutritionists and this book take the opposite view, read the article on unethical behavior of pharmacists. When there is a conflict of interest, promoting sales and keeping a healthy bottom line often win.

Twenty-Five Ways to Spot Quacks and Vitamin Pushers

Stephen Barrett, M.D.

Victor Herbert, M.D., J.D.

How can food quacks and other vitamin pushers be recognized? Here are 25 signs that should arouse suspicion.

1. When Talking about Nutrients, They Tell Only Part of the Story.

Quacks tell you all the wonderful things that vitamins and minerals do in your body and/or all the horrible things that can happen if you don't get enough. Many claim that their products or programs offer "optimal nutritional support." But they conveniently neglect to tell you that a balanced diet provides the nutrients people need and that the USDA food-group system makes balancing your diet simple.

2. They Claim That Most Americans Are Poorly Nourished.

This is an appeal to fear that is not only untrue, but ignores the fact that the main forms of bad nourishment in the United States are overweight in the population at large, particularly the poor, and under-nourishment among the poverty-stricken. Poor people can ill afford to waste money on unnecessary vitamin pills. Their food money should be spent on nourishing food.

It is falsely alleged that Americans are so addicted to "junk" foods that an adequate diet is exceptional rather than usual. While it is true that some snack foods are mainly "naked calories" (sugars and/or fats without other nutrients), it is not necessary for every morsel of food we eat to be loaded with nutrients. In fact, no normal person following the *U.S. Dietary Guidelines* is in any danger of vitamin deficiency.

3. They Recommend "Nutrition Insurance" for Everyone.

Most vitamin pushers suggest that everyone is in danger of vitamin deficiency and should therefore take supplements as "insurance." Some suggest that it is difficult to get what you need from food, while others claim that it is impossible. Their pitch resembles that of the door-to-door huckster who states that your perfectly good furnace is in danger of blowing up unless you replace it with his product. Vitamin pushers will never tell you who *doesn't* need their products.

4. They Say That Most Diseases Are Due to Faulty Diet and Can Be Treated with "Nutritional" Methods.

This simply isn't so. Consult your doctor or any recognized textbook of medicine. They will tell you that although diet is a factor in some diseases (most notably coronary heart disease), most diseases have little or nothing to do with diet. Common symptoms like malaise (feeling poorly), fatigue, lack of pep, aches (including headaches) or pains, insomnia, and similar complaints are usually the body's reaction to emotional stress. The persistence of such symptoms is a signal to see a doctor to be evaluated for possible physical illness. It is not a reason to take vitamin pills.

5. They Allege That Modern Processing Methods and Storage Remove all Nutritive Value from Our Food.

It is true that food processing can change the nutrient content of foods. But the changes are not so drastic as the quack, who wants you to buy supplements, would like you to believe. While some processing methods destroy some nutrients, others add them. A balanced variety of foods will provide all the nourishment you need.

Quacks distort and oversimplify. When they say that milling removes B-vitamins, they don't bother to tell you that enrichment puts them back. When they tell you that cooking destroys vitamins, they omit the fact that only a few vitamins are sensitive to heat. Nor do they tell you that these vitamins are easily obtained by consuming a portion of fresh uncooked fruit, vegetable, or fresh or frozen fruit juice each day. Any claims that minerals are destroyed by processing or cooking are pure lies. Heat does not destroy minerals.

6. They Claim That Diet Is a Major Factor in Behavior.

Food quacks relate diet not only to disease but to behavior. Some claim that adverse reactions to additives and/or common foods cause hyperactivity in children and even criminal behavior in adolescents and adults. These claims are based on a combination of delusions, anecdotal evidence, and poorly designed research.

7. They Claim That Fluoridation Is Dangerous.

Curiously, quacks are not always interested in real deficiencies. Fluoride is necessary to build decay-resistant teeth and strong bones. The best way to obtain adequate amounts of this important nutrient is to augment community water supplies so their fluoride concentration is about one part fluoride for every million parts of water. But *quacks usually oppose water fluoridation,* and some advocate water filters that remove fluoride. It seems that when they cannot profit from something, they may try to make money by opposing it.

8. They Claim That Soil Depletion and the Use of Pesticides and "Chemical" Fertilizers Result in Food That Is Less Safe and Less Nourishing.

These claims are used to promote the sale of so-called *"organically grown"* foods. If an essential nutrient is missing from the soil, a plant simply doesn't grow. Chemical fertilizers counteract the effects of soil depletion. Quacks also lie when they claim that plants grown with natural fertilizers (such as manure) are nutritionally superior to those grown with synthetic fertilizers. Before they can use them, plants convert natural fertilizers into the same chemicals that synthetic fertilizers supply. The vitamin content of a food is determined by its genetic makeup. Fertilizers can influence the levels of certain minerals in plants, but this is not a significant factor in the American diet. The pesticide residue of our food supply is extremely small and poses no health threat to the consumer. Foods "certified" as "organic" are not safer or more nutritious than other foods. In fact, except for their high price, they are not significantly different.

9. They Claim You Are in Danger of Being "Poisoned" by Ordinary Food Additives and Preservatives.

This is another scare tactic designed to undermine your confidence in food scientists and government protection agencies as well as our food supply itself. Quacks want you to think they are out to protect you. They hope that if you trust them, you will buy their "natural" food products. The fact is that the tiny amounts of additives used in food pose no threat to human health. Some actually protect our health by preventing spoilage, rancidity, and mold growth.

10. They Charge That the Recommended Dietary Allowances (RDAs) Have Been Set Too Low.

The RDAs have been published by the National Research Council approximately every five years since 1943. They are defined as "the levels of intake of essential nutrients that, on the basis of scientific knowledge, are judged by the Food and Nutrition Board to be adequate to meet the known nutrient needs of practically all healthy persons." Neither the RDAs nor the Daily Values listed on food labels are "minimums" or "requirements." They are deliberately set higher than most people need. The reason quacks charge that the RDAs are too low is obvious: if you believe you need more than can be obtained from food, you are more likely to buy supplements.

11. They Claim That under Stress, and in Certain Diseases, Your Need for Nutrients Is Increased.

Many vitamin manufacturers have advertised that "stress robs the body of vitamins." One company has asserted that, "if you smoke, diet, or happen to be sick, you may be robbing your body of vitamins." Another has warned that "stress can deplete your body of water-soluble vitamins . . . and daily replacement is necessary." Other products are touted to fill the "special needs of athletes."

While it is true that the need for vitamins may rise slightly under physical stress and in certain diseases, this type of advertising is fraudulent. The average American—stressed or not—is not in danger of vitamin deficiency. The increased needs to which the ads refer are not higher than the amounts obtainable by proper eating. Someone who is really in danger of deficiency due to an illness would be very sick and would need medical care, probably in a hospital. But these promotions are aimed at average Americans who certainly don't need vitamin supplements to survive the common cold, a round of golf, or a jog around the neighborhood! Athletes get more than enough vitamins when they eat the food needed to meet their caloric requirements.

Many vitamin pushers suggest that smokers need vitamin C supplements. Although it is true that smokers in North America have somewhat lower blood levels of this vitamin, these levels are still far above deficiency levels. In America, cigarette smoking is the leading cause of death preventable by self-discipline. Rather than seeking false comfort by taking vitamin C, smokers who are concerned about their health should stop smoking. Suggestions that "stress vitamins" are helpful against emotional stress are also fraudulent.

12. They Recommend "Supplements" and "Health Foods" for Everyone.

Food quacks belittle normal foods and ridicule the food-group systems of good nutrition. They may not tell you they earn their living from such pronouncements—via public appearance fees, product endorsements, sale of publications, or financial interests in vitamin companies, health-food stores, or organic farms.

The very term "health food" is a deceptive slogan. Judgments about individual foods should take into account how they contribute to an individual's overall diet. All food is health food in moderation; any food is junk food in excess. Did you ever stop to think that your corner grocery, fruit market, meat market, and supermarket are also health-food stores? They are—and they generally charge less than stores that use the slogan. By the way, have you ever wondered why people who eat lots of "health foods" still feel they must load themselves up with vitamin supplements? Or why so many "health food" shoppers complain about ill health?

13. They Claim That "Natural" Vitamins are Better than "Synthetic" Ones.

This claim is a flat lie. Each vitamin is a chain of atoms strung together as a molecule. With minor exception, molecules made in the "factories" of nature are identical to those made in the factories of chemical companies. Does it makes sense to pay extra for vitamins extracted from foods when you can get all you need from the foods themselves?

14. They Suggest That a Questionnaire Can Be Used to Indicate Whether You Need Dietary Supplements.

No questionnaire can do this. A few entrepreneurs have devised lengthy computer-scored questionnaires with questions about symptoms that could be present if a vitamin deficiency exists. But such symptoms occur much more frequently in conditions unrelated to nutrition. Even when a deficiency actually exists, the tests don't provide enough information to discover the cause so that suitable treatment can be recommended. That requires a physical examination and appropriate laboratory tests. Many responsible nutritionists use a computer to help evaluate their clients' diet. But this is done to make dietary recommendations, such as reducing fat content or increasing fiber content. Supplements are seldom necessary unless the person is unable (or unwilling) to consume an adequate diet.

Be wary, too, of questionnaires purported to determine whether supplements are needed to correct "nutrient deficiencies" or "dietary inadequacies." These questionnaires are scored so that everyone who takes the test is judged deficient. Responsible dietary analyses compare the individual's average daily food consumption with the recommended numbers of servings from each food group. The safest and best way to get nutrients is generally from food, not pills. So even if a diet is deficient, the most prudent action is usually diet modification rather than supplementation with pills.

15. They Say It Is Easy to Lose Weight.

Diet quacks would like you to believe that special pills or food combinations can cause "effortless" weight loss. But the only way to lose weight is to burn off more calories than you eat. This requires self-discipline: eating less, exercising more, or preferably doing both. There are about 3,500 calories in a pound of body weight. To lose one pound a week (a safe amount that is not just water), you must eat about five hundred fewer calories per day than you burn up. The most sensible diet for losing weight is one that is nutritionally balanced in carbohydrates, fats, and proteins. Most fad diets "work" by producing temporary weight loss—as a result of calorie restriction. But they are invariably too monotonous and are often too dangerous for long-term use. Unless a dieter develops and maintains better eating and exercise habits, weight lost on a diet will soon return.

The term "cellulite" is sometimes used to describe the dimpled fat found on the hips and thighs of many women. Although no medical evidence supports the claim, cellulite is represented as a special type of fat that is resistant to diet and exercise. Sure-fire *cellulite remedies* include creams (to "dissolve" it), brushes, rollers, "loofah" sponges, body wraps, and vitamin-mineral supplements with or without herbs. The cost of various treatment plans runs from a few dollars for a bottle of vitamins to many hundreds of dollars at a salon that offers heat treatments, massage, enzyme injections, and/or treatment with various gadgets. The simple truth about "cellulite" is that it is ordinary fat that can be lost only as part of an overall reducing program.

16. They Promise Quick, Dramatic, Miraculous Results.

Often the promises are subtle or couched in "weasel words" that create an illusion of a promise, so promoters can deny making them when the "feds" close in. False promises of cure are the quacks' most immoral practice. They don't seem to care how many people they break financially or in spirit—by elation over their expected good fortune followed by deep depression when the "treatment" fails. Nor do quacks keep count—while they fill their bank accounts—of how many people they lure away from effective medical care into disability or death.

Quacks will tell you that "megavitamins" (huge doses of vitamins) can prevent or cure many different ailments, particularly emotional ones. But they won't tell you that the "evidence" supporting such claims is unreliable because it is based on inadequate investigations, anecdotes, or testimonials. Nor do quacks inform you that megadoses may be harmful. Megavitamin therapy (also called *orthomolecular therapy*) is nutritional roulette, and only the house makes the profit.

17. They Routinely Sell Vitamins and Other "Dietary Supplements" as Part of Their Practice.

Although vitamins are useful as therapeutic agents for certain health problems, the number of such conditions is small. Practitioners who sell supplements in their offices invariably recommend them inappropriately. In addition, such products tend to be substantially more expensive than similar ones in drugstores —or even health-food stores. You should also disregard any publication whose editor or publisher sells dietary supplements.

18. They Use Disclaimers Couched in Pseudomedical Jargon.

Instead of promising to cure your disease, some quacks will promise to "detoxify," "purify," or "revitalize" your body; "balance" its chemistry or "electromagnetic energy"; bring it in harmony with nature; "stimulate" or "strengthen" your immune system; "support" or "rejuvenate" various organs in your body; or stimulate your body's power to heal itself. Of course, they never identify or make valid before-and-after measurements of any of these processes. These disclaimers serve two purposes. First, since it is impossible to measure the processes quacks allege, it may be difficult to prove them wrong. Moreover, if a quack is not a physician, the use of nonmedical terminology may help to avoid prosecution for practicing medicine without a license—although it shouldn't.

Some approaches to "*detoxification*" are based on notions that, as a result of intestinal stasis, intestinal contents putrefy, and toxins are formed and absorbed, which causes chronic poisoning of the body. This "autointoxication" theory was popular around the turn of the century but was abandoned by the scientific community during the 1930s. No such "toxins" have ever been found, and careful observations have shown that individuals in good health can vary greatly in bowel habits. Quacks may also suggest that fecal material collects on the lining of the intestine and causes trouble unless removed by laxatives, colonic irrigation, special diets, and/or various herbs or food supplements that "cleanse" the body. The falsity of this notion is obvious to doctors who perform intestinal surgery or peer within the large intestine with a diagnostic instrument. Fecal material does not adhere to the intestinal lining. Colonic irrigation is done by inserting a tube up to a foot or more into the rectum and pumping up to 20 gallons of warm water in and out. This type of enema is not only therapeutically worthless but can cause fatal electrolyte imbalance. Cases of death due to intestinal perforation and infection (from contaminated equipment) have also been reported.

19. They Use Anecdotes and Testimonials to Support Their Claims.

We all tend to believe what others tell us about personal experiences. But separating cause and effect from coincidence can be difficult. If people tell you that product X has cured their cancer, arthritis, or whatever, be skeptical. They may not actually have had the condition. If they did, their recovery most likely would have occurred without the help of product X. Most single episodes of disease end with just the passage of time, and most chronic ailments have symptom-free periods. Establishing medical truths requires careful and repeated investigation—with well-designed experiments, not reports of coincidences misperceived as cause-and-effect. That's why *testimonial evidence* is forbidden in scientific articles, is usually inadmissible in court, and is not used to evaluate whether or not drugs should be legally marketable. (Imagine what would happen if the FDA decided that clinical trials were too expensive and therefore drug approval would be based on testimonial letters or interviews with a few patients.)

Never underestimate the extent to which people can be fooled by a worthless remedy. During the early 1940s, many thousands of people became convinced that "glyoxylide" could cure cancer. Yet analysis showed that it was simply distilled water! [1] Many years before that, when arsenic was used as a "tonic," countless numbers of people swore by it even as it slowly poisoned them.

Symptoms that are psychosomatic (bodily reactions to tension) are often relieved by anything taken with a suggestion that it will work. Tiredness and other minor aches and pains may respond to any enthusiastically recommended nostrum. For these problems, even physicians may prescribe a placebo. A placebo is a substance that has no pharmacological effect on the condition for which it is used, but is given to satisfy a patient who supposes it to be a medicine. Vitamins (such as B12 shots) are commonly used in this way.

Placebos act by suggestion. Unfortunately, some doctors swallow the advertising hype or become confused by their own observations and "believe in vitamins" beyond those supplied by a good diet. Those who share such false beliefs do so because they confuse coincidence or placebo action with cause and effect. Homeopathic believers make the same error.

20. They Claim That Sugar Is a Deadly Poison.

Many vitamin pushers would have us believe that refined [white] sugar is "the killer on the breakfast table" and is the underlying cause of everything from heart disease to hypoglycemia. The fact is, however, that when sugar is used in moderation as part of a normal, balanced diet, it is a perfectly safe source of calories and eating pleasure. Sugar is a factor in the tooth decay process, but what counts is not merely the amount of sugar in the diet but how long any digestible carbohydrate remains in contact with the teeth. This, in turn, depends on such factors as the stickiness of the food, the type of bacteria on the teeth, and the extent of oral hygiene practiced by the individual.

21. They Display Credentials Not Recognized by Responsible Scientists or Educators.

The backbone of educational integrity in America is a system of accreditation by agencies recognized by the U.S. Secretary of Education or the Council on Postsecondary Recognition and Accreditation (CORPA). "Degrees" from nonaccredited schools are rarely worth the paper they are printed on. In the health field, there is no such thing as a reliable school that is not accredited.

Unfortunately, possession of an accredited degree does not guarantee reliability. Some schools that teach unscientific methods (chiropractic, naturopathy, acupuncture, and even quack nutritional methods) have achieved accreditation. Worse yet, a small percentage of individuals trained in reputable institutions (such as medical or dental schools or accredited universities) have strayed from scientific thought.

Since quacks operate outside of the scientific community, they also tend to form their own "professional" organizations. In some cases, the only membership requirement is payment of a fee. We and others we know have secured fancy "professional member" certificates for household pets by merely submitting the pet's name, address, and a check for $50. Don't assume that all groups with scientific-sounding names are respectable. Find out whether their views are scientifically based.

Some quacks are promoted with superlatives like "the world's foremost nutritionist" or "America's leading nutrition expert." There is no law against this tactic, just as there is none against calling oneself the "World's Foremost Lover." However, the scientific community recognizes no such titles. The designation "Nobel Prize Nominee" is also bogus and can be assumed to mean that someone has either nominated himself or had a close associate do so.

Some entrepreneurs claim to have degrees and/or affiliations to schools, hospitals, and/or professional that actually don't exist. The modern champion of this approach appears to be *Gregory E. Caplinger*, who claims to have acquired a medical degree, specialty training, board certification, and scores of professional affiliations—all from bogus or nonexistent sources.

22. They Offer to Determine Your Body's Nutritional State with a Laboratory Test or a Questionnaire.

Various health-food industry members and unscientific practitioners utilize tests that they claim can determine your body's nutritional state and—of course—what products you should buy from them. One favorite method is *hair analysis*. For $35 to $75 plus a lock of your hair, you can get an elaborate computer printout of vitamins and minerals you supposedly need. Hair analysis has limited value (mainly in forensic medicine) in the diagnosis of heavy metal poisoning, but it is worthless as a screening device to detect nutritional problems [2]. If a hair analysis laboratory recommends supplements, you can be sure that its computers are programmed to recommend them to everyone. Other tests used to hawk supplements include amino acid analysis of urine, muscle-testing (*applied kinesiology*), *iridology*, blood typing, "nutrient-deficiency" and/or lifestyle questionnaires, and *"electrodiagnostic" gadgets*.

23. They Claim They Are Being Persecuted by Orthodox Medicine and That Their Work Is Being Suppressed Because It's Controversial.

The "conspiracy charge" is an attempt to gain sympathy by portraying the quack as an "underdog." Quacks typically claim that the American Medical Association is against them because their cures would cut into the incomes that doctors make by keeping people sick. Don't fall for such nonsense! Reputable physicians are plenty busy. Moreover, many doctors engaged in prepaid health plans, group practice, full-time teaching, and government service receive the same salary whether or not their patients are sick—so keeping their patients healthy reduces their workload, not their income.

Quacks also claim there is a "controversy" about facts between themselves and "the bureaucrats," organized medicine, or "the establishment." They clamor for medical examination of their claims, but ignore any evidence that refutes them. The gambit "Do you believe in vitamins?" is another tactic used to increase confusion. Everyone knows that vitamins are needed by the human body. The real question is "Do you need additional vitamins beyond those in a well-balanced diet?" *For most people, the answer is no.* Nutrition is a science, not a religion. It is based upon matters of fact, not questions of belief.

Any physician who found a vitamin or other preparation that could cure sterility, heart disease, arthritis, cancer, or the like, could make an enormous fortune. Patients would flock to such a doctor (as they now do to those who falsely claim to cure such problems), and colleagues would shower the doctor with awards—including the extremely lucrative Nobel Prize! And don't forget, doctors get sick, too. Do you believe they would conspire to suppress cures for diseases that also afflict them and their loved ones? When polio was conquered, iron lungs became virtually obsolete, but nobody resisted this advancement because it would force hospitals to change. And neither will scientists mourn the eventual defeat of cancer.

24. They Warn You Not to Trust Your Doctor.

Quacks, who want you to trust them, suggest that most doctors are "butchers" and "poisoners." They exaggerate the shortcomings of our healthcare delivery system, but completely disregard their own—and those of other quacks. For the same reason, quacks also claim that doctors are nutrition illiterates. This, too, is untrue. The principles of nutrition are those of human biochemistry and physiology, courses required in every medical school. Some medical schools don't teach a separate required course labeled "Nutrition" because the subject is included in other courses at the points where it is most relevant. For example, nutrition in growth and development is taught in pediatrics, nutrition in wound healing is taught in surgery, and nutrition in pregnancy is covered in obstetrics. In addition, many medical schools do offer separate instruction in nutrition.

A physician's training, of course, does not end on the day of graduation from medical school or completion of specialty training. The medical profession advocates lifelong education, and some states require it for license renewal. Physicians can further their knowledge of nutrition by reading medical journals and textbooks, discussing cases with colleagues, and attending continuing education courses. Most doctors know what nutrients can and cannot do and can tell the difference between a real nutritional discovery and a piece of quack nonsense. Those who are unable to answer questions about dietetics (meal planning) can refer patients to someone who can—usually a registered dietitian.

Like all human beings, doctors sometimes make mistakes. However, quacks deliver mistreatment most of the time.

25. They Encourage Patients to Lend Political Support to Their Treatment Methods.

A century ago, before scientific methodology was generally accepted, valid new ideas were hard to evaluate and were sometimes rejected by a majority of the medical community, only to be upheld later. But today, treatments demonstrated as effective are welcomed by scientific practitioners and do not need a group to crusade for them. Quacks seek political endorsement because they can't prove that their methods work. Instead, they may seek to legalize their treatment and force insurance companies to pay for it. One of the surest signs that a treatment doesn't work is a political campaign to legalize its use.

References

1. Young JH, McFayden RE. The Koch Cancer Treatment. *Journal of the History of Medicine* 53:254–284, 1998.
2. Hambidge KM. *Hair analyses:* Worthless for vitamins, limited for minerals. *American Journal of Clinical Nutrition* 36:943–949, 1983.

This article was condensed from *The Vitamin Pushers: How the Health Food Industry Is Selling Americans a Bill of Goods.*

Yet Another Study—Should You Pay Attention?
How to know when to take health research news with a grain of salt

Hot Dogs Cause Cancer? Researchers Say Yes

New warnings revive fears about the danger of eating hot dogs, particularly among children

Study Links Hot Dogs, Cancer Ingestion by Children Boosts Leukemia Risk, Report Says

SO WENT headlines in the *Los Angeles Times,* the *New York Times,* and the *Washington Post* back in June of 1994. They came on the heels of three studies published simultaneously in a cancer research journal.

One of the studies found that children who eat more than 12 hot dogs a month have nine times the normal risk of developing childhood leukemia. The second suggested that children born to mothers who eat at least one frank a week during pregnancy have double the normal risk of developing brain tumors. The third traced brain tumors in children to *fathers* who ate hot dogs before conception. The risk of leukemia to children born of fathers who consumed hot dogs regularly was 11 times normal.

The problem: the three studies—and most certainly all the media commentary they attracted—were riddled with scientific holes.

To be sure, many of the reports in newspapers and other media outlets did point out weaknesses in the studies. But those weaknesses were strung between unnecessarily alarming headlines and warnings from researchers who, perhaps, had themselves experienced something of a knee-jerk reaction to the research. For instance, the concluding paragraph of the *New York Times* article leaves readers with this quoted advice about frankfurters from the former director of a cancer research center: "Reduce consumption of them as much as you can. They are a source of a possible cancer risk. I would not expose my children to it. It's like secondhand smoking."

Therein lies the difficulty at the heart of the matter. If scientists can't always look at research with a cool eye, how in the world are *you* supposed to? Following, **four questions to ask yourself as you read about study results or hear about them on the news.** They should help you put the latest reports into perspective as you try to make informed decisions about how to improve or maintain your lifestyle habits.

1 *What are the actual numbers as opposed to the relative numbers?* Let's say the hot dog research was airtight and children who eat franks more than a dozen times each month really are nine times (900 percent) more likely to get leukemia than children who eat them less often. The question is, how likely are children to develop leukemia to begin with?

They have a 0.3-in-1,000 chance. If you multiplied that number by nine to get the risk for children who have more than a dozen franks every month, the answer comes to roughly 2.5 in 1,000.

The point here is that even if something is many times more likely to happen under certain circumstances, that doesn't mean its potential influence is great enough to warrant changing the way you live your life.

Adding to the mathematical irrelevance of the findings is that there were only 17 children out of hundreds in the study who ate more than 12 franks each month—much too few to make any declarations about the dangers of hot dogs for the general population.

2 *What type of study was it?* There are three major types of human research—clinical trials, epidemiologic studies, and population-based intervention trials—and each has inherent strengths and limitations.

Clinical trials A clinical trial is an experiment conducted in a controlled setting, often a hospital, where researchers give a group of people treatment—such as a supplement, drug, or diet—and then measure their response.

Clinical trials are believed to yield very accurate results that can help establish cause-and-effect relationships between various substances or lifestyle activities and specific health outcomes. However, they tend to be conducted on restricted groups of people that include, for instance, just one age group, sex, or race. That allows the scientists to keep the study environment more "air-tight" so that variations within the population being studied don't confound the results. However, it means the results are not necessarily generalizable to all people. Clinical trials often need to be repeated in different groups with different genetic makeups and lifestyles before a recommendation for the general public can reliably be made.

Epidemiologic studies
Epidemiologic studies look at much larger groups of people than clinical trials—up to tens of thousands of subjects. These are not experiments in which researchers control a certain aspect of the subjects' lives but, rather, make *observations* of free-living populations in which they search for relationships between lifestyle or genetic factors and the risk for chronic diseases. Harvard University's Nurses' Health Study, which looks at the lifestyles of some 90,000 women, is an example of epidemiologic research.

Because epidemiologic research is generally conducted on large groups of people, the results tend to be more generalizable to the population at large. However, epidemiology virtually never proves cause and effect; it can only make *associations* on which other researchers might then decide to base a clinical trial to test whether "X" lifestyle actually leads to "Y" condition.

Granted, the more people in the study and the more tightly controlled it is for various lifestyle factors, the higher the chance that there really is something to any association found. But still, one can never automatically assume that an association proves a cause.

To show just how tenuous links brought to light in epidemiologic studies can be, scientists who published research on aspirin and heart disease in the prestigious journal *The Lancet* pointed out that according to one of their findings, people born under the signs of Gemini and Libra are likely to be harmed by taking aspirin rather than helped. If that piece of their research were serious science, the conclusion might be drawn by some that astrological influences directly affect health. The researchers highlighted the association specifically to point out the mistakes that could be made in viewing epidemiologic associations as fact.

Population-Based Intervention Trials Sort of a cross between an epidemiologic study and a clinical trial, a population-based intervention trial is a project in which large numbers of people live freely rather than in a controlled setting but are given either a treatment or a placebo and then observed to see whether a specific outcome occurs. A study of 29,000 male Finnish smokers that was released a few years ago, in which those who took beta-carotene turned out to be more likely to develop lung cancer than those who didn't, is an example of an intervention trial.

The strength of such studies is that, like epidemiologic research, they can observe thousands of people. The drawback is that they cannot be as well-controlled as clinical trials. Thus, it may not always be the treatment that's having the effect (or the full effect) but something in the subjects' lifestyles that the scientists didn't account for.

3 *Does the study stand alone, or are its results corroborated by other pieces of research?* A single study hardly ever tells the whole story. While the goal of the media is to turn a piece of research into news—or at least to make news sound exciting—the goal of scientists is to add *incrementally* to a body of knowledge. In fact, before a scientist makes a recommendation, there must be supportive evidence from a variety of approaches so that the strengths of all of them combined compensate for the weaknesses in any single one. Clinical and epidemiologic studies are not the only kinds of investigations necessary. There is also research conducted with tissue cultures and with laboratory animals—which often doesn't make the front page or the 6 o'clock news.

Consider the hot dog research. The scientists who conducted it commented that perhaps chemicals in hot dogs called nitrites cause leukemia. One way they could test that theory would be to "contaminate" normal cells in the laboratory with various doses of nitrites and see whether the cells mutated in such a way as to suggest that inside the body, the mutations would develop into leukemia.

They could also feed various doses of hot dogs—or of nitrites themselves—to laboratory animals and see if hot dog-nourished animals developed leukemia at a faster rate than those fed other meats. Cell culture studies and animal studies would also be necessary to help determine why hot dog-eating mothers raised their children's risk of developing brain cancer two-fold while hot dog-eating fathers raised the risk 11-fold. After all, for 9 months, a developing fetus is directly affected by everything its mother eats. Thus, without any clues to a plausible mechanism for how a father's frankfurter consumption could have so much more of an effect than a mother's, the numbers remain in the realm of fluke findings, and the hot dog hypothesis remains just that.

4 *Was the study published in a peer-reviewed journal?* Peer review is the process by which experts in a particular field review a study before it is accepted for publication in order to ensure that it was conducted appropriately. It is their express role to poke holes in the study's design or the researchers' interpretations. Only if they deem the study scientifically "clean" do the publication's editors print it. The journal in which the hot dog-leukemia research was published, *Cancer Causes and Control*, is not peer-reviewed. If it were, the research, riddled as it is with inconsistencies and faulty methodology, probably never would have made it into print.

Mini-Glossary of Research Terms

Placebo-controlled: If a clinical trial or population-based intervention trial is placebo-controlled, that means there is a group similar to the treatment group that is given a mock pill, or placebo. The effect on the placebo group allows researchers to tell whether the actual treatment is having an effect or whether it's just the fact that their subjects are being treated; sometimes just being given a "sugar pill" provides a psychological boost that yields beneficial results.

Double-blind: A double-blind trial is one in which neither the study participants nor the researchers heading the study know who is getting the real treatment and who is getting the placebo until the experiment is over. As a result, the subjects can't knowingly alter their lifestyles during the trial to make the treatment more or less effective, and the researchers are prevented from reading into findings in order to come up with "expected" results.

Prospective study: In a prospective epidemiologic study, scientists look at a group of people at a specific point (or points) in time and then wait to see who gets what diseases before making associations between lifestyle and risk of illness. Harvard's Nurses' Health Study is prospective.

Retrospective study: In a retrospective study, researchers compare people with a disease or other condition to a similar group of people who aren't affected and then look backwards in time to see what differences in their lifestyles might have contributed to the different outcomes in their health status. Some retrospective studies are designed better than others. In the retrospective study that looked at pregnant women's consumption of hot dogs, mothers with teenage children were asked to recall what they ate as many as 14 years ago. (Can you remember what you ate last week?)

Article 51

ALTERNATIVE MEDICINE— THE RISKS OF UNTESTED AND UNREGULATED REMEDIES

WHAT is there about alternative medicine that sets it apart from ordinary medicine? The term refers to a remarkably heterogeneous group of theories and practices—as disparate as homeopathy, therapeutic touch, imagery, and herbal medicine. What unites them? Eisenberg et al. defined alternative medicine (now often called complementary medicine) as "medical interventions not taught widely at U.S. medical schools or generally available at U.S. hospitals."[1] That is not a very satisfactory definition, especially since many alternative remedies have recently found their way into the medical mainstream. Medical schools teach alternative medicine, hospitals and health maintenance organizations offer it,[2] and laws in some states require health plans to cover it.[3] It also constitutes a huge and rapidly growing industry, in which major pharmaceutical companies are now participating.[4]

What most sets alternative medicine apart, in our view, is that it has not been scientifically tested and its advocates largely deny the need for such testing. By testing, we mean the marshaling of rigorous evidence of safety and efficacy, as required by the Food and Drug Administration (FDA) for the approval of drugs and by the best peer-reviewed medical journals for the publication of research reports. Of course, many treatments used in conventional medicine have not been rigorously tested, either, but the scientific community generally acknowledges that this is a failing that needs to be remedied. Many advocates of alternative medicine, in contrast, believe the scientific method is simply not applicable to their remedies. They rely instead on anecdotes and theories.

In 1992, Congress established within the National Institutes of Health an Office of Alternative Medicine to evaluate alternative remedies. So far, the results have been disappointing. For example of the 30 research grants the office awarded in 1993, 28 have resulted in "final reports" (abstracts) that are listed in the office's public on-line data base.[5] But a Med-line search almost six years after the grants were awarded revealed that only 9 of the 28 resulted in published papers. Five were in 2 journals not included among the 3500 journal titles in the Countway Library of Medicine's collection.[6-10] Of the other four studies, none was a controlled clinical trial that would allow any conclusions to be drawn about the efficacy of an alternative treatment.[11-14]

It might be argued that conventional medicine relies on anecdotes, too, some of which are published as case reports in peer-reviewed journals. But these case reports differ from the anecdotes of alternative medicine. They describe a well-documented new finding in a defined setting. If, for example, the *Journal* were to receive a paper describing a patient's recovery from cancer of the pancreas after he had ingested a rhubarb diet, we would require documentation of the disease and its extent, we would ask about other, similar patients who did not recover after eating rhubarb, and we might suggest trying the diet on other patients. If the answers to these and other questions were satisfactory, we might publish a case report—not to announce a remedy, but only to suggest a hypothesis that should be tested in a proper clinical trial. In contrast, anecdotes about alternative remedies (usually published in books and magazines

From *The New England Journal of Medicine*, September 17, 1998, pp. 839–841. © 1998 by the Massachusetts Medical Society. All rights reserved. Reprinted by permission.

for the public) have no such documentation and are considered sufficient in themselves as support for therapeutic claims.

Alternative medicine also distinguishes itself by an ideology that largely ignores biologic mechanisms, often disparages modern science, and relies on what are purported to be ancient practices and natural remedies (which are seen as somehow being simultaneously more potent and less toxic than conventional medicine). Accordingly, herbs or mixtures of herbs are considered superior to the active compounds isolated in the laboratory. And healing methods such as homeopathy and therapeutic touch are fervently promoted despite not only the lack of good clinical evidence of effectiveness, but the presence of a rationale that violates fundamental scientific laws—surely a circumstance that requires more, rather than less, evidence.

Of all forms of alternative treatment, the most common is herbal medicine.[15] Until the 20th century, most remedies were botanicals, a few of which were found through trial and error to be helpful. For example, purple foxglove was found to be helpful for dropsy, the opium poppy for pain, cough, and diarrhea, and cinchona bark for fever. But therapeutic successes with botanicals came at great human cost. The indications for using a given botanical were ill defined, dosage was arbitrary because the concentrations of the active ingredient were unknown, and all manner of contaminants were often present. More important, many of the remedies simply did not work, and some were harmful or even deadly. The only way to separate the beneficial from the useless or hazardous was through anecdotes relayed mainly by word of mouth.

All that began to change in the 20th century as a result of rapid advances in medical science. The emergence of sophisticated chemical and pharmacologic methods meant that we could identify and purify the active ingredients in botanicals and study them. Digitalis was extracted from the purple foxglove, morphine from the opium poppy, and quinine from cinchona bark. Furthermore, once the chemistry was understood, it was possible to synthesize related molecules with more desirable properties. For example, penicillin was fortuitously discovered when penicillium mold contaminated some bacterial cultures. Isolating and characterizing it permitted the synthesis of a wide variety of related antibiotics with different spectrums of activity.

In addition, powerful epidemiologic tools were developed for testing potential remedies. In particular, the evolution of the randomized, controlled clinical trial enabled researchers to study with precision the safety, efficacy, and dose effects of proposed treatments and the indications for them. No longer do we have to rely on trial and error and anecdotes. We have learned to ask for and expect statistically reliable evidence before accepting conclusions about remedies. Without such evidence, the FDA will not permit a drug to be marketed.

The results of these advances have been spectacular. As examples, we now know that treatment with aspirin, heparin, thrombolytic agents, and beta-adrenergic blockers greatly reduces mortality from myocardial infarction; a combination of nucleoside analogues and a protease inhibitor can stave off the onset of AIDS in people with human immunodeficiency virus infection; antibiotics heal peptic ulcers; and a cocktail of cytotoxic drugs can cure most cases of childhood leukemia. Also in this century, we have developed and tested vaccines against a great many infectious scourges, including measles, poliomyelitis, pertussis, diphtheria, hepatitis B, some forms of meningitis, and pneumococcal pneumonia, and we have a vast arsenal of effective antibiotics for many others. In less than a century, life expectancy in the United States has increased by three decades, in part because of better sanitation and living standards, but in large part because of advances in medicine realized through rigorous testing. Other countries lagged behind, but as scientific medicine became universal, all countries affluent enough to afford it saw the same benefits.

Now, with the increased interest in alternative medicine, we see a reversion to irrational approaches to medical practice, even while scientific medicine is making some of its most dramatic advances. Exploring the reasons for this paradox is outside the scope of this editorial, but it is probably in part a matter of disillusionment with the often hurried and impersonal care delivered by conventional physicians, as well as the harsh treatments that may be necessary for life-threatening diseases.

Fortunately, most untested herbal remedies are probably harmless. In addition, they seem to be used primarily by people who are healthy and believe the remedies will help them stay that way, or by people who have common, relatively minor problems, such as backache or fatigue.[1] Most such people would probably seek out conventional doctors if they had indications of serious disease, such as crushing chest pain, a mass in the breast, or blood in the urine. Still, uncertainty about whether symptoms are serious could result in a harmful delay in getting treatment that has been proved effective. And some people may embrace alternative medicine exclusively, putting themselves in great danger. In this issue of the *Journal*, Coppes et al. describe two such instances.[16]

Also in this issue, we see that there are risks of alternative medicine in addition to that of failing to receive effective treatment. Slifman and her colleagues report a case of digitalis toxicity in a young woman who had ingested a contaminated herbal concoction.[17] Ko reports finding widespread inconsistencies and adulterations in his analysis of Asian patent medicines.[18] LoVecchio et al. report on a patient who suffered central nervous system depression after ingesting a substance sold in health-food stores as a growth hormone stimulator,[19] and Beigel and colleagues describe the puzzling clinical course of a patient in whom lead poisoning developed after he took an Indian herbal remedy for his diabetes.[20] These are without doubt simply examples of what will be a rapidly growing problem.

What about the FDA? Shouldn't it be monitoring the safety and efficacy of these remedies? Not any longer, according to the U.S. Congress. In response to the lobbying efforts of the multibillion-dollar "dietary supplement" industry, Congress in 1994 exempted their products from FDA regulation.[21,22] (Homeopathic remedies have been exempted since 1938.[23]) Since then, these products have flooded the market, subject only to the scruples of their manufacturers. They may contain the substances listed on the label in the amounts claimed, but they need not, and there is no one to prevent their sale if they don't. In analyses of ginseng products, for example, the amount of the active ingredient in each pill varied by as much as a factor of 10 among brands that were labeled as containing the same amount.[24] Some brands contained none at all.[25]

Herbal remedies may also be sold without any knowledge of their mechanism of action. In this issue of the *Journal*, DiPaola and his colleagues report that the herbal mixture called PC-SPES (PC for prostate cancer, and *spes* the Latin for "hope") has substantial estrogenic activity.[26] Yet this substance is promoted as bolstering the immune system in patients with prostate cancer that is refractory to treatment with estrogen.[27] Many men taking PC-SPES have thus received varying amounts of hormonal treatment without knowing it, some in addition to the estrogen treatments given to them by their conventional physicians.

The only legal requirement in the sale of such products is that they need not be promoted as preventing or treating disease.[28] To comply with that stipulation, their labeling has risen to an art form of double-speak (witness the name PC-SPES). Not only are they sold under the euphemistic rubric "dietary supplements," but also the medical uses for which they are sold are merely insinuated. Nevertheless, it is clear what is meant. Shark cartilage (priced in a local drugstore at more than $3 for a day's dose) is promoted on its label "to maintain proper bone and joint function," saw palmetto to "promote prostate health," and horse-chestnut seed extract to "promote... leg vein health." Anyone can walk into a health-food store and unwittingly buy PC-SPES with unknown amounts of estrogenic activity, plantain laced with digitalis, or Indian herbs contaminated with heavy metals. Caveat emptor. The FDA can intervene only after the fact, when it is shown that a product is harmful.[28]

It is time for the scientific community to stop giving alternative medicine a free ride. There cannot be two kinds of medicine—conventional and alternative. There is only medicine that has been adequately tested and medicine that has not, medicine that works and medicine that may or may not work. Once a treatment has been tested rigorously, it no longer matters whether it was considered alternative at the outset. If it is found to be reasonably safe and effective, it will be accepted. But assertions, speculation, and testimonials do not substitute for evidence. Alternative treatments should be subjected to scientific testing no less rigorous than that required for conventional treatments.

MARCIA ANGELL, M.D.
JEROME P. KASSIRER, M.D.

References

1. Eisenberg D. M., Kessler R. C., Foster C., Norlock F. E., Calkins, D. R., Delbanco T. L. Unconventional medicine in the United States—prevalence, costs, and patterns of use. N. Engl J Med 1993;328:246–52.

2. Spiegel D., Stroud P., Fyfe A. Complementary medicine. West J Med 1998;168:241–7.

3. Cooper R. A., Stoflet S. J. Trends in the education and practice of alternative medicine clinicians. Health Aff (Millwood) 1996;15(3):226–38.

4. Canedy D. Real medicine or medicine show? Growth of herbal remedy sales raises issues about value. New York Times. July 23, 1998:D1.

5. National Institutes of Health, Office of Alternative Medicine. Grant award and research data. Bethesda, Md.: Office of Alternative Medicine. (See: http://altmed.od.nih.gov/oam/research/grants.)

6. Chou C. K., McDougall J. A., Ahn C., Vora N. Electrochemical treatment of mouse and rat fibrosarcomas with direct current. Bioelectromagnetics 1997;18(1):14–24.

7. Olson M., Sneed N., LaVia M., Virella G., Bonadonna R., Michel Y. Stress-induced immunosuppression and therapeutic touch. Alternative Ther Health Med 1997;3(2):68–74.

8. Shaffer H. J., LaSalvia T. A., Stein J. P. Comparing Hatha yoga with dynamic group psychotherapy for enhancing methadone maintenance treatment: a randomized clinical trial. Alternative Ther Health Med 1997;3(4):57–66.

9. Walker S. R., Tonigan J. S., Miller W. R., Corner S., Kahlich L. Intercessory prayer in the treatment of alcohol abuse and dependence: a pilot investigation. Alternative Ther Health Med 1997;3(6):79–86.

10. Richardson M. A., Post-White J., Grimm E. A., Moye L. A., Singletary S. E., Justice B. Coping, life attitudes, and immune responses to imagery and group support after breast cancer treatment. Alternative Ther Health Med 1997;3(5):62–70.

11. Reid S. A., Duke L. M., Allen J. B. Resting frontal electroencephalographic asymmetry in depression: inconsistencies suggest the need to identify mediating factors. Psychophysiology 1998;35(4):389–404.

12. Crawford H. J., Knebel T., Kaplan L., et al. Hypnotic analgesia. 1. Somatosensory event-related potential changes to noxious stimuli and 2. Transfer learning to reduce chronic low back pain. Int J Clin Exp Hypn 1998;46:92–132.

13. Shannahoff-Khalsa D. S., Beckett L. R. Clinical case report: efficacy of yogic techniques in the treatment of obsessive compulsive disorders. Int J Neurosci 1996;85:1–17.

14. Prasad K. N., Hernandez C., Edwards-Prasad J., Nelson J., Borus T., Robinson W. A. Modification of the effect of tamoxifen, cis-platin, DTIC, and interferon–α2b on human melanoma cells in culture by a mixture of vitamins. Nutr Cancer 1994;22:233™45.

15. Brody J. E. Alternative medicine makes inroads, but watch out for curves. New York Times. April 28, 1998:F7.

16. Coppes M. J., Anderson R. A. Egeler R. M., Wolff J. E. A. Alternative therapies for the treatment of childhood cancer. N Engl J Med 1998;339:846–7.

17. Slifman N. R., Obermeyer W. R., Aloi B. K., et al. Contamination of botanical dietary supplements by *Digitalis lanata*. N Engl J Med 1998;339:806–11.

18. Ko R. J. Adulterants in Asian patent medicines. N Engl J Med 1998;339:847.

19. LoVecchio F., Curry S. C., Bagnasco T. Butyrolactone-induced central nervous system depression after ingestion of RenewTrient, a "dietary supplement." N Engl J Med 1998;339:847–8.

20. Beigel Y., Ostfeld I. Schoenfeld N. A. leading question. N Engl J Med 1998;339:827–30.

21. Wittes B. FDA exemption sought for self-help medicines. The Recorder. October 7, 1994:2.

22. Dietary Supplement Health and Education Act of 1994. (Public Law 103-417.)

23. Wagner M. W. Is homeopathy 'new science' or 'new age'? Sci Rev Alternative Med 1997;1(1):7–12.

24. Herbal roulette. Consumer Reports. November 1995:698.

25. Cui, J., Garle M., Eneroth P., Björkhem I. What do commercial ginseng preparations contain? Lancet 1994;344:134.

26. DiPaola R. S., Zhang H., Lambert G. H., et al. Clinical and biologic activity of an estrogenic herbal combination (PC-SPES) in prostate cancer. N Engl J Med 1998;339:785–91.

27. Anticancer botanicals that work supportively with chemotherapy: PCSpes. Alternative Medicine Digest. November 1997:84–5.

28. Love L. A. The MedWatch Program. Clin Toxicol 1998;36:263–7.

The Mouse that Roared:

Health Scares on the Internet

The World Wide Web is a tremendous resource for consumers and others who want an additional outlet to help them take control of their health. "The Internet is full of important, even lifesaving, medical information," stated Randolph Wykoff, M.D., M.P.H., of the U.S. Food and Drug Administration (FDA). But, not all Internet information passes the test of the Hippocratic oath. Enter: Doctor Deception who now makes house calls.

On occasion, some not-so-sound information spoils a wealth of excellent information on the Internet. With a click of the mouse, a word-of-mouth phenomenon can be multiplied exponentially via the World Wide Web or electronic mail and result in questionable nutrition, food safety and health stories being sent directly to your computer. In the age of the Internet and instantaneous global communication—in tandem with an increasing interest in nutrition's relation to health—it is not surprising that anyone with a modem can send consumers and others into a food and health panic.

Most of us have heard at least a few of the following myths that have been started and perpetuated on the Web: the great kidney harvest caper; the antibacterial sponge made with agent orange; the fluorescent lights that leach vitamins from your body; the cancer-causing shampoo, and dozens, maybe hundreds more.

These would all be simply entertaining if everyone recognized them as practical jokes, the mantras of unhappy people, or simply misunderstandings given life on the Internet. But not everyone can recognize these tall tales as fiction.

The Bias Belt
Some of the most egregious myths come from legitimate sounding individuals who have fallen in love with their theories. They believe they are serving the public by warning them of dire health consequences as the result of touching, smelling, eating or drinking a perfectly safe product. Many consumers are confused and unwittingly oblige in the scam by forwarding the frightening electronic mail or referencing the site to family, friends and associates believing they are doing them a service. And, receiving one of these reports from a family member or friend adds to its alleged authenticity.

A recent *TIME Magazine* article (April 26, 1999) sums it up well: "The Web is praised as a wondrous educational tool, and in some respects it is. Mostly though, it appears to be a stunning advance in the shoring up of biases, both benign (one's own views) and noxious (other views)."

In most cases, there is no harm intended by those who position their opinions as facts. In other instances, the sly intent of the author may be relatively easy for health professionals, who have a strong science background, to detect. But, for some consumers with little frame of reference to tell fact from fiction, it can be misleading.

For example, an innocent Web surfer looking for information about dietary fats may stumble across one of several Web sites spreading fear and confusion about a frequently used cooking oil. With a masthead featuring a skull and crossbones, or the headline: "Canola Oil: Deadly for the Human Body!," such sites may cause baseless consumer concern. If the consumer does not seek unbiased information, he or she will miss the real story: canola oil, a safe, monounsaturated oil, can help lower blood cholesterol levels when substituted for saturated fats in the diet.

Where Did You Hear That?
"At one time, doctors were the primary source of health information for

consumers, but in the late 1990s the paradigm for securing this type of information changed," remarked Fergus Clydesdale, Ph.D., University of Massachusetts. Now, for both consumers and health professionals, the primary source of information is the news media. This information source replaces the traditional physician-patient relationship for consumers. For health professionals, media accounts now precede the medical journals and attendance at academic meetings. Often, a consumer first raises an issue with his or her health professional by asking about a story that ran in an on-line story, the local paper or on the evening TV news before health professionals have even received their journals.

A recent telephone survey conducted by Schwarz Pharma, Inc., and reported in the *American Journal of Public Health,* noted that approximately 29 percent of Americans have turned to the Internet for medical information—a number that, although not high compared to other media outlets, is likely to grow.

According to the *1997 Nutrition Trends Survey* conducted by The American Dietetic Association (ADA), 57 percent of consumers named television as their main source of nutrition information, followed by magazines at 44 percent and newspapers at 23 percent. Doctors and dietitians were at just 9 and 5 percent, respectively (see graph).

The same ADA survey, however, found that the tables were turned in terms of credibility. Information from doctors and dietitians/nutritionists was found to be "more valuable" (52%) than that from television news and newspaper articles (24% and 21%, respectively). The Internet may follow this same pattern of delivery versus credibility—the Internet or World Wide Web was found to be the least believable source of medical and health news according to respondents in the 1997 report, *Americans Talk About Science and Medical News* from the National Health Council. While the Internet can be a valuable source for scientifically accurate health information, it can also be a frontier town with no sheriff for assuring the truth of the information presented.

John Renner, M.D., of the National Council for Reliable Health Information remarked, "There is a health information shock factor on the Internet because there is so much information, both good and bad, marvelous and terrible. We've moved from a small library of information with a friendly librarian, to a huge warehouse with lots of people offering information," he continued. Consumers have not faced this situation before. The problem is the public can be deceived—believing that because they have seen something on the Web, it must be true.

A perfect example of how the public can be misled is a recent Internet article by a Nancy Markle that has taken on a "cyberlife" of its own. The article alleges that aspartame (a sweetener found in food and beverages) causes lupus, multiple sclerosis (MS) and other diseases and conditions, none of which has any scientific validity. Highly respected health professional organizations were fraudulently associated with the story, and numerous vulnerable people were needlessly frightened by this scientifically false allegation.

One of the marvels of the Internet is that as easily as you can receive *inaccurate* information, you can search for and find *accurate* information. If consumers were concerned about the alleged aspartame connection with MS, they could check the Multiple Sclerosis Foundation's Internet site for accurate information. David Squillacote, M.D., senior medical advisor of the MS Foundation wrote in his response to the Internet scare, "This series of allegations by Ms. Markle are almost totally without foundation. They are rabidly inaccurate and scandalously misinformative." Fortunately, numerous reliable organizations, Internet sites and publications have refuted this particular epidemic of hysteria and provided additional context for consumers.

The FDA's website is an excellent source for accurate information. Consumers wishing to counteract or confirm the aspartame story can find the following information from the FDA which could allay their fears: "After reviewing scientific studies, the FDA determined in 1981 that aspartame was safe for use in foods.... To date, the FDA has not determined any consistent pattern of symptoms that can be attributed to the use of aspartame, nor is the agency aware of any recent studies that clearly show safety problems."

What's a Cyber-Citizen to Do?

How can consumers judge the validity of information received via electronic

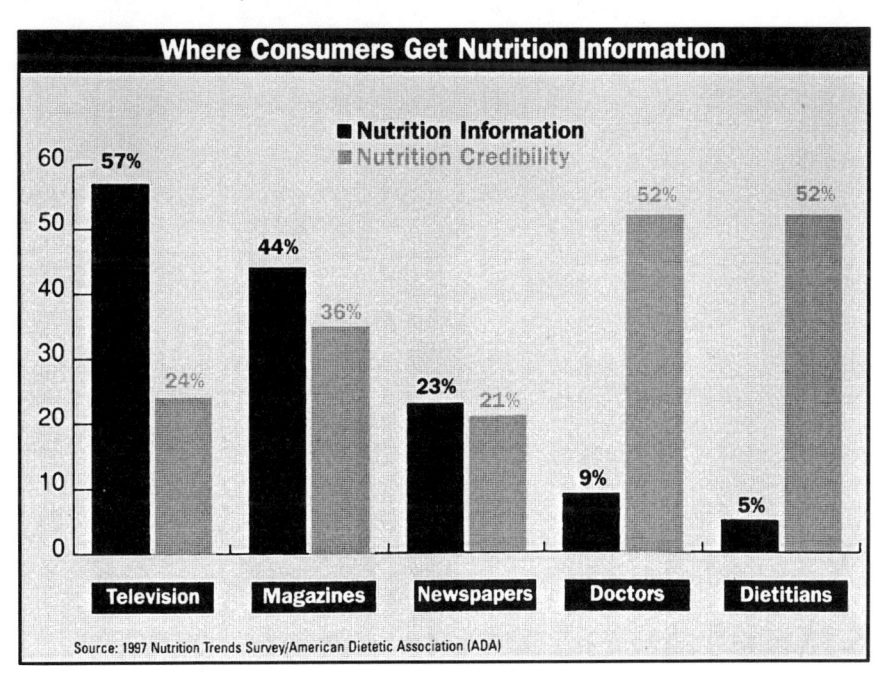

Where Consumers Get Nutrition Information

Source	Nutrition Information	Nutrition Credibility
Television	57%	24%
Magazines	44%	36%
Newspapers	23%	21%
Doctors	9%	52%
Dietitians	5%	52%

Source: 1997 Nutrition Trends Survey/American Dietetic Association (ADA)

6 ❖ HEALTH CLAIMS

mail or popping up in a Web search? The foremost guideline for sorting the "trash" from the "treasure" is—just because something is printed on the Internet does not mean that it is true or credible.

Unfortunately for most of us, the best defense against nutrition misinformation and quackery on the Internet is in-depth scientific knowledge. Since not everyone has the level of scientific awareness or advanced degrees necessary to judge the validity of every story, the following tactics may be useful:

- Ask questions. Anecdotes and one individual's personal story are not scientific evidence.
- Look at the source of the information. A professional medical organization or government agency such as the American Academy of Family Physicians or the U.S. Department of Agriculture is more likely to have reliable information than an unknown person or group of people.
- If the story mentions a specific health condition, such as diabetes or breast cancer, search the Internet for reputable health professional organizations and foundations devoted to that disease. An example would be the American Diabetes Association or the American Cancer Society.
- Watch out for use of buzzwords like "conspiracy" and "poison."
- Don't take assertions at face value—give the other side of the issue the benefit of the doubt. Do your homework and call or e-mail appropriate health professional organizations to get a balanced picture.
- Consult with your doctor, a registered dietitian or other health professional.

The Internet has been a boon to consumers who want research and information on voluminous issues and topics at the tip of their fingers. It has also empowered many people to find health information to help them improve their well-being. Nevertheless, the ease of Web publishing has also given an unregulated forum to unreliable sources. Careful scrutiny and a healthy dose of skepticism are still necessary to determine what applies to you and what may need a second opinion.

Internet sources for sound nutrition and health information

- Tufts University Nutrition Navigator
  http://navigator.tufts.edu
- The American Dietetic Association
  http://www.eatright.org
- The International Food Information Council Foundation http://ificinfo.health.org
- Medline
  http://www.nlm.nih.gov/databases/freemedl.html
- National Institutes of Health
  http://www.nih.gov
- The U.S. Food and Drug Administration
  http://vm.cfsan.fda.gov
- Mayo Health Oasis (of the Mayo Clinic)
  http://www.mayohealth.org
- Johns Hopkins Health Information
  http://www.intelihealth.com/IH/ihtIH
- World Health Organization
  http://www.who.int
- Food & Agriculture Organization
  http://www.fao.org
- Government healthfinder
  http://www.healthfinder.gov

Uprooting herbal myths

Some herbal remedies do seem to work. But misconceptions about herbs can lead to disappointment—or danger.

The notion of herbal remedies used to evoke images of faraway lands, mystical healers, and exotic shops scented with incense. But today, herbal products are moving headlong into the mainstream. Bayer Corporation, maker of *Bayer Aspirin* and *One-A-Day* vitamins, is launching a line of *One-A-Day Specialized Supplements*, which combined herbs with vitamins or minerals. Other corporate giants, including American Home Products, SmithKline Beecham, and Warner-Lambert, have their own herbal-supplement lines either in the works or already on the shelves. And the products won't be tucked away in some obscure corner of the local health-food store; they'll be sold in supermarkets, large retail chains, and major drugstores, right alongside the conventional over-the-counter drugs.

The herbal-image makeover stems partly from recent research showing that some remedies—such as feverfew for migraine, ginger for nausea, saw palmetto for symptoms of prostate enlargement, and St. John's wort for minor depression—may indeed be at least mildly effective. Those findings help dispel one myth about herbal remedies: that they're all based on nothing more than folklore or Eastern traditions, with little or no scientific support.

But the upgraded image of herbal remedies may help perpetuate the opposite—and potentially more harmful—type of misconception, which glorifies herbs, overstates their benefits, and obscures their possible risks. Here are six such myths.

1. Myth: Herbs are natural, so they must be safe and effective.

Truth: "Natural" is hardly synonymous with "safe"—just think of hemlock or poisonous mushrooms. And while most herbal remedies are believed to be benign at least in the short run, there are numerous exceptions.

Probably all herbs have the potential to cause allergic reactions, and many herbs can produce side effects, such as stomach upset or diarrhea from saw palmetto or feverfew. Overdosing or overuse can lead to greater danger. Taking high doses of ephedra (ma huang), for example, can cause high blood pressure, heart palpitations, stroke, seizure, and even death. Taking licorice or cascara sagrada bark for more than a few weeks can deplete potassium levels and, in turn, cause muscle weakness and potentially deadly heart-rhythm irregularities. Moreover, certain herbs can harm people with certain diseases, or interact dangerously with conventional drugs.

> **'Natural' is not synonymous with 'safe'—just think of hemlock.**

Some herbal products may be contaminated with pesticides or toxic chemicals, such as arsenic, mercury, and lead; that's most often found in chopped-plant products and various Asian remedies. Other herbal products, usually pills or extracts, may be illegally spiked with potentially harmful prescription drugs, including steroids and diazepam *(Valium)*.

"Natural" is not synonymous with "effective," either. Herb enthusiasts claim that the multiple compounds in plant remedies work in a synergistic, or mutually enhancing way, and that "natural" compounds are absorbed more readily than synthetic ones. But while herbs do contain numerous compounds, their effect often stems from a single active ingredient—such as kawain for the calming effect of kava kava, or capsaicin for the pain-relieving effect of hot pepper. Moreover, the body can't tell whether the compound comes straight from a plant or is synthesized in a lab. Once scientists replicate the chemical structure of a "natural" substance, the copy has exactly the same effect on the body. For example, salicin and its synthetic twin salicylic acid, the active ingredient in early aspirin-like products, are equally effective, both for headaches and for inflammation. Acetylsalicylic acid—a derivative developed to reduce side effects and used today in all aspirin products—also works equally well. However, you'd have to drink about 10 cups of white-willow-bark tea or take dozens of capsules before you'd get enough salicin to equal the amount of acetylsalicylic acid in a single standard aspirin tablet.

2. Myth: Herbs must be safe and effective because they've been used for thousands of years.

Truth: Traditional healers never knew about the risks of many herbs, for two reasons. Certain health problems—such as cancer caused by chemicals in borage, coltsfoot, comfrey, life root, and sassafras root—may not show up for years, so it's hard to pin them on the herb without a long-term study. Other serious problems occur too infrequently to be noticed except by a large study or by gathering numerous isolated case reports.

As for effectiveness, people have used such herbs as alfalfa, chaparral, goldenseal, pennyroyal, and yucca for centuries. But modern research has debunked many of their purported benefits—and confirmed none of them.

3. Myth: You don't need to tell your doctor you're taking herbs.

Truth: In one survey, three out of four people who took herbal supplements said that they never told their doctor. That's unwise.

Adverse reactions to herbs may go undiagnosed—and mistreated—if your doctor doesn't know what you're taking. That's particularly worrisome for people who have a chronic disease. For example, echinacea may aggravate rheumatoid arthritis or other disorders caused by misdirected immune activity; eleuthero may send blood pressure soaring in people with hypertension; and devil's claw root may make gastric or duodenal ulcers worse.

Further, some herbs may interact harmfully with the drugs your doctor prescribes. Herbal laxatives such as flaxseed, guar gum, and psyllium can slow the absorption of most medications. Garlic, ginger, and ginkgo biloba may inhibit clotting, which could cause excessive bleeding if you're taking other, more powerful blood thinners such as aspirin or warfarin *(Coumadin)*. And ginseng and gotu kola may lower blood sugar excessively in people taking conventional diabetic drugs to control sugar levels.

4. Myth: If the label says an herb works, there must be some scientific evidence that it does.

Truth: The label for one saw palmetto supplement says it "promotes prostate and urinary well-being." Another, for goldenseal, says it helps "reduce inflammation of mucous membranes." Most makers of herbal products now make such claims—and they almost never have to provide any proof.

Since passage of the Dietary Supplement Health and Education Act of 1994, the Food and Drug Administration has had to allow such unproven claims, provided the label describes only how the product affects the body's "structure or function," rather than promising to treat or prevent any disease. Of course, men wouldn't care about their "urinary well-being" if they weren't really hoping to treat symptoms of an enlarged prostate; nor would people care about "inflammation of mucous membranes" if they didn't have a head cold. While the maker is supposed to have some substantiation for the claims, the FDA rarely asks to see it.

5. Myth: All products that say they contain a particular herb are essentially the same.

Truth: The same herb often comes in several different forms: a tea, an alcohol-and-water tincture, a pill, even a patch. But not all forms produce the same effects. Tea made from saw palmetto probably has no health benefits, since the active compounds don't dissolve in water. And while the active chemical in ginkgo, white hollow bark, or milk thistle does dissolve, even the strongest tea is probably too weak to do any good.

Further, different parts of the same herb can have different effects. Dandelion leaves may act as a diuretic, the roots as a laxative. While the Chinese eat ginkgo seeds, only ginkgo leaves contain the active compounds—and only *processed* ginkgo leaves are safe to take internally. And sassafras remedies are made from the root, the one part of the plant that's potentially carcinogenic.

Finally, the potency and purity of individual plants can differ appreciably, depending on how and where they're grown and how they're stored and handled.

More and more manufacturers are trying to standardize their products by combining batches and isolating the active compounds. But manufacturers often disagree on which ingredients to include and what dose to use. Analyses of ginseng and St. John's wort products have found radically different amounts of the active ingredients in different brands. And it's often impossible to spot the difference, since manufacturers are required to list only the plant and the part used, not the name or amount of the supposedly active ingredient. Even if they did list it, there's no guarantee you'd get what the label says, since no government agency or other independent group monitors the potency and purity of herbal products.

6. Myth: There's not much you need to know about how to take herbs.

Truth: All conventional medications are sold in standardized doses and provide information about the appropriate use, side effects, and precautions. Moreover, prescription drugs are taken under a doctor's guidance.

There are no such safeguards in the largely unregulated herbal jungle. So you may need to know even more about herbal remedies than you do about medications. Unfortunately, information about herbs can be just as unreliable as their quality. For a few good sources, see the sidenote at right.

Summing up

While some studies have suggested that certain herbs may be beneficial, romanticizing all "natural" remedies and ignoring their potential risks can lead to disappointing—or dangerous—results. Herbs can cause allergic reactions, side effects, and drug interactions, especially if you take too much of the herb or use it for too long. And because herbal remedies are virtually unregulated, you can't rely on their potency or purity—or on the claims made on the label. To use herbs as safely and effectively as possible:

■ Tell your doctor about any herbal remedies—and any other dietary supplements or nonprescription drugs—that you take.
■ Consult your doctor *before* taking herbal remedies if you have a chronic disease or if you are taking medications.
■ Avoid herbal remedies if you're pregnant, may become pregnant, or are breastfeeding; give them to children only under a doctor's supervision.
■ Consult a reliable source of information about dosages and precautions (see sidenote below).
■ If you suspect a problem, stop immediately and call your doctor. To report adverse effects, contact the FDA's MedWatch program (see sidenote).

For more information

■ "Herbs of Choice," by Varro Tyler, Ph.D. Haworth Press, 1994. $39.95, hardcover; $14.95, softcover. Call 800-342-9678. An update, "Tyler's Herbs of Choice," prepared by James Robbers, Ph.D., may be available for $49.95 (hardcover) by the end of the year.
■ American Herbal Products Association's Botanical Safety Handbook. $39.95. Call CRC Press at 800-272-7737.
■ World Health Organization. Comprehensive reports on 28 herbs. Price and publication date not yet determined, but should be available by the end of this year or early next year. Call 518-436-9686. (E-mail: *qcorp@compuserve.com*)
■ The U.S. Pharmacopeia (USP). Free fact sheets on a few common herbs; comprehensive reports for $25 each. Material on more herbs may be available soon. Call 301-816-8223. *(www.usp.org/did/mgraphs/botanica/index.htm)*
■ FDA MedWatch monitoring program. To report adverse effects, call 800-FDA-1088. *(www.fda.gov/medwatch/report/consumer/consumer.htm)*

Herbal Weight Loss Tea: Beware the Unknown Brew

June Grell, age 37, died suddenly in the night in her bed in San Rafael, California, on July 20, 1991, leaving an anguished, angry husband and a 2-year-old son.

On the previous night, June and Christopher Grell were relaxing at home, looking at old photos and playing with their child. Then June did something she had been doing for weeks, she drank a cup of Laci Le Beau Super Dieter's Tea. The next morning Chris let his wife sleep late. At 11:00 AM he and his son went to wake her. "She didn't wake up," he said, in a telephone interview.

Grell, an attorney, has been crusading ever since to get herbal diet teas off the market, to warn consumers away from the teas, to get required warning labels.

Another death associated with the same tea is that of Debbie Helphrey, 20, of Palm Harbor, Florida. Trying to lose weight in anticipation of her brother's return from the service, she drank a cup of tea every night before she went to bed. Her mother said she drank it regularly for several months, and was experiencing cramps and loose bowels as a result. She said, "Many of Debbie's friends drank this tea. They all thought it was healthy because it was purchased at a health food store."

Another user wrote the Food and Drug Administration (FDA), "On Oct. 6, 1993, I purchased a box of Laci Le Beau Super Dieter's Tea and consumed several cups the following morning... I began experiencing abdominal cramping... During the next half hour the cramping became intense and I began to feel nauseated and light-headed... I began fainting, vomiting, and experiencing breathing difficulties and extreme fluctuations in body temperature. I was in excruciating pain, my stomach became grossly distended, and I was unable to remain conscious and coherent for any length of time... relief (diarrhea) came by evening."

By June of 1995, the FDA had received reports of the deaths of at least four women who drank Laci Le Beau Super Dieter's Tea. From different parts of the country, the women were described as being rigorous dieters, who had been using the senna-laced diet tea several times a week for around 2 years. All died suddenly, and three of the four had cardiac effects.

Debbie's father says, "She wanted to be in this special dress and it was a little tight... she was on a strict diet. The night of her brother's homecoming party, Debbie went into cardiac arrest and was rushed to the hospital, where doctors ran a battery of tests." He recalls them running in to the waiting room, asking, "What has she done to reduce her potassium to such a low level?"

"I don't trust like I used to trust," said one tea drinker. "Anybody can market anything and say it's pure, it's natural, and we have no way of knowing."

Dangerous laxatives and more

Every herbal dealer seems to market still another weight loss tea, unregulated as to ingredients and nonstandardized as to potency, of course. There are Trim-Maxx, 24-Hour Diet Tea, Ultra Slim Tea, Seelect Senna Leaf Tea, Super Fatbuster Tea, Super Dieter's Tea, Original Slim Tea, Fasting Tea, Uncle Lee's Body Slim Dieter Tea, Herb Tea Diet and Cleansing Program, Alvita Trim-Time Thermogenic Tea, Sou Tsian Tea, Diet Partner Herb Tea by Celestial Seasonings, Diet-Max Diet Tea which "gently cleanses the system," Elegant Jasmine Slim Tea, and others.

Many contain drugs that have powerful, toxic effects. If used often or in excess amounts, herbal diet teas that contain senna, aloe, buckthorn, rhubarb root, cascara, castor oil, and other plant-derived laxatives can cause harmful effects, including diarrhea, nausea, vomiting, stomach cramps, chronic constipation, fainting, dehydration, mineral imbalances and deficiencies, and even death. Chronic use can impair colon function. Other potentially harmful ingredients in some teas are Ma huang, locust plant, wymote, ginseng, honeysuckle, and chaparral.

Since the teas are currently being regulated as foods, the exact amounts of laxative herb in each tea are unknown, as are the potential effects of mixing different laxative herbs. Dosage varies widely.

The main ingredient in Laci Le Beau Super Dieter's Tea is senna. The tea contains 50 percent senna leaves, according to the FDA inspection report, as well as chaparral, which the agency warns is hazardous. Senna has a powerful laxative effect. When sold as a nonprescription drug, over the counter, senna must carry the warning, "Laxative products should not be used for a period longer than 1 week unless directed by a doctor." However, this warning need not appear on herbal teas, which evade regulation because they are "food supplements." Instead, directions urge the user to "stay in shape" by using the tea regularly, or to increase dosage over time if the "cleansing" effects wear off. One advertisement urges, "The more diet tea you drink, the more weight you lose."

Among the most severe problems associated with diet teas, says the FDA, are dehydration and electrolyte disorders, such as low blood potassium, a condition that can cause paralysis, irregular heartbeat, and death. Being undernourished or dieting increases the risk.

Longer brewing time increases the potency of herbal tea—and its potential deadlines. Mrs. Helphrey recalls that her daughter Debbie would steep the tea for a long time, "She left the tea bag in boiling water until the water was lukewarm."

Recently, Debbie Helphrey's 1991 death certificate was amended to show Laci Le Beau Super Dieter's Tea as the underlying cause of her death. Dated June 4, 1998, the amended medical certification of death lists the immediate cause of death as "anoxic encephalopathy, due to cardiac arrhythmias, due to electrolyte imbalance, due to (or as a consequence of) use of Super Dieter's Tea."

Earlier reports hesitated to blame the tea directly. In a letter to the FDA, the medical examiner had said, "It is my opinion that there was an association between [Debbie's] death and the tea. I do not, however, know if this was a direct cause and effect relationship due to some toxic effect of the tea, or whether the tea was just part of a weight reduction program which failed to provide proper nutrients."

Warning labels urged

In response to the Grell campaign, dozens of complaints were filed in California by consumers about adverse effects they suffered from diet teas. As of January 1, 1997, state law requires a warning label on all herbal products that have a laxative effect. The warning must include the statement: "Do not use if you have or develop diarrhea, loose stools, or abdominal pain."

However, there is no federal regulation, although the industry has agreed to label teas with "appropriate consumer information" on a voluntary basis, and the FDA says it will monitor this labeling.

Canada has banned the sale of 57 herbs and requires warning labels on five more.

But, in dealing with herbal fraud, the FDA is an agency that often seems to operate with one hand tied behind its back. In the mid-1990s, the FDA charged that Laci Le Beau tea was an unproven new drug and prohibited its interstate commerce. But the company simply changed the label to avoid drug-like statements and continued marketing the tea as a food. This transition from mislabeled drug to health food happens often, says Stephen Barrett, MD, co-author of *The health robbers: a close look at quackery in America*. He writes, "Companies in the health food industry market products with explicit therapeutic claims. When and if FDA tells them to stop, they back off—but try to retain as much of the original purpose as they can without making a frank claim."

In 1995, an Advisory Panel to the FDA recommended that warnings be required on certain herbal teas, especially "those that contain stimulant laxative substances, such as senna, aloe, rhubarb root, buckthorn, cascara, and castor oil." The committee looked at what they considered drug claims on boxes of Laci, Trim-Maxx, 24-Hour Diet Tea, Ultra Slim Tea, and Seelect Senna Leaf Tea. The advisory panel members were unanimous in their opinion that the teas presented a health risk and should be labeled with warnings. They found most of the teas mentioned "flushing" or "cleansing" effects that seemed to be metaphors for laxative and diuretic effects.

The panel wanted to know why the FDA did not consider the teas as drugs, because they contain the same materials as over-the-counter laxatives, and often in higher concentrations. The agency explained that it is the claim made, not the product itself, that often makes the legal distinction between foods and drugs, especially in the case of the laxative herbs.

Unfortunately, FDA regulation of herbal teas falls into the gray area between food and drugs. The FDA regards herbal teas that are consumed for their taste and aroma only (not for medical purposes) as foods. Thus they are unregulated, as long as they do not claim to promote weight loss on the label—even though the name obviously suggests this very claim.

Senator Orrin G. Hatch, of Utah, a leading defender of the health food industry, argues against regulating food supplements. He is on the committee that oversees the FDA, and said on the ABC News Primetime Live broadcast (November 24, 1994): "I don't know what more power you want to give to the FDA. I'm not about to give them power over an industry that has done a good job with little hazard, with little problems, with little hurt to mankind, just because a bunch of extremists on one side, who are in the minority, believe that every thing ought to be regulated to death."

Yet, an article in the FDA Consumer,[1] offers the startling conclusion that: "For American herbal tea drinkers it might be best to play safe and heed the old proverb about those who gather wild mushrooms, 'There are old mushroom hunters, and there are bold mushroom hunters. But there are no old, bold mushroom hunters.'"

Note: Health professionals are requested to report serious adverse reactions related to dieter's teas and similar products to MedWatch at 1-800-FDA-1088.

Reference

1. Snider S. Herbal teas and toxicity. FDA Consumer, May 1991:31–33.

5 Nutrition Topics that Are Not All They're Cracked Up to Be

1 Creatine Claims have been flying that creatine supplements can burn body fat and build lean muscle tissue—quickly. But they're not true.

Granted, creatine, which is both made in the body and supplied by animal foods such as meat and fish, becomes important when muscles need short, quick bursts of energy for activities like sprinting or strength training. Under those circumstances, a fuel known as ATP is used up by the muscles in seconds, and creatine is part of a compound that replenishes the ATP stores as they are exhausted. That extends the burst of energy for a few more seconds, allowing for an extra repetition or two with weights or the couple of seconds of speed needed at the end of a sprint. Creatine is also thought to indirectly delay the production of lactic acid, a byproduct of physical exertion that not only causes an uncomfortable burning sensation but also contributes to muscle fatigue.

But it doesn't miraculously increase muscle mass. And whether creatine *supplements* contribute to any beneficial effect whatsoever is very much up in the air. Research to date suggests that if there are any potential benefits, they are limited to serious, elite athletes for whom the edge of a few extra seconds or a very small amount of extra strength could make a difference. They would not be of particular value in endurance activities like running or swimming or in recreational sports. In fact, creatine supplements might actually slow down the recreational athlete because they are believed to increase the uptake of water by muscle cells, causing weight gain.

On top of all that, no one knows whether taking creatine supplements regularly is safe. Most of the studies on the compound have involved college-age or slightly older men who were in excellent physical condition. Even less is known about the effect of creatine supplementation in women. That's why the American College of Sports Medicine firmly states that "further study is necessary before any conclusions can be reached regarding the safety of long-term creatine supplementation."

2 Algae At least one brand of this supplement purportedly produces feelings of increased energy and vitality; alleviation of stress, anxiety, and depression; relief from fatigue, allergies, poor digestion, and sluggishness; and improved memory and mental clarity. Don't believe any of it.

The health benefits ascribed to algae are almost wholly anecdotal, that is, based on personal reports of people who use it—and in many cases sell it. Scientific research demonstrating any usefulness is virtually nonexistent.

The lack of scientific validity should come as no surprise. The cardinal sign of health quackery is the promise that a single product can treat a multitude of ills. Such overblown claims have been used to sell everything from snake oil to swampland. In this case, they're being used to sell pond scum; algae is essentially scum that floats on brackish waters.

If algae were simply useless, it would be bad enough. But there is also concern among legitimate health professionals that some strains of algae can be toxic. Users have reported nausea, diarrhea, weakness, numbness, and tingling of the extremities.

3 Liquid Meal Replacements Advertisements for liquid meal replacements, sometimes referred to as meals-in-a-can, have indicated that the milkshake-like beverages provide solid nutrition for people too harried to sit down to eat. But it's not so simple.

True, doctors and dietitians have long recommended such drinks to patients who are too sick to meet their nutrition needs with a regular diet. For instance, bedridden hospital patients who can't swallow often receive liquid meal replacements through a tube passed from the nose down into the stomach. Some of these very same liquid meals, in fact, are now showing up on supermarket shelves.

But there's nothing that makes them particularly healthful. An eight-ounce can racks up as many as 250 calories and nine grams of fat, nearly identical to the fat and calorie content of an eight-ounce chocolate milkshake.

To be sure, these products also contain a number of vitamins and minerals. But you could get the same effect by popping a multivitamin/mineral

6 ❖ HEALTH CLAIMS

pill and washing it down with a milkshake chaser.

Moreover, these beverages are not truly full meal replacements because they don't provide many of the health-promoting substances found in traditional foods, namely fiber and the beneficial phytochemicals found in vegetables and fruits.

That doesn't mean it's a nutrition crime to have, say, Carnation Instant Breakfast or Ensure once in a while if you like the taste (which many people do not). But they should not take the place of real food on a regular basis.

4 Lactose Intolerance Ads for products that make it easier for lactose intolerant people to digest dairy foods can make it seem as if intolerance to lactose, the sugar in milk, is running rampant. It's not. In fact, the results of a survey conducted last year show that one in three people who think they are lactose intolerant really are not.

Granted, the majority of human beings—notably blacks of African descent, those of Asian ancestry, many people whose first language is Spanish, Native Americans, and Jews—tend to be lactose maldigesters, meaning they don't properly digest milk sugar. But relatively few people suffer such symptoms as gas, bloating, stomach cramps, and diarrhea upon consumption of reasonable amounts of milk (a half cup to a cup at a time), ice cream (a half cup at a time), and so on.

Even many people who feel sick after eating dairy products can handle more than they think they can—if they space their dairy items several hours apart and eat other foods along with milk-based ones. Furthermore, because hard or aged cheeses like cheddar and Swiss contain less lactose than milk itself, they are generally fairly easy to tolerate. Yogurt with active cultures tends to be tolerated rather well, too. The cultures, or bacteria, in yogurt contain enzymes that digest lactose on their own.

Then, too, there appears to be a "use it or lose it" aspect to handling lactose. Research suggests that people who have trouble digesting milk sugar get better at handling it by not avoiding dairy products altogether. Consider that schoolchildren in Colombia who experienced unpleasant symptoms when milk was first introduced at their school were able to tolerate it without incident six months later.

Finally, don't underestimate the power of the old adage that "believing makes it so." That is, even just assuming that milk disagrees with you can cause symptoms. But gradually adding milk back into the diet can wear down the power of the belief.

If having some dairy products some of the time fails, consider buying lactose-free milk; or droplets that you can add to milk to do the lactose digesting for you; or tablets to take before eating, say, an ice cream cone or other dairy food. That will allow you to enjoy it without symptoms, and, of course, to get the calcium and other valuable nutrients that milk products provide.

5 Dehydration It seems everyone's carrying around a water bottle these days, perhaps in no small part because dire warnings of dehydration abound. Consider one view expressed in the media recently that many Americans may be "drinking themselves to dehydration" because they drink too little water and too many caffeinated beverages that "rob the body of water."

To be sure, there are a variety of reasons not to consume too much caffeine. But fluid loss is not one of them. The fact is that the body regulates fluid balance very well, even in people who drink a lot of coffee every day. Granted, when your water comes from caffeinated beverages, you will urinate more than when you drink the same amount of plain water, juice, or milk. But you will still retain an adequate supply of water in your body. Indeed, the more coffee you drink on a regular basis, the more your body will be able to compensate for caffeine's effect by holding onto a greater proportion of the water that the coffee contains.

Note, too, that for most people, thirst is a very good indicator of when to drink fluids; you don't need to count how many cups you are drinking each day. The only exceptions are the elderly, whose thirst mechanisms may be blunted; people engaging in heavy physical activity, particularly in hot weather; and anyone who tends to suffer from kidney stones. It would be a good idea for individuals in those groups to make sure to drink at least eight cups of fluid a day—in the form of water, juice, milk, lemonade, decaffeinated coffee or tea, and so on.

Much of the material here is adapted from the *Tufts University Health & Nutrition Letter's* "Ask Tufts Experts" section of the PHYS Web site, located at www.phys.com.

Pyruvate: Just the Facts

Why there's less than meets the eye

by Joseph P. Cannon

Every year a new batch of weight-loss products is touted to melt off excess pounds and increase muscle mass with minimal effort. This year is no different. One thing that's new, however, is that one new weight-loss product actually has scientific studies published in reputable journals that are alleged to back up its claims. The product is called pyruvate.

As promoted in health-food stores and in radio commercials, scientific evidence is supposed to show that pyruvate can:

- Enhance weight loss by 37% over dieting alone
- Enhance fat loss by 48% over dieting alone
- Decrease appetite
- Increase muscle endurance
- Inhibit the regaining of fat once dieting stops
- Increase metabolism

Pyruvate (also known as pyruvic acid) is a three-carbon compound generated as the end product of glycolysis, one of the body's energy-generating pathways. During the early 1980s, research showed that pyruvate could prevent fatty buildup in rat livers from chronic alcohol use. It was probably these studies that inspired University of Pittsburgh researcher Ronald Stanko to investigate whether pyruvate might also work as a weight-loss product. To date, Stanko is responsible for practically all of the studies on pyruvate and also holds the U.S. patent on "Pyruvate +," a form of pyruvate sold through Med Pro Industries.

The vast majority of studies done on pyruvate have in reality been mixtures of pyruvate and dihydroxyacetone, another three-carbon metabolite formed during glycolysis. Dihydroxyacetone is also found in over-the-counter pyruvate formulations but is rarely mentioned on the labels.

To date, Stanko is responsible for practically all of the studies on pyruvate and also holds the U.S. patent on "Pyruvate +."

Science and Wishful Thinking

How well, though, does scientific research support the claims made for pyruvate?

Claim # 1: Enhances weight loss. There are few studies on pyruvate and its effects on weight loss. Those that have been done suggest that pyruvate works under laboratory conditions, but its effect is not very impressive. In one study, for example, obese women (defined as weighing over 200 pounds) added 30 grams of pyruvate to a 1000-calorie/day liquid diet for 21 days. This resulted in 37% more weight loss and 48% more fat loss compared to control subjects who were on the 1000-calorie/day diet only (*American Journal of Clinical Nutrition* 56:630–635, 1992).

These figures seem impressive until one looks at the actual pounds of weight and fat lost. Specifically, the 37% enhancement in weight loss amounts to an average of only 3.5 pounds difference between the group taking the pyruvate and the one not taking it. With respect to the 48% increase in fat loss, this too is misleading because only 3.2 pounds more fat were lost in those consuming pyruvate.

In a second study, obese women were placed on a 500-calorie/day diet for 21 days, with some of the women supplementing with 16 grams of pyruvate and 12 grams of dihydroxyacetone (*American Journal of Clinical Nutrition* 55:771–776, 1992). Again, women supplementing with pyruvate did lose significantly more fat and weight than those not supplementing, but those using pyruvate lost an average of only 1.98 pounds more weight and 1.76 pounds more fat. It's important to note that these weight-loss studies took place under controlled laboratory conditions. No published peer-reviewed study to date has ever been conducted in real-life situations where calorie intake is not strictly controlled.

Claim #2: Decreases appetite. This claim is based on only one study—a study that was performed not on humans but on laboratory rats. In this investigation, laboratory rats were allowed to eat as much food as they wanted. At the end of the study, researchers found that the rats that received pyruvate and dihydroxyacetone consumed less food than rats not receiving the supplements (*Journal of Clinical Nutrition* 53:847–853, 1991). To date, however, such a study has never been performed on humans.

Claim #3: Increases muscle endurance. There is only one published peer-reviewed study suggesting that pyruvate can increase muscle endurance—and the only published study done on men (*Journal of Applied Physiology* 68[1]: 119–124, 1990). This is the study that is most quoted to people interested in increasing their exercise ability. The study showed that a mixture of 25 grams of pyruvate and 75 grams of dihydroxyacetone taken for 7 days increased triceps endurance by 20%.

Of course, until other studies are done, this study should be considered preliminary. What's more, this study did not look at traditional aerobic conditioning like jogging or bicycling but rather at how long the triceps muscle (on the back of the upper arm) took to totally exhaust itself. Muscles other than the triceps as well as those undergoing different types of exercise might react differently, so it's unknown how these results might translate over to exercising individuals. This problem is even mentioned in the study in light of the fact that one of the participants had a *reduced* triceps endurance capacity following ingestion of pyruvate. Therefore, individuals looking to pyruvate to enhance their exercise ability should save their money until more research is conducted in this area.

Claim #4: Inhibiting the regaining of fat once dieting stops. Everybody knows that when one stops dieting and goes back to old eating habits, that weight slowly creeps back. Anything that could slow this process would certainly appeal to dieters who fall off the wagon. But the claim that pyruvate can suppress appetite is based on only one published peer-reviewed study (*International Journal of Obesity* 20:925–930, 1996).

In this investigation, obese women (average weight 228 pounds) went on a 310-calorie/day diet for 21 days. Following this, they then went on a three-day high-calorie diet to purposely regain the weight. Some women used a mixture of 15 grams of pyruvate and 75 grams of dihydroxyacetone during the dieting process. After the study, it was found that those women who didn't receive any pyruvate regained an average of 6.38 pounds of weight, while women who used pyruvate regained an average of 3.96 pounds of weight. This amounts to only a 2.42-pound difference between the groups. With respect to the regaining of fat, women not using pyruvate regained an average of 3.96 pounds of fat while those using the pyruvate regained an average of 1.76 pounds of fat. Again, this amounts to only a 2.2-pound difference between them.

There is only one published peer-reviewed study suggesting that pyruvate can increase muscle endurance.

Claim # 5: Increases metabolism. Much hype surrounds the claim that pyruvate can increase one's metabolism and therefore help one lose weight. Unfortunately there is no solid evidence to support this claim. Earlier studies in rats did show that pyruvate increased resting metabolism (the number of calories used at rest), but these results have never been confirmed in human studies. In fact, in the most recently published pyruvate study, the group of people who did *not* receive pyruvate had a higher resting metabolism at the end of the study than those who did receive the pyruvate. Therefore, the idea that pyruvate enhances human metabolism remains speculative at best.

With respect to side effects, the literature to date seems to show that pyruvate is relatively safe with the most noticeable problems being occasional diarrhea, loose or softened stools, and a rumbling sound in the gut which is caused by gas passing through the intestines. At the present time, nobody is sure of the physiological mechanism of action of the pyruvate/dihydroxyacetone mixture and how it relates to weight loss or any other reported claim.

All of the published peer-reviewed studies done to date except one have been either conducted on obese women on very restrictive diets or on laboratory rats. Therefore, results obtained from these populations may not indicate what would be gained from humans under more real-life situations where food intake is not strictly controlled. Also, the subjects in the studies consumed very large amounts of pyruvate and dihydroxyacetone, far in excess of the dose of 3 to 5 grams per day recommended in over-the-counter products. To date, no published peer-reviewed research exists showing that the 3- to 5-gram dose will produce the same effects as the higher dosages used in the studies.

Popular Hype

One prominent false claim that one is likely to encounter is "pyruvate is backed up by 25 years of extensive scientific research" (J. B. Roufs, *Muscle and Fitness,* December 1996). While it's true that research on pyruvate does appear in prestigious scientific journals, the fact is that there were no studies on pyruvate and weight loss published before 1986 or after 1996. That's only 10 years, not 25. Furthermore, if one were to look just at the human studies using pyruvate, then this number is even further reduced to only six years.

Some people selling pyruvate give out free audiotapes that boast of pyruvate's supposed amazing abilities. In one of these tapes, the person selling pyruvate (who is identified as a physician) states that when you are using pyruvate, "You are in the fat-burning mode—even when you are not exercising." This is very interesting because when you are resting, you are already in the "fat-burning mode." At rest, approximately 70% of the calories you derive energy from are coming from fat with the remaining 30% coming from carbohydrates (sugars).

Some people claim that pyruvate is an antioxidant. As is mentioned in a recent review of pyruvate in *Medicine and Science in Sport and Exercise* (30: 837–843, 1998), some evidence hints that pyruvate might act as an antioxidant. But only three studies show that pyruvate acts as an antioxidant—and these studies were conducted not on humans but on rodent hearts. More research is necessary to determine the efficacy of pyruvate's antioxidant action in humans.

Claims that pyruvate aids in cardiac function are prevalent. But there is absolutely no published peer-reviewed evidence that either pyruvate or dihydroxyacetone aids the heart in pumping blood more effectively. In fact, those studies that did record pyruvate's effect on heart functions found no change after use. Therefore, if you have any cardiac abnormalities, pyruvate is not the answer to your problems. You are best served by following medical advice.

Pyruvate is also supposed to build muscle. There is no published peer-reviewed scientific evidence showing that pyruvate can build muscle tissue. In the only study of exercise and pyruvate ever conducted, no mention was made regarding pyruvate having any effect on muscular strength or hypertrophy. This claim seems to be specifically targeting those individuals interested in weight lifting and bodybuilding.

Joseph P Cannon is an exercise physiologist and an NSCA-certified personal trainer.

Are Health Food Stores Better Bets Than Traditional Supermarkets?

THE DOOR SWINGS OPEN, and over a terra-cotta tile floor you step, passing between two rows of lush, fragrant flowers at the peak of their bloom. Straight ahead, extending the color scheme found in the fragrant blossoms, lie red and green apples, artfully arranged next to smooth, round oranges and lovely-looking vegetables.

No, you haven't happened onto a Martha Stewart set. You've entered a supermarket-size natural foods store owned by Austin, Texas-based Whole Foods Market, which operates almost 100 outlets in more than 20 states. In Boston, it's called Bread & Circus, although depending on where you live, you may know it as Whole Foods, Fresh Foods, Wellspring Group, Bread of Life, or Merchant of Vino.

Whatever name it goes by, it's the present-day version of a health food store, specializing in organic fruits and vegetables, nutrition supplements, and myriad grains, beans, rice, and granola sold in bulk. And it's not alone. A company called Wild Oats owns 59 stores in 16 states and Canada with names like Alfalfa's, Capers, and Uptown Whole Foods. And many areas have local health food supermarkets of their own.

Make no mistake. These are not the crunchy-granola counterculture hangouts of yore. They're big business supermarketing, with collective sales in the billions of dollars a year.

The question for the consumer, of course, is whether picking up your groceries in them means eating more healthfully than if you go to a traditional supermarket. To find out, we did some comparison shopping.

Organically terrific

Organically grown fruits and vegetables, farmed without pesticides, herbicides, and fungicides, have not been shown to be more nutritious than other produce. No matter what methods are used to raise crops, they will have the same abundance of vitamins, minerals, fiber, and other phytochemicals important to good health.

But organic fruits and vegetables are definitely better for the planet—keeping toxic chemicals out of ground water supplies, stemming soil deterioration via crop rotation, and safeguarding farm workers and livestock from potentially harmful compounds. If those issues are a concern for you and you want to take a stand through your food purchases, today's health food markets offer a much greater variety of organic foods than traditional supermarkets.

Not only can you buy everything from beautiful-looking organic Romaine lettuce and asparagus to organic oranges and apples, you can also purchase tomato sauce made only with organically grown ingredients, organic applesauce, organic olive oil, and the list goes on.

Meat, fish, and poultry are "organic" in these stores, too. Granted, as markets like Bread & Circus plainly point out, the U.S. Department of Agriculture presently does not recognize the term "organic" in relation to meat production, but meats offered in health food markets are raised on organic feed. The meat is also produced without the use of drugs such as growth hormones and antibiotics.

Cutting back on the routine use of antibiotics in animals can help stem the development of super-strength bacteria that then prove resistant to the antibiotics used to treat infections in humans. Consider that more than 40 percent of the antibiotics produced in this country are used in animals, and many of them are the same as or similar to antibiotics used in humans. The more that various bacteria are exposed to antibiotics, the greater the chance they will mutate to forms that make them immune to the drugs' effects. The upshot: the drugs lose their effectiveness.

Of course, meat produced without antibiotics, as well as other foods made with the environment in mind, all come with a price. And it's a hefty one. A 25-ounce jar of Whole Foods organic applesauce costs $2.99, while a 23-ounce jar of Mott's, housed on the same shelf for the faint of pocketbook, retails for $1.49. (In a regular supermarket, we found the same-size jar of Mott's for just $1.29.)

Similarly, a 10-ounce package of Organic Cascadian Farm Chopped Spinach costs $2.39, while a 10-ounce package of Birds Eye Spinach in the same freezer case goes for 99 cents (67 cents in the regular store). And a pound of bottom round rump roast: a rather astounding $4.59 (as compared to $2.39 in the traditional market).

Supplementally disappointing

If the availability of organic foods is the high (albeit expensive) point of natural foods markets, their large supplement sections are the low point. Mixed in with the multivitamins and other potentially helpful tables are some of the most bogus products making some of the most outlandish claims we've ever seen.

The label on the bottle of Hot Flash tables we found at Bread & Circus, for instance, promises that the supplement "helps reduce hot flash frequency." We doubt it. Yes, it contains a small amount of soy concentrate, which preliminary research suggests might help reduce the symptoms of menopause. But the $9.99 bottle (which contains only 15 days' worth of tables) is basically an unproven concoction of ingredients that includes licorice root extract and dong quai. Neither of those substances have been scientifically proven to help quell hot flashes.

Another health food store we visited, Wild Harvest, offers KidCalm, a "St. John's Wort Complex for your child's emotional well-being and nervous system function" (we don't even know all the science relating to St. John's wort in adults). It also contains more than 2,000 percent of the recommended level of vitamin B_6 for children four to eight years old, with 50 milligrams of kava root and 100 milligrams of valerian root extract mixed in. How those substances in those proportions can be good for a child is a mystery. Scientists are only now beginning to take a rigorous look at herbs like kava and valerian.

In the same section appears Fat Defense, "an effective natural formula for weight management" with ingredients like garcinia cambogia extract and gymnema sylvestre powder (benefits unproven). The cost: $14.79 for 10 to 20 days' worth of tablets, or up to about $500 a year—enough to join a health club and lose weight via a *proven* method.

We inquired about the training of the "nutrition manager" at Wild Harvest, whose store position was printed on his name tag. His response was that he had been doing it for six years. "It," it turned out, was working at other stores that sell supplements, such as GNC. He also told us he learned about nutrition from vendors who supply the products— that is, people who stand to make money off the sale of supplements.

Mixed messages

Scorecard so far: for the environmentally concerned consumer who wants a wide selection of organic foods, a plus. But a big minus for the minefield of scientifically unproven potions.

On some issues, however, the takeaway points are less obvious, and they often occur in the aisles with packaged goods. Consider, for instance, that in the "National Selections" section of Wild Harvest, a pound of Davinci spaghetti imported from Italy is 99 cents. Yet just across the aisle in "Traditional Groceries," *two* pounds of Ronzoni spaghetti (made in the U.S.) cost $1.19.

Other than in price, we couldn't see any difference between the two products. The wheat used to produce the Italian spaghetti was not organic. In fact, the ingredients on the Italian and American packages were identical. Both listed semolina wheat and the same five nutrients added for enrichment. The extra cost for the Italian spaghetti, it seemed, could be chalked up solely to its cachet as a European product and the fact that it had to be shipped thousands of miles over the Atlantic Ocean.

Consider, too, that a health food supermarket might stock ruby red, fresh, organic raspberries in early April, which is great for people who want to eat the widest variety possible of delicious produce. But a placard above some raspberries that we saw in one store indicated that they had been shipped from Chile, which seemed to go against the store's own commitment to the environment. A company with a deep concern for ecologically sound food practices might prefer to ask people to wait until summer, when raspberries can be grown locally (and therefore don't have to use up fuel resources in being shipped thousands of miles), or to choose frozen raspberries grown closer to home.

Other products also have the aura of being produced with the planet in mind but come with a compromise that isn't necessarily apparent at first glance. For instance, health food supermarkets make it easy to buy many items in bulk, which allows you not only to buy just the amount you need but also cuts down on wasteful packaging that clutters landfills. But they also sell products like 15-ounce packages of frozen split pea soup that contain just two servings. Granted, the soup is organic, but it seems to us that any store that professes to help safeguard the environment would not sell two servings of a product that's so easy to package in large quantities.

In addition, there's the "all natural" burst printed on many products in health food stores. It *sounds* better for

6 ❖ HEALTH CLAIMS

you, but it doesn't necessarily signify any extra health benefits. All Natural Born Free Vanilla Pecan Chip Cookies, for example, are made with "no refined sugar." But the so-called raw sugar they contain (and the sugar used in the chocolate chips) is nutritionally equivalent to refined table sugar: all have 16 calories a teaspoon and virtually no other nutrients. Similarly, while the "frosted crisps and puffs of brown rice" in Rice Twice Cereal come "naturally," the rice is glazed with honey—again, the nutritional equivalent of sugar.

Making it particularly difficult to see all sides of products in health food emporiums is the fact that the stores are so undeniably pleasant to shop in. In fact, for sheer entertainment value, they're matchless. As mentioned earlier, they're beautiful, with wide aisles and attractive displays. And the employees in these markets tend to act less like store clerks and more like wait staff at a restaurant that prides itself on service. Furthermore, at least at the Bread & Circus we visited, there were lots of delicious free samples of food—baby carrots with pepper Parmesan dip in the produce section; tortilla chips with parsley, scallion and red pepper hummus in the takeout section; cookie pieces in the bakery section, and so on. You could leave literally stuffed without spending a cent.

But while these stores are a feast for both the stomach and the senses (even wandering past the glistening displays of fresh striped bass, rainbow trout, salmon fillets, and monkfish in the seafood section is entertaining), the bottom line is that you have to read labels carefully, just like you would in a traditional supermarket. And, if the health of the planet is on your mind and you're looking at two servings of organic, packaged, frozen soup, it pays to think past the "organic/all natural" burst on the front and decide whether, for $2.99, you're being as good to Mother Earth—and to yourself—as the box suggests.

The Unethical Behavior of Pharmacists

How to market dubious supplements and unproven remedies

by Stephen Barrett, MD

Most pharmacists who work in retail pharmacies have a serious potential conflict of interest. On the one hand, they are professionals, expected to be knowledgeable about drugs and to dispense them in a responsible and ethical manner. On the other hand, their income depends on the sale of products. Before the FDA's OTC (Over-the-Counter) Drug Review drove most of the ineffective ingredients out of OTC drug products, few pharmacists protested or attempted to protect their customers from wasting money on products that were ineffective, unnecessary, or irrationally formulated.

During the mid-1980s, two dietitians examined the labels of vitamin products at five pharmacies, three groceries, and three health-food stores in New Haven, CT. Products were considered appropriate if they contained between 50% and 200% of the U.S. RDAs and no more than 100% of others for which Estimated Safe and Adequate Daily Dietary Intakes exist. Only 16 out of 105 (15%) of the multivitamin/mineral products met these criteria (*Journal of the American Dietetic Association* 87:341–343, 1987).

Today the situation appears worse. Although OTC drugs are generally effective, nearly all pharmacies still carry irrational supplements, and many stock dubious herbal and homeopathic products as well. Chain drugstores are more likely to do so than individually owned stores.

Marketing Ploys

Pharmacy schools appear to teach the facts needed to advise people that "nu-

> *Nearly all pharmacies still carry irrational supplements, and many stock dubious herbal and homeopathic products as well.*

trition insurance" is rarely needed, that "stress" supplements are a scam, and that doses above the RDAs are seldom appropriate. Yet pharmacists throughout America seem content to sell supplements to people who don't need them. Their professional journals rarely contain articles criticizing the fraud involved, and their trade publications talk mainly about vitamin promotion. In fact, most pharmacy trade publications carry articles urging pharmacists to compete with health-food retailers by using similar propaganda techniques!

Many pharmacies display posters or flyers telling what vitamins do in the body. Some also list the problems that occur with nutrient deficiencies. These items are obviously intended to promote sales by inducing customers to think that (a) if a little is good, more is better, and/or (b) if they have any of the symptoms listed, a vitamin might be the answer to their problem.

Many vitamin promoters suggest that being busy, skipping meals, or "eating on the run" places people at risk for dietary deficiency. According to this notion, busy people don't take the time to consume nourishing food. These claims are misleading because preparing or eating a balanced diet takes no more time than preparing or eating an unbalanced diet.

Major vitamin manufacturers and trade associations play a significant role in spreading misinformation. During the early 1980s, for example, Hoffman-La Roche advertised that "busy" people should take supplements. An article in a pharmacy trade publication later revealed that these ads were intended to influence pharmacists (who advise many customers) as well as the general public. During the same period, until stopped by the New York State Attorney General, Lederle Laboratories marketed Stresstabs with misleading claims that "stress robs the body of nutrients."

In 1989, the Council for Responsible Nutrition (CRN), a nutritional supplement industry association that mainly represents large manufacturers, began advertising that virtually everyone has a "vitamin gap." During the mid-1980s, market research had found that most Americans felt they were getting adequate nutrition from their diet. CRN's "Vitamin Gap" campaign was designed to convince people that supplements were still needed. First it falsely suggested that vitamins could help against stress. Then it falsely suggested that most Americans were not getting enough in their diet.

Lederle used the "vitamin gap" theme in a Centrum ad in the June 1997

Journal of the American Dietetic Association. Centrum is a sensibly formulated multivitamin/multimineral product that costs about 10¢ per day. However, the ad suggested that the majority of Americans are not getting the nutrients they need in their diet and should use Centrum to bridge the alleged "gaps." According to the ad: "Statistics show that 9 out of 10 Americans don't get all the nutrients they need from what they eat, and, in fact, are missing out on important vitamins and minerals."

This statement was based on an analysis of data collected between 1976 and 1980 from the Second National Health and Nutrition Examination Survey. The survey found that only 9% of the participants remembered consuming the recommended five portions of fruits and vegetables on the day covered by the survey (*American Journal of Public Health* 80:1443–1449, 1990). This does not mean that people who reported less were deficient in vitamins or minerals. Dietary surveys that measure nutrient intake for a single day or even a few days are not suitable for determining the overall quality of an individual's diet. Adequate nutrient intake can be achieved with fewer than the "recommended" number of portions of fruits and vegetables. Furthermore, Americans are eating more fruits and vegetables than they did 20 years ago. CRN used the same faulty reasoning to justify its original campaign.

CRN has produced two brochures that the National Association of Chain Drug Stores distributed to retail pharmacies. One contains a chart of "the health benefits of vitamins and minerals" and subtly suggests that many people don't get enough. Both refer to research developments and speculations that higher-than-RDA levels of various nutrients might help prevent disease. Both state that "appropriate use of nutritional supplements should be part of a healthy lifestyle," but neither provides the information an individual would need to judge whether supplementation makes sense. Both are posted to CRN's Web site (**http://www.crnusa.org/Consumer.htm**)

Investigative Reports

If asked directly for advice, most pharmacists will answer to the best of their ability. However, many are poorly informed.

In 1985, reporters from *Consumer Reports* magazine visited 30 drugstores in Pennsylvania, Missouri, and California. The reporters complained of feeling tired or nervous, and asked whether a vitamin product might help. Seventeen were sold a vitamin product, and one was sold an amino acid preparation. Only 9 of the 30 pharmacists suggested

> *If asked directly for advice, most pharmacists will answer to the best of their ability. However, many are poorly informed.*

Making Up for Lost Revenues

Pharmacy trade publications, such as *Natural Pharmacist*, suggest that "natural products" offer opportunities to make up for prescription drug revenues lost as a result of managed care and other cost-containment programs. One pharmacy supplier aligned with this trend is The JAG Group of San Clemente, California. According to its Web site (**http://www.jagenterprises.com/servmain.htm**), "natural products offer profit margins greater than those for prescription drugs." JAG's comprehensive program features:

- Product lines that typically produce a 100% markup or more.
- A three-day seminar covering "the importance of wellness" and how to "use natural products to prevent and/or improve chronic disease states."
- WellStore Software designed as a sales and marketing tool to: (1) capture customer information, including e-mail address, (2) categorize products to market directly to customer needs, (3) provide thank-you notes to encourage loyalty, (4) provide product information to print for customers, and (5) track patient-health histories to create fee-for-service revenue.
- Pharmacist Plus™ Software with causes, signs, and symptoms of 223 common ailments and specific dietary, homeopathic, and herbal recommendations. (I believe that providing such information to customers would be outside the scope of pharmacy practice and would constitute the illegal practice of medicine and would violate state laws against theft by deception. Furthermore, homeopathic products have no proven effectiveness.)
- Drug Depletion Software telling "what supplements patients need to replace vital nutrients that are depleted by many of the prescription drugs they are taking." (I do not believe there are many situations in which this is important.)
- Nutritional Analysis Software (an electronic nutritionist) to allow the pharmacist to charge a fee for providing consultations to patients—including assessment of "nutritional needs that best fit your patient's gender, age, lifestyle, analysis of food intake and identification of nutritional deficiencies" and "recommendations for optimum nutrient levels to maintain good health." (I do not believe any software can do this.)
- A TV commercial, radio spots, newspaper and yellow page ads, doctor letters, and a column that can be published under the pharmacist's own name.
- A personalized Internet Web page, which adds the pharmacist to a list of "complementary and natural healthcare practitioners worldwide" so that "when someone searches for a natural healthcare practitioner, they will find you." (I do not believe that pharmacists are qualified or legally permitted to be "natural healthcare practitioners.")
- An in-store display unit designed to let customers see a variety of products, books, and services in one place.
- Answers to questions needed "when a customer is standing in front of you" or when "you want to know about a new fad or product your customer just asked you about."
- "The best experts in the fields of pharmacy, natural products, and complementary medicine available" by picking up the phone or accessing the Internet.—SB

that a doctor be consulted (*Consumer Reports* 51:170–175, 1986).

In 1987, two pharmacy school professors sent a questionnaire to 1000 pharmacists in the Detroit metropolitan area and received 197 responses. Among the 116 who identified their five most-common reasons for recommending vitamins or minerals, 66 (56%) listed fatigue and 57 (49%) listed stress (*Journal of Clinical Pharmacy and Therapeutics* 15:141–146, 1990). Neither reason is valid. In response to a question about homeopathy, 27.4% said it was "useful," 18.3% judged it "useless," and 54.3% "didn't know" (*Journal of Clinical Pharmacy and Therapeutics* 15:131–139, 1990).

What Happened to Ethics?

Merlin Nelson, MD, Pharm.D., coauthor of the above-mentioned survey, has asked pharmacists why they promote and sell food supplements to healthy individuals who don't need them. He concluded: "The most common reason is greed. Advertising creates a demand that the pharmacist can supply and make a profit. 'If I don't sell them, they'll just go to my competition down the street,' is a common response. Pharmacists are apparently more interested in a sale than in the patient's welfare. . . .

"Rather than just recommending a multivitamin to patients concerned about obtaining enough vitamins in their diet, pharmacists should offer sound nutritional advice or provide referrals to experts in nutrition such as registered dietitians" (*American Pharmacy* NS28(10) 34–36, 1988).

Pharmacists are also the only recognized health professionals who sell tobacco products, which cause more death and years of lost life than any other consumer product. Although some pharmacists have stopped, the majority do not consider tobacco sales unethical. Nelson is one of only a handful of pharmacists who have criticized the misleading promotions of supplement manufacturers. As far as I can tell, no professional pharmacy organization has ever done so.

The American Pharmaceutical Association's code of ethics does not state that pharmacists have a duty to prevent dubious products from lining their shelves. Five states have laws declaring it illegal for pharmacists to sell ineffective products, but these laws have never been applied to the sale of OTC products.

I believe that pharmacists have as much of an ethical duty to discourage use of inappropriate products as physicians do to advise against unnecessary surgery or medical care. Very few pharmacists do so. Pharmacy journal editors ignore this problem. Hospital-based pharmacists generally exhibit a higher standard of practice, but very few of them are speaking out about the problems described in this article.

Stephen Barrett, MD, is a retired psychiatrist who resides in Allentown, Pennsylvania. His 44 books include The Vitamin Pushers: How the "Health Food" Industry Is Selling America a Bill of Goods.

Unit 7

Unit Selections

59. **FAO Releases Annual State of Food and Agriculture Report Showing Worldwide Number of Hungry People Rising Slightly,** Food and Agriculture Organization of the United Nations
60. **Special Programme for Food Security at the Food and Agriculture Organization,** Journal of Family and Consumer Sciences
61. **Starvation Syndrome in Africa,** Frances M. Berg
62. **How to Measure Malnutrition,** Healthy Weight Journal
63. **Hunger and Food Insecurity,** Katherine L. Cason

Key Points to Consider

❖ Should more be done about hunger in the United States? Whose responsibility is it, that of the government or of the private sector? How could you help?

❖ What should be the roles of the United States and other developed countries in solving world hunger? To what extent should countries be expected to solve their own problems?

❖ What criteria would you use to decide when to help another country and how much?

❖ How well has the Food and Agriculture Organization (FAO) addressed concerns about hunger and malnutrition in its World Food Summit? What else would you have included or expressed differently? Why?

DUSHKIN ONLINE Links   www.dushkin.com/online/

35. **Population Reference Bureau**
    http://www.prb.org
36. **World Health Organization**
    http://www.who.ch
37. **WWW Virtual Library: Demography & Population Studies**
    http://demography.anu.edu.au/VirtualLibrary/

These sites are annotated on pages 4 and 5.

World Hunger and Malnutrition

If you give me a fish, I will eat for a day And
you will have my thanks, and I'll be on my way.
If you teach me to fish, you'll bring me dignity,
For I can feed myself, through all eternity.
—*Don Ferrens, 1990*

Officials from nearly 200 nations met in Rome at the World Food Summit in 1996. They declared that all people have the right to be free from hunger through access to safe, nutritious, and culturally acceptable food. In making this declaration, officials pledged to cooperate in providing a political environment within which economic and social policies could deliver this promise. A strong emphasis was placed on changing world trade policies as the key to improving food access, but no binding agreement was signed.

There was, moreover, disagreement with the conclusions of the World Food Summit. Meeting nearby were representatives of a variety of secular and religious organizations that work directly with people. They claimed that food security is not a supply problem that can be solved by controlling the population growth of undeveloped countries and expanding agriculture in the industrialized world, as the Summit had declared. Rather, they contended, food security is a demand problem, to be solved by distributing food more fairly, reducing overconsumption by affluent nations, and improving sustainable smallholder agriculture.

Periodically, reports are issued that identify the extent of hunger and malnutrition around the world and categorize the primary contributing factors to these conditions. Yet, even these reports may be contradictory, and some argue that the data used are both flawed and inadequate, that we simply don't know what the nutritional needs of people are.

Few will argue, however, either that the amount of hunger and malnutrition is insignificant or that we have found ways to reduce them significantly. In the first article, the UN Food and Agriculture Organization (FAO) indicates that the total number of the chronically malnourished has risen to 828 million, an increase of 6 million in a 4-year period. Asia has the largest number of undernourished people, while the highest percentage of malnourished people is in sub-Saharan Africa.

International food programs have worked hard to meet emergency food needs caused by floods in Bangladesh, war in Kosovar and Angola, and famines and droughts elsewhere. More than 80 countries rely heavily on the World Food Program. The United States is its largest donor and will supply a million metric tons of wheat this year through this program alone.

There also is little disagreement over the costs of hunger and malnutrition. A 1998 fact sheet from the UNICEF states that "Malnutrition contributes to over 6 million child deaths each year, 55 percent of the nearly 12 million deaths among children under 5 in developing countries." Malnourished children live out their lives with disabilities and weakened immune systems. As adults they are more subject to heart disease, diabetes, and hypertension. Their motivation and curiosity are dulled, reducing the exploratory activities that result in normal mental and cognitive development. In turn, this robs their countries of innovative and rational leadership and undermines the world struggle for peace and equality.

Hunger and malnutrition result from too few calories or low intakes of nutrients. The lack of a single nutrient can result in an obvious deficiency such as goiters or rickets. Mild to moderate deficiencies that are hardly observable but that significantly impair health are just as likely. The causes are complex. They follow war and environmental disasters. They are a consequence of discrimination against women, who often lack access to education and good information and have difficulty finding gainful employment. They result from too little purchasing power and poor distribution of the food that is available. And they are found in all corners of the world.

But hunger is more than a physical phenomenon. An article describing the starvation syndrome as experienced by the Ik in Africa vividly portrays the emotional impact when food is severely deprived. Hunger respects no geographical boundaries, and although it is most common in Africa, it is known on every continent and in every country. Famines have been frequent throughout history, and they bring an acute focus to hunger. Between 1845–1850, the Irish potato famine resulted in thousands of deaths and huge numbers of immigrants to the United States. Millions of Ethiopians and other citizens of Africa have died during recent years. China has faced periodic famines throughout the nineteenth and twentieth centuries. India now claims to be self-sufficient in food production; but it has not solved the problem of chronic hunger.

In spite of decidedly greater wealth, hunger is also visible in developed countries. Among the poor in the United Kingdom, increased risks of premature births, obesity, and hypertension can be documented. Stunting among young children in the Russian Federation increased from 9 to 15 percent in a recent 2-year period. Even in the United States, an estimated 4 percent of households experience hunger, and malnutrition among the elderly is considered a serious national epidemic. Experts say that U.S. hunger differs from hunger in developing countries in that its cause is poverty uncomplicated by natural disasters, war, or an undeveloped economy. More Americans go to bed hungry than did in the mid-1980s, and the likelihood of this occurring is greater when the head of household is female and if the family is black or Hispanic.

Food programs that are intended to supplement the family's food budget sometimes become the primary source of food. WIC (a supplemental nutrition program for women, infants, and children) in particular has been documented to be extremely cost-effective, saving $3 in potential medical costs for every $1 spent, according to the General Accounting Office. But even federal food assistance programs such as WIC and food stamps do not reach all of the needy. Paradoxically, food stamp rolls have declined 28 percent since 1994, even as soup kitchens and food pantries have multiplied all over the country. It is argued that recent welfare reforms may have left many people unaware of their eligibility.

It would be unfair to leave the impression that no global progress is evident. Bolivia is the first country to declare that iodized salt has virtually eliminated iodine deficiency as a public health problem. Food fortification programs elsewhere are saving children from deficiencies. Community volunteer programs in a number of countries are monitoring growth rates, promoting breast feeding, and reducing malnutrition. And many local efforts are successfully assisting small farmers to increase and improve their food production.

Article 59

FAO RELEASES ANNUAL STATE OF FOOD AND AGRICULTURE REPORT SHOWING WORLDWIDE NUMBER OF HUNGRY PEOPLE RISING SLIGHTLY; WARNS OF SLOWER ECONOMIC GROWTH IN MOST DEVELOPING COUNTRIES

Rome, November 26—The number of undernourished people in the world has increased since the early 1990s, mainly because there has been little progress in reducing poverty, according to new estimates released today in the annual UN Food and Agriculture Organization report, The State of Food and Agriculture 1998 (SOFA 98). The report notes the rise in the number of hungry people, despite significant reductions in hunger and malnutrition in several developing regions.

"The total number of chronically undernourished people in developing countries is now estimated to be 828 million for the 1994–96 period" up from 822 million for 1990–92, according to the report. In addition to weather-related crop damage leading to less domestic food availability in many countries, the problem was compounded by foreign exchange constraints that prevented the import of food to make up the domestic shortfall. Other factors involved in the growing numbers of hungry people include the growth in the

Editor's note: See related article, which follows on page 212.

total population and changing demographics that result in a larger proportion of that population being young, which leads to changes in minimum dietary requirements.

However, the overall percentage of malnourished as a part of the world population has declined over the same period from 20 to 19 percent, the report says, adding that this has not been sufficient to compensate for population growth.

SOFA 98 warns that global financial turmoil now threatens the earlier economic gains, including improved food security, made by many Asian and Latin American countries. Its negative effects on household incomes, employment and prospects for agricultural production and trade could lead to greater food insecurity for millions of people.

"Efforts to meet the World Food Summit goal of reducing, by at least half, the 1996 number of hungry people in the world by the year 2015 are all the more urgent," said Mr. Jacques Vercueil, Director of FAO's Agriculture and Economic Development Analysis Division that produced SOFA 98. "In East Asia and Southeast Asia, there are 258 million malnourished people. In South Asia, in 1994–96, there were 254 million undernourished people, up from 237 million in 1990–92," said Vercueil.

"In sub-Saharan Africa," he said, "the number of hungry is also increasing. Our most recent data on Africa south of the Sahara show an increase in malnour-

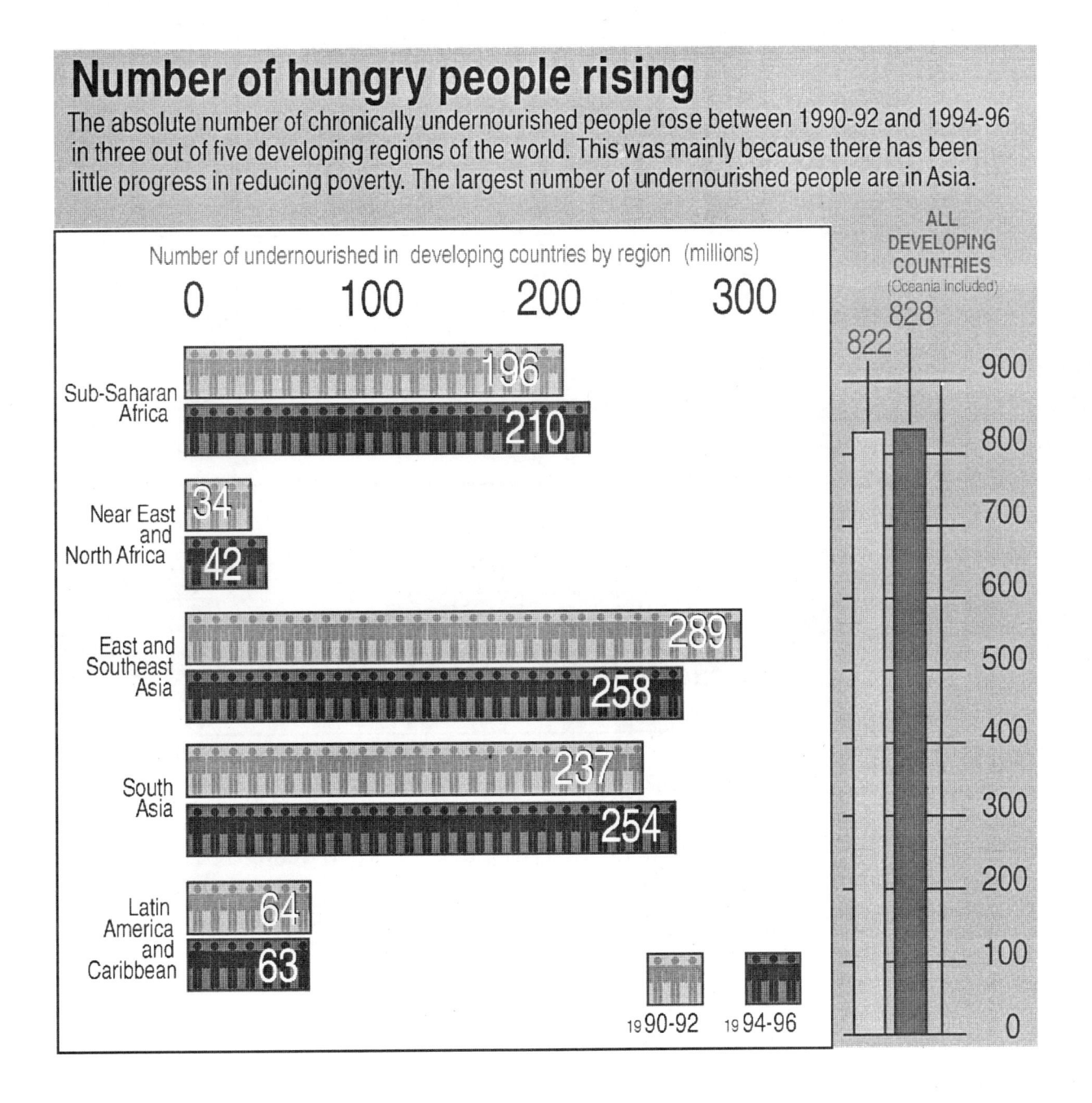

Number of hungry people rising

The absolute number of chronically undernourished people rose between 1990-92 and 1994-96 in three out of five developing regions of the world. This was mainly because there has been little progress in reducing poverty. The largest number of undernourished people are in Asia.

Number of undernourished in developing countries by region (millions)

Region	1990-92	1994-96
Sub-Saharan Africa	196	210
Near East and North Africa	34	42
East and Southeast Asia	289	258
South Asia	237	254
Latin America and Caribbean	64	63

ALL DEVELOPING COUNTRIES (Oceania included): 822 (1990-92), 828 (1994-96)

7 ❖ WORLD HUNGER AND MALNUTRITION

ished people from 196 million in 1990–92 to 210 million in 1994–96.

"SOFA 98 also shows that the widening gap in income distribution in many parts of the world is also an important factor in undernourishment," Mr. Vercueil said.

"The largest absolute numbers of undernourished people are in Asia," according to SOFA 98, while the largest proportion of the population that is undernourished is in sub-Saharan Africa.

"More striking," says the report, "is the fact that, contrary to the overall tendency in the developing countries as a whole, the poorest group of countries has not been able to reduce the number or percentage of undernourished since 1969–71."

Globally, SOFA 98 says, "The number of countries facing food emergencies rose from 29 in mid-1997 to 36 in mid-1998, mainly owing to the effects of the El Niño weather phenomenon." Since going to press, that number has risen to 40, according to FAO's Global Information and Early Warning System.

In a special feature on Feeding the World's Cities, SOFA 98 says, "Over the next 20 years, 93 percent of urban growth will occur in the cities of the developing world. Some of these cities are already huge: the world now has more than 20 megacities with a population of more than 10 million each, while 50 years ago only New York City could claim that distinction." Dhaka in Bangladesh has a population of 9 million

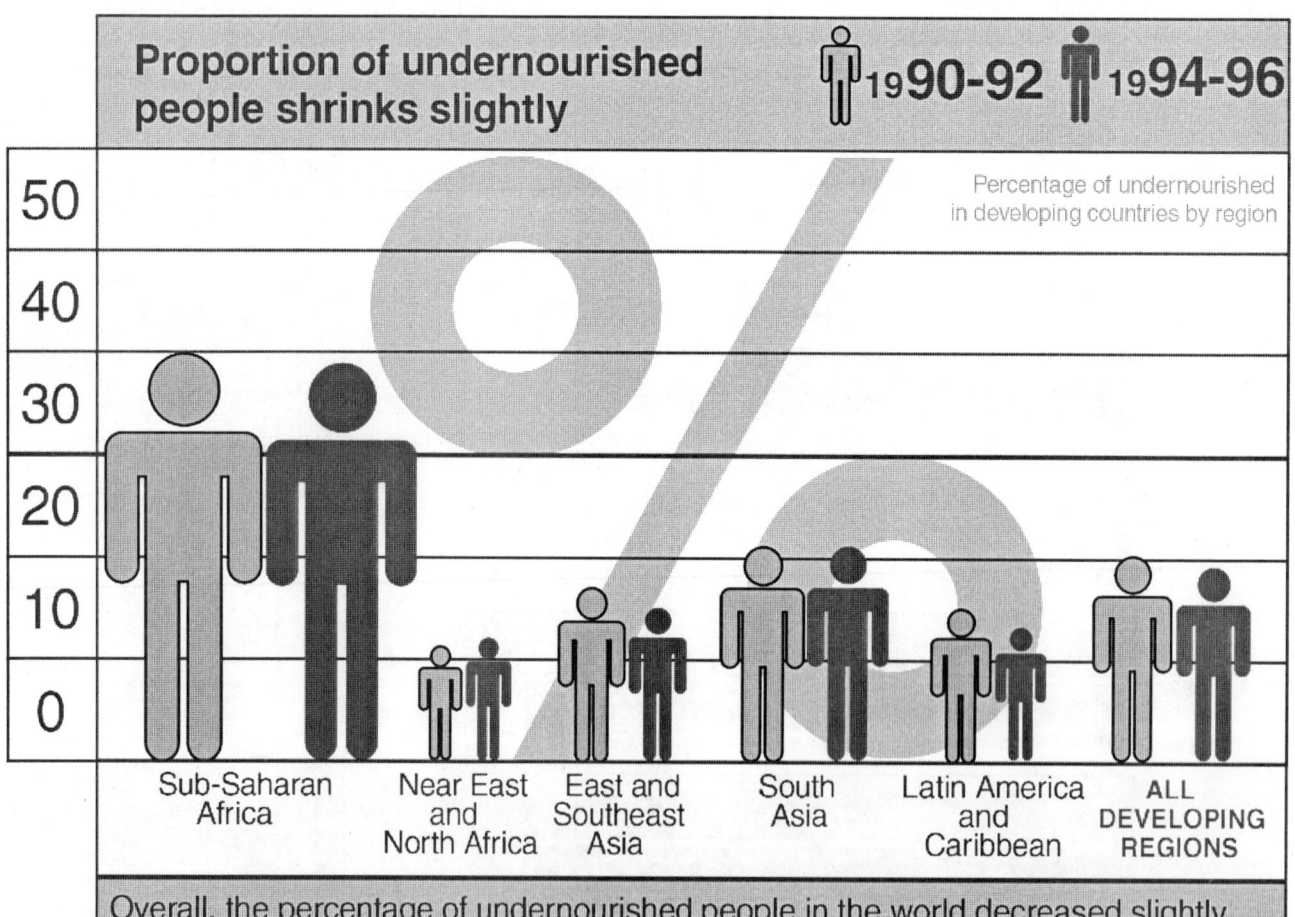

Proportion of undernourished people shrinks slightly — 1990-92 ▮ 1994-96

Percentage of undernourished in developing countries by region

Region	1990-92	1994-96
Sub-Saharan Africa	~30	~33
Near East and North Africa	~8	~10
East and Southeast Asia	~17	~13
South Asia	~22	~22
Latin America and Caribbean	~15	~13
ALL DEVELOPING REGIONS	~20	~18

Overall, the percentage of undernourished people in the world decreased slightly between 1990-92 and 1994-96. But this total decrease masks regional and national increases. Regionally, the Near East and North Africa and South Asia give most cause for concern.

59. FAO Releases Annual State of Food and Agriculture Report

and is growing at an annual rate of 5 percent, adding 1,300 people as city residents every day.

It is a huge task to feed a city of several million people, says SOFA 98. "A city of 10 million people—for example Manila, Cairo or Rio de Janeiro—may need to import at least 6,000 tonnes of food per day. This requires much coordination among producers, transporters, market managers and retailers in stores, on the street and in open-air markets. By 2005, more than 50 percent of the world's population will be urban and food insecurity will become an increasingly urban problem. Consumer needs and the responsibilities of both government and private operators as well as marketing facilities are just some of the issues examined in the SOFA 98 feature. . . .

SOFA 98 can be purchased from the FAO Sales and Marketing Group, Information Division (fax: 39 06 57 05 33 60)—E-mail: Publications@fao.org.

For further information call FAO Information Officer John Riddle at: 39 06 57 05 32 59, or e-mail him at john.riddle@fao.org

Also, please visit the FAO Website at http://www.fao.org/

Article 60

SPECIAL PROGRAMME

FOR FOOD SECURITY AT THE FOOD AND AGRICULTURE ORGANIZATION

Food security is defined by the Food and Agriculture Organization (FAO) as access by all people at all times to the food needed for a healthy and active life. Achieving food security means ensuring that sufficient food is available, that supplies are relatively stable, and that those in need of food can obtain it. Although over the years, governments, with support from FAO and other development agencies, have addressed food security and its related elements in many ways, today some 800 million people in developing countries—about 20% of their total population—are chronically undernourished. With a growing world population—the present figure of 5.7 billion is expected to rise to 8.3 billion by the year 2025—this situation will worsen unless very determined and well-targeted actions are taken to improve food security.

Chronic undernutrition and food insecurity are principally caused by
- low productivity in agriculture, frequently caused in part by policy, institutional, and technological constraints;
- high seasonal and year-to-year variability in food supplies, often the result of unreliable rainfall and insufficient water for crop and livestock production; and
- lack of off-farm employment opportunities, contributing to low and uncertain incomes in urban and rural areas.

The causes and consequences of food insecurity and poverty are inextricably linked.

One way to break the vicious circle of poverty and food insecurity is to increase agricultural productivity, particularly where gains can be achieved by small farmers who are often among the poorest. As the world's population and living standards rise, the need for food will grow, and the availability of underused, arable land will continue to decrease. Therefore, it is important to intensify production on land with agricultural potential currently in use, using sustainable methods, rather than to encroach on land that is only marginally suitable for cultivation.

In 1994, FAO's director-general initiated a review of the organization's priorities, programs, and strategies. This review concluded that
- improving food security should be reaffirmed as the organization's top priority and
- that there was an urgent need for the organization's programs to focus more sharply on increasing food production, improving stability of supplies, and generating rural employment, thereby contributing to more accessible supplies.

The director-general therefore proposed that FAO should launch a Special Programme for Food Security (SPFS), focused on low-income food-deficit countries (LIFDCs)—the countries least able to meet their food needs with imports.

This approach was endorsed by the World Food Summit held in Rome in November 1996, which called for concerted efforts at all levels to raise food production and increase access to food in 86 LIFDCs, with the objective of cutting the present number of malnourished people in the world by half by the year 2015. The plan of action adopted by the summit concludes that to reduce hunger, action is required in the following areas: ensuring enabling conditions, improving access to food, producing food, increasing the role of trade, dealing adequately with disaster, and investing in food security.

SPFS draws from Agenda 21, unanimously adopted at the 1992 United Nations Conference on Environment and Development (UNCED), held in Rio de Janeiro, which states in Chapter 14.6, "The major thrust of food security . . . is to bring about a significant increase in agricultural production in a sustainable way and to achieve a substantial improve-

---

Editor's note: See previous related article on page 208.

60. Special Programme for Food Security

ment in people's entitlement to adequate food and culturally appropriate food supplies." As populations continue to grow, pressure on arable land steadily increases. "Agriculture has to meet this challenge (of rapidly increasing population), mainly by increasing production on land already in use and by avoiding further encroachment on land that is only marginally suitable for cultivation" (Chapter 14.1).

The SPFS is an FAO initiative unanimously approved by the 106th Session of the FAO Council in June 1994. The SPFS commenced its operations in late 1994. A budget of US$10 million was provided for the 1996–1997 biennium and for the 1998–1999 biennium.

The main objective of the SPFS is to help LIFDCs to improve their national food security—through rapid increases in productivity and food production and by reducing year-to-year variability in production—on an economically and environmentally sustainable basis. The underlying assumption is that in most LIFDCs, viable and sustainable means of increasing food availability exist but are not realized because of a range of constraints that prevent farmers from responding to needs and opportunities. By working with farmers and other stakeholders to identify and resolve such constraints—whether they are of a technical, institutional, or policy nature—and to demonstrate ways of increasing production, the SPFS should open the way for improved productivity and broader food access.

The SPFS is founded on the concepts of national ownership, a participatory approach, environmental awareness and sensitivity, and regard for the role of women. The SPFS is expected to contribute substantially to the implementation of the World Food Summit Plan of Action for food security in the 86 LIFDCs at the individual, household and national levels.

For more information, visit the FAO web site at (http://www.fao.org).

Mongolian farmers begin to feel the benefits of SPFS

Mongolia is one of the latest countries to sign up under the SPFS. An LIFDC because of its harsh natural environment and its transitional economy, Mongolia is still essentially a pastoral nation. Since the collapse of the Soviet Union, there has been a dramatic decline in agricultural production. Land planted to cereals shrank from 900 000 ha in 1990 to some 250 000 ha in 1997. Similar declines in vegetable and potato production are reported, together with a 60 percent reduction in irrigated area. Vegetable consumption fell from around 25 kg per capita during the 1980s, to just 9 kg per capita in 1994/95.

Work under the Special Programme began in identified priority areas with:

- minor rehabilitation of four selected small-scale irrigation schemes;
- demonstrations of inexpensive, small-scale sprinkler technology;
- training of farmers in improved water management and irrigated horticultural practices;
- diversification into beekeeping, poultry keeping, vegetable processing and home gardening;
- constraints analysis.

Results after the first season were highly encouraging. All the minor rehabilitation works were completed on schedule and below the estimated cost. Some 33 farmers, more than half of whom were women, were supplied with simple portable irrigation sprinkler sets and pumps to irrigate 0.86 ha each. The systems work well and farmers are enthusiastic about how easy they are to use.

The main vegetables grown were carrot, turnip, cucumber and cabbage, together with smaller quantities of potato, watermelon and tomato. Some new vegetables were introduced, including - courgette, green pepper, radish, dill, aubergine, lettuce and spinach. More than 800 m^2 of plastic sheet was distributed and farmers made their own frames from wood and other local materials. Compost was supplied to farmers as no mineral fertilizer is available. Locally produced hand tools are used for weeding. Preliminary estimates indicate that on average in 1998 the SPFS farmers earned 69 percent more than they did in 1997.

Under the Diversification component, vegetable processing was the most successful activity, with large quantities of cucumber, cabbage, carrot and tomato pickled in vinegar, either for household consumption during winter or for sale at the market, where they fetch up to ten times their fresh value. Underground storage spaces for increased production have also been constructed by many farmers. The stores are big enough to hold 5–10 tons of produce and are kept at between +2°C and –5°C by small stoves. Root crops like potatoes, turnips and carrots store most successfully and even cabbages keep for up to three or four months.

An interim report produced by the Mongolian Agriculture University indicates that the main constraints to improving production were lack of mineral fertilizer and agro-chemicals, inadequate financing for seasonal inputs and marketing problems.

Source: SPFS-FAO

Starvation Syndrome in Africa

by Frances M. Berg, MS

Starving people can lose their sense of humanity and behave in hostile, cruel ways as they struggle to survive, says anthropologist Colin M. Turnbull, in his book *The Mountain People*. Turnbull describes the dehumanization of an African hunting tribe as it deteriorated through a period of drought and starvation in the mid- 1960s. Forbidden by the Uganda government to hunt game in the newly established Kidepo National Park, their major hunting ground, the Ik tried with little success to farm and forage for food in the barren mountains adjoining the park.

Drought and starvation made them a strange and heartless people, mistrustful, their days occupied with constant competition and the search for food.

As starvation advanced, children and the elderly were abandoned, or even forcefully thrown out of their homes. The starving Ik came to fear and distrust each other. They seldom spoke. Cruelty took the place of love as their culture broke down. They lost all sense of moral obligation, their religion, rituals, and spirituality. Men and women went out alone to forage for food, returning empty-handed to avoid sharing with crying children, fragile parents, or spouses.

Turnbull contrasts the Ik with other hunter societies he studied in Africa that display "the intense love that is so truly a part of ordinary African life... kindness, generosity, consideration, affection, honesty, hospitality, compassion, and charity. Traits that help them in the hunt, but were luxuries to starving individuals. None of these were present in the starving Ik."

These people would be kind, generous, and friendly if they could afford it, he suggests, but as starvation progressed during the 2 years he spent with them, basic survival instincts took over. Reduced to desperate hunger and fight for survival, they became as "unfriendly, uncharitable, inhospitable, and generally mean as people can be."

In the crisis for survival there was no social life, no religion, no friendship or love, only mistrust and fear between members of a village, without regard to family or kinship. Isolated from one another, each family was separated in its own walled compound within the village fortress walls. In the family, there was mistrust between man and wife, and between parents and their children. Each family was divided: husbands, wives, and children remorselessly avoided helping one another find food.

"The lack of any sense of moral responsibility toward each other, the lack of any sense of belonging to, needing, or wanting each other, showed up daily and most clearly in what otherwise would have passed for family relationships," writes Turnbull.

A mother would force her child out, to go and live with the younger group of foraging children at the age of 3. Before this, the mother seemed to care only grudgingly for her child, and laughed if the toddler was hurt. In starvation, Turnbull observed, anyone who could not take care of himself or herself was a burden and hazard to the survival of others.

He tells of one mother who left her baby on the ground where it was carried off by a predator. "The mother was delighted. She was rid of the child and no longer had to carry it about and feed it, and still further this meant that a leopard was in the vicinity and would be sleeping the child off and thus be an easy kill. The men set off and found the leopard, which had consumed all of the child except part of the skull; they killed the leopard and cooked it and ate it, child and all."

In another example, he observed the callousness of a father named Giriko whose son, about age 10, developed an intestinal blockage. Giriko was amused and would call people to look at the boy's distended belly. It became a favorite topic for jokes because ultimately the boy could neither eat nor drink. It hurt when he lay down, so he spent most of the time on his hands and knees, even at night, his bloated stomach hanging down and resting on the ground. This boy had a father, two mothers, and three sisters—but not one helped to lift him when he struggled to move. The response when he died was neither surprise nor interest.

What was true for parent-child was true for husband-wife or brother-sister. They stole from each other, laughed at another's misfortune, and refused help or food when needed.

Foraging bands of children

Children lived in two age-level bands—a younger group about 3 to 7 years, and a senior band 8 to 12 years. These bands foraged out each morning in search of food. Within the band they found some protection from other bands, lions, and leopards, but each child hunted his or her own food alone. In this time of hunger, they ate mostly figs that had been partially eaten by baboons, a few berries, certain bark that was edible but sometimes made them feel sick. When really hungry they swallowed earth or even pebbles.

The children often were cruel to each other, with no adults offering protection or guidance. The younger band members were bullied and beaten, and in time they became the bullies and the beaters.

One girl called Adupa was especially picked on and often beaten and teased. As she grew hungrier, her stomach grew more and more distended, her legs and arms more spindly. Her reactions became slower and slower. When she managed to find food—fruit peels, skins, bits

---

Adupa's playmates attacked her with cries of excitement, fun, and laughter, snatched the food, and beat her savagely over the head.

---

of bone, half-eaten berries—she held it in her hand and looked at it with wonder and delight, savoring its taste before she ate it. Her playmates caught on quickly and would watch, even putting tidbits in her way, then as she raised her hand to her mouth, they attacked her with cries of excitement, fun, and laughter, snatched the food, and beat her savagely over the head. Adupa pleaded to be taken in by her parents and sometimes brought them food that she had scrounged, but they drove her out. When they saw she was dying, her parents did take her in, then went out and closed the opening tightly so she could not get out, promising to bring her food. Instead, they went away for several days. She was dead when they returned, and they threw her body out "as one does the riper garbage, a good distance away."

The Ik showed no concern for others, indeed, there was little emotion of any kind except for a detached kind of cruelty. The Ik dismissed love as idiotic and highly dangerous.

"I had seen no evidence of family life such as is found almost everywhere else in the world. I had seen no sign of love, with its willingness to sacrifice. I had seen little that I could even call affection... I had never seen an Ik anywhere near tears of sorrow—only the children's tears of anger, malice and hate," Turnbull reports.

Loveless humor

"There simply was not room in the life of these people for such luxuries as family and sentiment and love. So close to the verge of starvation, such luxuries could mean death," Turnbull explains.

Perversely, they found entertainment and even joy in the misfortune of others, says Turnbull. "Cruelty was with them, in their humor, in their interpersonal relations, in their thoughts and reflections. Yet, so utter was their isolation, as individuals, that I do not think they thought of their cruelty as affecting others."

They laughed at each other and even at themselves when they fell over from hunger. He describes how men would watch with eager anticipation as a child crawled toward the fire, then burst into gay and happy laughter as it plunged a skinny hand into the coals. This was one of the few times he observed parental affection—the mother would glow with pleasure to hear such joy occasioned by her child and pull it tenderly out of the fire.

Anyone falling down was good for a laugh too, especially if he were old, weak, or blind. Those who watched seemed content to let things happen and just enjoy them. They conserved their energy and did not intervene.

In work, such as making rope or spears, people would gather and watch each other in the pleasurable prospect of being able to enjoy someone else's misfortune, in the hope of being able to criticize, says Turnbull. Rope making offered endless opportunity for criticism and ridicule. "Other Ik would stop their own work and look, with hope and anticipation. If the rip was clean, work was resumed, but if the bark tore at a knot or where a branch had been cut too close or not close enough, there were howls of laughter... Eyes flick hungrily from the ripping bark to the face, so as to be able to detect the first sign of splitting and the subsequent expression of anger or frustration..."

As starvation progressed, there seemed to be increasingly less that could be called social life, Turnbull says. There was simply no community of interest, familial or economic, social or spiritual. He had not believed people could behave this way, and searched for evidence of love almost from the beginning. "But love implies mutuality, a willingness to sacrifice the self. The Ik, however, do not value emotion above survival, and they are without love." He considers whether love is a luxury, only for those who have plenty.

Each person was simply alone, living in isolation, seldom speaking. "It was this very acceptance of individual isolation that made love almost impossible. Contact, when made, was usually for a very specific and practical purpose having to do with food and the filling of a stomach, a single stomach. Such contacts were temporary and contextual... The last possibility was affection, which may be a forerunner to love."

If people did go off to seek food together, their goodwill was quickly dispelled by acrimony in division of the spoils, if communally acquired, "or by the sheer envy of seeing anyone else eating food even if it was acquired by his own solitary effort... More often all three forces were at work—acrimony, envy and suspicion—and that was not fertile ground for the seeds of affection."

How to Measure Malnutrition

For simplicity, weight is often used as a measure of malnutrition. The United Nations Food and Agriculture Organization (FAO) recently adopted body weight as the standard to measure nutritional status and starvation worldwide.[1] A body mass index of 18.5 is defined as the cutoff point for "chronic energy deficiency" in adults. Weights below this level are highly correlated with starvation, deficiencies of the immune system, illness, morbidity, and mortality, according to the 1995 FAO report *Body Mass Index: A measure of chronic energy deficiency in adults*. Thus, a BMI of 18.5 is regarded as the lower limit of healthy weight. (It is acknowledged that some healthy people may weigh less than this, particularly if they are tall and thin.) Far greater attention needs to be paid to adult underweight, as physical effectiveness and the ability to withstand illness and stress is severely compromised, says the report.[2]

Protein-calorie malnutrition, especially in older persons, is usually based on such measures as weight, loss of weight, serum concentrations of proteins produced by the liver, anthropometric measurements, grip strength, anergy, immunologic functions, low cholesterol, low albumin, nutritional risk index, and may also include dysphoria (sadness), eating problems, and shopping problems. Historic weight loss is known to be an excellent measure of nutritional depletion in persons who do not have a disease of water metabolism. Low albumin and cholesterol concentrations usually indicate both malnutrition and excessive cytokine production. The gold standard for the diagnosis of protein-energy malnutrition in older persons is the MiniNutritional Assessment (MNA) initially developed at the University of Toulouse in France in collaboration with Nestlé in Lausanne, Switzerland. Two other screening tests for older persons are the Nutrition Screening Initiative DETERMINE and SCALES.[3,4]

Body Mass Index Chart for Lower Body Weights

Height (ins.)	Body Mass Index		
	17	18	19
	Weight (lbs.)		
60	85	90	95
62	90	100	105
64	100	105	110
66	105	115	120
68	110	120	125
70	120	125	130
72	125	135	140

Adapted from Guidelines for Adolescent Preventive Services. AMA 1995.

References

1. Body Mass Index: a measure of chronic energy deficiency in adults. United Nations Food and Agriculture Organization, 1995.
2. Berg F. World starvation: weight may be best tool to measure malnutrition. Healthy Weight Journal 1995; 9:47–49.
3. Souba W. Nutritional support. Drug Ther 1997; 336: 41.
4. Morley J. Anorexia of aging: physiologic and pathologic. Am J Clin Nutr 1997; 66:760–773.

HUNGER AND FOOD INSECURITY

KATHERINE L. CASON, Ph.D, R.D.
Associate Professor, Department of Family and Youth Development
Clemson University

ABSTRACT
Approximately 30 million Americans, including 11 million children, currently experience hunger and food insecurity. Assistance programs and policies help alleviate poverty and food insecurity; however, the rate of hunger and malnutrition has increased. Recent welfare reform legislation decreases funding for assistance. Approaches are needed to achieve long-term food security in our communities. Family and consumer scientists can help through education, food-recovery programs, cost-effectiveness program assessments, and public issues education.

According to data released by the U.S. Census Bureau in September 1997, 36.5 million Americans, or 13.7% of the population, lived in poverty in 1996. Poverty is a high priority on the agendas of many economists and politicians; yet no one has been able to overcome the problems and obstacles associated with this social disease.

Living in poverty often means that individuals are victims of hunger (Clancy & Bowering, 1992). Living below the poverty line puts tremendous strains on a household budget, adversely affecting the ability to purchase a nutritionally adequate diet (Clancy & Bowering, 1992). Hunger and the broader issue of food security have been a public concern in the United States since our nation's inception. One of the earliest underlying goals of public policy (still in effect) is to assure an adequate supply of safe, nutritious food at reasonable cost (Voichick & Drake, 1994). Recent studies suggest at least 30 million Americans, including 11 million children, currently experience food insecurity (Wehler, Scott & Anderson, 1996).

Food security can be defined as access by all people at all times to enough food for an active, healthy life. Food security includes a ready availability of nutritionally adequate and safe foods and an ability to acquire acceptable foods in socially acceptable ways (Hamilton et al., 1997). The complex issues surrounding food insecurity encompass physiological, social, and economic dimensions. Food, or lack of it, is a determinant of human development, health, and behavior. Its absence affects a community's economy, taxes its resources, and influences its social policies (Breglio, 1992).

Those who experience food insecurity may try to avoid hunger by decreasing the size of meals, skipping meals, or not eating any food for one or more days. When food is severely limited, these methods for avoiding hunger are ineffective (Klein, 1996).

Lack of food, and the subsequent undernutrition, affects physiological functioning in every stage of the life cycle. Most adversely affected are the fetus, pregnant and lactating women, children, and older adults. According to the Community Childhood Hunger Identification Project (CCHIP), hungry children suffer from two to four times as many individual health problems as low-income children whose families do not experience food shortages. Only 44% of low-income children consumed at or above 100% of the Recommended Dietary Allowance (RDA) for calories (USDA, 1989).

Failure to grow over time is a consequence of undernutrition. Inadequate food intake limits the ability of children to learn about the world around them (Center on Hunger, Poverty and Nutrition Policy, 1993). When children are chronically undernourished, their bodies attempt to conserve energy by shutting down "nonessential" bodily functions, leaving energy available for vital organs and growth. If any energy remains, it can be used for social activity and cognitive development. When the body conserves energy, decreased activity levels and increased apathy soon follow. This in turn affects social interactions, inquisitiveness, and overall cognitive functioning. In comparison to nonhun-

> **Anxiety, negative feelings about self-worth, and hostility toward the outside world can result from chronic hunger and food insecurity**

gry children, hungry children are more than four times as likely to suffer from irritability; more than 12 times as likely to report dizziness; and almost three times as likely to suffer from concentration problems (Food Research and Action Center [FRAC], 1991).

In the United States, iron deficiency anemia is still common in infants and young children between 6 months and 3 years, and again during adolescence. About twice as many 4- to 5-year-old African American children have iron deficiency as Mexican American or Caucasian children. The most common causes of anemia in childhood are inadequate intakes of iron, infection, and lead poisoning. Among children 12 to 36 months of age with iron deficiency anemia, 20.6% were from low-income families (Fomon, 1993).

Pregnant women who are undernourished are more likely to experience low birth weight babies. These infants are more likely to suffer delays in their development and are more likely to experience behavior and learning problems later in life. The infant mortality rate is closely linked to inadequate quantity of quality in the diet of the infant's mother (U.S. Department of Health and Human Services [USDHHS], 1994).

Older adults are also at increased risk of suffering health consequences as a result of food insecurity and hunger. Older adults have a number of risk factors that place them at an increased risk for developing malnutrition. Among these risk factors are diseases such as chronic lung disease, heart disease, neurological diseases; disabilities, functional impairments; sensory losses; poor dental health; multiple medication use; therapeutic diets; and social isolation. Malnutrition in older adults can result in loss of muscle mass, which can lead to disabilities that affect levels of independence. Malnutrition can also compromise the immune function, increasing susceptibility to infections (Codispoti & Bartlett, 1994).

Insecurity about whether a family will be able to obtain enough food to avoid hunger also have an emotional impact on children and their parents. Anxiety, negative feelings about self-worth, and hostility toward the outside world can result from chronic hunger and food insecurity (World Hunger Year, 1994).

FOOD ASSISTANCE PROGRAMS

During the 1960s, food security became a high-priority issue at all levels of the government. Government officials and influential leaders, the media, and the general public could no longer ignore the issue of hunger (Egan, 1980).

Several programs were implemented in the 1960s and early 1970s, including the Food Stamp Program; the Special Supplemental Program for Women, Infants and Children (WIC); the Community Food and Nutrition Program; and the Expanded Food and Nutrition Education Program (EFNEP) within the Cooperative Extension Service Program. The media has labeled these years the "War on Hunger" (Voichick & Drake, 1994).

During the 1980s, hunger increased primarily due to a combination of economic factors and resulting cuts in federal assistance programs (FRAC, 1991). In the early 1990s, advocates were hopeful about the renewed interest among elected leaders in improving programs that feed people. The historic passage of the Mickey Leland Childhood Hunger Relief Act in August 1993 helped to improve benefits to food stamp families and improve access for those who had been unable to participate in the Food Stamp Program. The president and Congress committed to place the Special Supplemental Nutrition Program for Women, Infants, and Children (WIC) on track for full funding by 1996, and Congress made funding available to start and expand the School Breakfast and Summer Food Programs (Uvin, 1994).

Food Stamp Program

The Food Stamp Program puts food on the table for some 9 million households and 22 million individuals each day. It provides low-income households with coupons or electronic benefits used like cash at most grocery stores to ensure access to a healthy diet. The current program structure was implemented in 1977 with a goal of alleviating hunger and malnutrition by permitting low-income households to obtain a more nutritious diet through normal channels of trade. It provided more than $19 billion in benefits in 1997 (FRAC, 1997).

The Food Stamp Program began as a federal assistance program designed to help farmers dispose of surplus food products. While assistance to farmers remains a part of the program, the current objective is to help low-income families increase their food purchasing power and achieve a nutritionally adequate diet (Social Security, 1996). However, CCHIP data and other sources indicate that food stamps are not used by millions of people who appear eligible to participate in them due to barriers to participation, lack of information about eligibility, and inadequate funding. Survey results consistently show food stamp benefits are not sufficient to protect many low-income families from experiencing hunger (FRAC, 1998). The *Third Report on Nutrition Monitoring in the United States (1995)* indicates that individuals receiving food stamps have less than adequate diets than those low-income individuals who do not receive food stamps. The report suggests that such risk factors as obesity, hypertension, and high serum cholesterol are major concerns for low-income individuals and place them at higher risk for developing chronic diseases due to inadequate diets. The lack of improvement in adequacy of the diets of food stamp recipients suggests that food stamp recipients would benefit from nutrition education; yet nutrition education is not a mandatory component of the program (Joy & Doisy, 1996).

Since 1986, USDA funds have been available for development and implementation of nutrition education programs; however, only 21 states have instituted such programs. Evaluation of the program is at the discretion of each state (Joy & Doisy, 1996).

National School Lunch Program (NSLP)

The National School Lunch Program was created by Congress 50 years ago as a measure of national security, to safeguard the health and well-being of the nation's children. The NSLP provided meals to 25.1 million children in 1997. Of the more than 26 million children participating in the lunch program, 14.6 million low-income children receive free or reduced price lunches daily (FRAC, 1997).

School Breakfast Program

The School Breakfast Program was established by Congress, initially as a temporary measure through the Child Nutrition Act of 1966 in areas where children had long bus rides to school and in areas where mothers were in the workforce. Permanent authorization in 1975 assisted schools in the provision of a nutritious morning meal to children. In 1997, more than 7 million children and 67,063 schools participated in the School Breakfast Program; 86% were from families with low incomes (FRAC, 1997).

Summer Food Service Program

The Summer Food Service Program was created by Congress in 1968. It is an entitlement program designed to provide funds for eligible sponsoring organizations to serve nutritious meals to low-income children when school is not in session. In the summer of 1996, the program served more than 2.2 million children at more than 28,000 sites operated by more than 3,400 sponsoring organizations nationwide (FRAC, 1997).

Child and Adult Care Feeding Program (CACFP)

The CACFP was founded in 1968 to provide federal funds for meals and snacks to licensed public and nonprofit child-care centers and family and group child-care homes for preschool children. Funds are also provided for meals and snacks served at after-school programs for school-age children, and to adult day-care centers serving chronically impaired adults or people over the age of 60. In 1966, CACFP served more than 2.6 million children daily, providing approximately 1.5 billion meals and snacks; and served more than 40,000 elderly persons in the Adult Day Care portion of the program (FRAC, 1997).

The Special Supplemental Program for Women, Infants, and Children (WIC)

WIC was established by Congress as a pilot program in 1972 and authorized as a national program in 1975. WIC is a federally funded, preventive nutrition program that provides nutritious foods, nutrition education, and access to health care to low-income pregnant women, new mothers, and infants and children at nutritional risk. The WIC program appropriation in fiscal year 1997 was $3.7 billion, which the USDA estimated would serve approximately 7.4 million participants (FRAC, 1997).

The Expanded Food and Nutrition Education Program (EFNEP)

EFNEP is administered by the Cooperative State Research Education and Extension Service of the U.S. Department of Agriculture, in cooperation with state Cooperative Extension Services in the 55 U.S. states and territories. In 1968, EFNEP was federally initiated by the USDA Extension Service with $10 million (from Section 32 of An Act to Amend the Agricultural Adjustment Act). In 1970, EFNEP received funding under the Smith-Lever Act; in 1977, under the Food and Agriculture Act; and in 1981, under the Agriculture and Food Act.

Since the program's inception, EFNEP paraprofessionals have taught limited-resource families how to improve dietary practices and become more effective managers of their available resources. The paraprofessionals provide intensive nutrition education to individuals and groups in a variety of nonformal education settings, including homes, community centers, housing complexes, WIC offices, and churches.

While EFNEP is not a food-assistance program, it is an effective educational program with a mission to reduce food insecurity. EFNEP teaching is tailored to the needs, interests, financial resources, age, ethnic backgrounds, and learning capabilities of participants.

EFNEP's objectives are to improve diets and nutritional welfare for the total family; to increase knowledge of the essentials of human nutrition; to increase the ability to select and buy food that satisfies nutritional needs; to improve practices in food production, storage, preparation, safety, and sanitation; to increase ability to manage food budgets and related resources such as food stamps.

Personal Responsibility and Work Opportunity Reconciliation Act of 1996

The Personal Responsibility and Work Opportunity Reconciliation Act of 1996 (PRWORA) is the most comprehensive welfare reform program since the Social Security Act of the 1930s. The PRWORA has far-reaching implications in a number of programs. The act fundamentally reforms the Food Stamp Program, Supplemental Security Income (SST) for children, the Child Support Enforcement Program, and benefits for legal immigrants. The act modifies the child nutrition programs and provides cuts in the Social Service Block Grants (SSBG).

The act features decreases in funding for programs for low-income children and families and requires structural changes in the Aid to Families with Dependent Children (AFDC) program. The act converts AFDC and Job Opportunities and Basic Skills (JOBS) into the Temporary Assistance to Needy Families (TANF) block grant. Family assistance is limited to 5 years, while granting states the option to limit assistance for a shorter time period.

The PRWORA significantly reduced funding for food assistance programs and represented a sharp reversal from

Hunger and the broader issue of food security have been a public concern in the United States since our nation's inception.

the trends of the early 1990s. This 1996 legislation contains numerous, significant structural changes to the Food Stamp Program, public assistance programs in general, to the Summer Food Program, and the Child and Adult Care Food Program. Start-up and expansion funds for the School Breakfast and Summer Food Programs were eliminated by this legislation. Entire classes of people have been eliminated from eligibility for the Food Stamp Program. For example, unemployed, childless individuals aged 18 to 50 years can receive food for only 3 of every 36 months.

> **Up to one fifth of America's food goes to waste each year, with an estimated 130 pounds of food per person ending up in landfills.**

Cuts in food assistance programs are likely to cause an increase in hunger and food insecurity. State and local governments and private charities, enlisted to make up for federal cutbacks and budget restraints, are increasingly unable to shoulder the burden. Many states, in financial crisis, have previously made severe cuts in human services programs.

RECOMMENDATIONS AND IMPLICATIONS FOR FAMILY AND CONSUMER SCIENTISTS

The physical, psychological, social, and economic tolls of food insecurity are both interconnected and interdependent. While important work has been conducted to redefine and clarify terms related to hunger and food security, redefinition of the solution to food insecurity is needed.

Family and consumer scientists understand the complexity of food security issues and their interrelatedness with other social, economic, and environmental problems that affect the individual, the family, and society.

Strengthen the Safety Net

The most immediate and direct way to reduce hunger and food insecurity is to strengthen the array of food assistance programs in place. The benefits of food assistance programs such as Food Stamps, WIC, School Breakfast Program, and the Summer Food Service Program have not been fully realized because a large percentage of eligible households are not participating. Barriers exist that prevent those needing and wanting assistance from receiving the services. Little research has been conducted that identifies the barriers and possible methods to reduce them. Extensive needs assessment, which includes addressing the social diagnosis phase of Green and Kreuter's PRECEDE-PROCEED planning framework (1991) is needed. Social diagnosis allows the researcher to determine the target population's perceptions of its own needs or quality of life through multiple information-gathering activities. There are only a few methodologies that allow the emic point of view emphasized in social diagnosis. The focus group method provides an ideal venue for eliciting emic data, and it is proven to be effective in collecting this type of information (Dignan, 1995). Family and consumer scientists can work to increase awareness, identify barriers through focus group techniques, and make recommendations to policy makers and program directors on ways to reduce barriers to participation.

Education

The importance of education in resolving the food security issue has been recognized by researchers as well as policy makers. Education is necessary to elicit changes in behavior that will lead to improved food security. While nutrition and family food economics education is provided by some states as a part of the food assistance programs, it is not a mandatory component of all of the available programs. The nutrition education programs offered through the Food Stamp Program, EFNEP, and WIC need to be enhanced and adequately funded to meet the needs of all low-income families and youth. Family and consumer scientists have a direct role in the provision of innovative nutrition education targeted at health promotion and disease prevention. Professionals serve as advocates to provide support for public policy and legislation that promotes cost-effective food assistance programs that require nutrition education for participants.

Food Recovery

Food recovery is a creative way to decrease hunger in America. It supplements the federal food assistance programs by making better use of a food source that already exists. Up to one fifth of America's food goes to waste each year, with an estimated 130 pounds of food per person ending up in landfills. The annual value of this wasted food is approximately $31 billion. It is estimated that about 49 million people could have been fed by these lost resources (USDA, 1996).

Food recovery is the collection of wholesome food for distribution to those who are hungry. Gleaning, the gathering of food after harvest, dates back to biblical times. Today the terms gleaning and food recovery cover a variety of different efforts. Gleaning refers to the collection of crops from farmers' fields that have been mechanically harvested or from fields where it is not economically profitable to harvest. Food rescue refers to the collection of perishable food from wholesale and retail stores, and prepared and processed food from the food processors and food service industry. Family and consumer scientists can actively support and participate in food recovery programs. They can assist diverse agencies and community-based groups to work together to establish local hunger programs, administer food-recovery programs, and coordinate gleaning efforts. Family and consumer scientists provide a national network of practical science-based knowledge; an important contribution may be education and training for recipients, staff, and volunteers working with food recovery. Information may be provided on food preparation and handling, nutrition, food preservation and safety, dietary guidance, and balanced meal planning.

Cost Effectiveness Analysis and Impact Assessment

The cost effectiveness of food assistance programs must be assessed so that program directors can modify the programs to best meet the needs of those receiving benefits. Family and consumer scientists are positioned to conduct or participate in research on the cost effectiveness of food assistance programs, to assist in the evaluation of nutrition education programs designed to alleviate food insecurity, and to monitor the effects of welfare reform in their communities.

The PRWORA is in its early stages of implementation, and scholars and policy makers have not assessed its impact on welfare recipients. Examination of how the PRWORA and subsequent changes in policies and programs affect food security is important research. Assessment of the impacts of PRWORA implementation on food security of families and children will provide a better understanding of program benefits as well as adverse effects on those in poverty. This information is crucial for program planning and management. These issues are very important in making public policy decisions that address the food security problems associated with poverty.

Public Issues Education

Public policy shapes and directs actions to achieve defined societal goals. It may be adopted and implemented formally through government action or adopted informally through common practice and assumptions. Public policy provides direction for personal and group behavior based on values and beliefs as well as government and economic systems. Public policy decisions affect food security and nutritional well-being of the population. There is a need for broad public participation in policy decisions that affect food security. Family and consumer scientists can assist communities in this process through building societal capacity to understand and address this critical issue. The democratic political process works when citizens believe that they have sufficient power to negotiate for their own rights and interests. As people develop their public leadership skills and gain access to information, they are better able to achieve food security for themselves and their communities. Family and consumer scientists can facilitate a greater awareness and understanding of the food security situation in communities throughout the nation.

SUMMARY

Despite all the programs implemented and legislation designed to reduce poverty and its consequences, hunger and food insecurity will continue to be critical issues in the next century. Hunger and food insecurity have serious, complex effects. Clearly, new approaches are necessary to achieve long-term food security in our communities.

Family and Consumer Science professionals can work for policy changes that would increase cost effectiveness and decrease barriers to participation in food assistance programs, provide intensified education about hunger, and help to shape public policy at the local, state, and national levels. Aggressive action is needed to bring an end to hunger and to achieve food security for all citizens.

References

Breglio, V. J. (1992). *Hunger in America: The voter's perspective*. Lanham, MD: Research/Strategy/Management (RMS).

Center for Hunger, Poverty and Nutrition Policy. (1993). *The link between nutrition and cognitive development in children*. Medford, MA: Tufts University.

Clancy, K. L., & Bowering, J. (1992). The need for emergency food: Poverty problems and policy responses. *J Nutr Ed., 24*, 12S–17S.

Codispoti, C. L., & Bartlett, B. J. (1994). *Food and nutrition for life: Malnutrition and older Americans*. Washington, DC: National Aging Information Center. (Publication No. NAIC–12).

Dignan, M. B. (1995). *Measurement and evaluation of health education*. Springfield, IL: C. C. Thomas Publisher.

Egan, M. (1980). Public health nutrition services: Issues today and tomorrow. *JADA, 77*, 423–427.

Federation of American Societies for Experiment Biology, Life Sciences Research Office. (1995). *Third Report on nutrition monitoring in the United States*. Washington, DC: U.S. Government Printing Office.

Fomon, S. J. (1993). *Normal nutrition of infants*. St. Louis, MO: Mosby.

Food Research and Action Center (FRAC). (1991). *Community Childhood Hunger Identification Project: A survey of childhood hunger in the United States*. Washington, DC.

Food Research and Action Center (FRAC). (1997). *Community Childhood Hunger Identification Project: A survey of childhood hunger in the United States*. Washington, DC.

Green, L. W., & Kreuter, M. W. (1991). *Health promotion planning: An educational and environmental approach* (2nd ed.). Mountain View, CA: Mayfield.

Hamilton, W. L., Cook, J. T., Thompson, W. W., Buron, L. F., Frongillo, E. A., Olson, D. M., & Wehler, C. A. (1997). *Household food security in the United States in 1995*. Washington, DC: U.S. Department of Agriculture Food and Consumer Service.

Joy, A. B., & Doisy, C. (1996). Food stamp nutrition education program: Assisting food stamp recipients to become self-sufficient. *J Nutr Ed., 28*, 123–126.

Klein, B. W. (1996). Food security and hunger measures: Promising future for state and local household surveys. *Family Econ Nutr Rev, 9*, 31–37.

U.S. Department of Agriculture. (1989). *Nationwide Food Consumption Survey, continuing survey of food intakes by individuals, low income women 19–50 years and their children, 1–5 years, 4 days*. (NFCF, CSFII Report 85-4). Hyattsville, MD: U.S. Government Printing Office.

U.S. Department of Agriculture. (1996). *A citizen's guide to food recovery*. Washington, DC: U.S. Government Printing Office.

U.S. Department of Health and Human Services. (1994). *Healthy People 2000 review 1993*. (DHHS Publication No. PHS 94-1232-1). Hyattsville, MD: U.S. Government Printing Office.

Uvin, P. (1994). The state of world hunger. *Nutr Rev., 52*, 151–1161.

Voichick, J., & Drake, L. T. (1994). Major stages of U.S. Food and Nutrition Policy Development Related to Food Security. In: *Food security in the United States: A guidebook for public issues education*. Washington, DC: USDA Cooperative Extension System.

Wehler, C. A., Scott, R. I., & Anderson, J. J. (1996). *The Community Childhood Hunger Identification Project: A survey of childhood hunger in the United States*. Washington, DC: Food Research and Action Center.

World Hunger Year. (1994). *Reinvesting in America: Hunger and poverty wheel*. New York: Reinvesting in America.

Glossary

Absorption The process by which digestive products pass from the gastrointestinal tract into the blood.
Acid/base balance The relationship between acidity and alkalinity in the body fluids.
Amino acids The structural units that make up proteins.
Amylase An enzyme that breaks down starches; a component of saliva.
Amylopectin A component of starch, consisting of many glucose units joined in branching patterns.
Amylose A component of starch, consisting of many glucose units joined in a straight chain, without branching.
Anabolism The synthesis of new materials for cellular growth, maintenance, or repair in the body.
Anemia A deficiency of oxygen-carrying material in the blood.
Anorexia nervosa A disorder in which a person refuses food and loses weight to the point of emaciation and even death.
Antioxidant A substance that prevents or delays the breakdown of other substances by oxygen; often added to food to retard deterioration and rancidity.
Arachidonic acid An essential polyunsaturated fatty acid.
Arteriosclerosis Condition characterized by a thickening and hardening of the walls of the arteries and a resultant loss of elasticity.
Ascorbic acid Vitamin C.
Atherosclerosis A type of arteriosclerosis in which lipids, especially cholesterol, accumulate in the arteries and obstruct blood flow.
Avidin A substance in raw egg white that acts as an antagonist of biotin, one of the B vitamins.

Basal metabolic rate (BMR) The rate at which the body uses energy for maintaining involuntary functions such as cellular activity, respiration, and heartbeat when at rest.
Basic four The food plan outlining the milk, meat, fruits and vegetables, and breads and cereals needed in the daily diet to provide the necessary nutrients.
Beriberi A disease resulting from inadequate thiamin in the diet.
Beta-carotene Yellow pigment that is converted to vitamin A in the body.
Biotin One of the B vitamins.
Bomb calorimeter An instrument that oxidizes food samples to measure their energy content.
Buffer A substance that can neutralize both acids and bases to minimize change in the pH of a solution.

Calorie The energy required to raise the temperature of one gram of water one degree Celsius.
Carbohydrate An organic compound composed of carbon, hydrogen, and oxygen in a ratio of 1:2:1.
Carcinogen A cancer-causing substance.
Catabolism The breakdown of complex substances into simpler ones.
Celiac disease A syndrome resulting from intestinal sensitivity to gluten, a protein substance of wheat flour especially and of other grains.
Cellulose An indigestible polysaccharide made of many glucose molecules.
Cheilosis Cracks at the corners of the mouth, due primarily to a deficiency of riboflavin in the diet.
Cholesterol A fat-like substance found only in animal products; important in many body functions but also implicated in heart disease.
Choline A substance that prevents the development of a fatty liver; frequently considered one of the B-complex vitamins.
Chylomicron A very small emulsified lipoprotein that transports fat in the blood.
Cobalamin One of the B vitamins (B$_{12}$).
Coenzyme A component of an enzyme system that facilitates the working of the enzyme.
Collagen Principal protein of connective tissue.
Colostrum The yellowish fluid that precedes breast milk, produced in the first few days of lactation.

Cretinism The physical and mental retardation of a child resulting from severe iodine or thyroid deficiency in the mother during pregnancy.

Dehydration Excessive loss of water from the body.
Dextrin Any of various small soluble polysaccharides found in the leaves of starch-forming plants and in the human alimentary canal as a product of starch digestion.
Diabetes (diabetes mellitus) A metabolic disorder characterized by excess blood sugar and urine sugar.
Digestion The breakdown of ingested foods into particles of a size and chemical composition that can be absorbed by the body.
Diglyceride A lipid containing glycerol and two fatty acids.
Disaccharide A sugar made up of two chemically combined monosaccharides, or simple sugars.
Diuretics Substances that stimulate urination.
Diverticulosis A condition in which the wall of the large intestine weakens and balloons out, forming pouches where fecal matter can be entrapped.

Edema The presence of an abnormally high amount of fluid in the tissues.
Emulsifier A substance that promotes the mixing of foods, such as oil and water in a salad dressing.
Enrichment The addition of nutrients to foods, often to restore what has been lost in processing.
Enzyme A protein that speeds up chemical reactions in the cell.
Epidemiology The study of the factors that contribute to the occurrence of a disease in a population.
Essential amino acid Any of the nine amino acids that the human body cannot manufacture and that must be supplied by the diet, as they are necessary for growth and maintenance.
Essential fatty acid A fatty acid that the human body cannot manufacture and that must be supplied by the diet, as it is necessary for growth and maintenance.

Fat An organic compound whose molecules contain glycerol and fatty acids; fat insulates the body, protects organs, carries fat-soluble vitamins, is a constituent of cell membranes, and makes food taste good.
Fatty acid A simple lipid—containing only carbon, hydrogen, and oxygen—that is a constituent of fat.
Ferritin A substance in which iron, in combination with protein, is stored in the liver, spleen, and bone marrow.
Fiber Indigestible carbohydrate found primarily in plant foods; high fiber intake is useful in regulating bowel movements, and may lower the incidence of certain types of cancer and other diseases.
Flavoprotein Protein containing riboflavin.
Folic acid (folacin) One of the B vitamins.
Fortification The addition of nutrients to foods to enhance their nutritional values.
Fructose A six-carbon monosaccharide found in many fruits as well as honey and plant saps; one of two monosaccharides forming sucrose, or table sugar.

Galactose A six-carbon monosaccharide, one of the two that make up lactose, or milk sugar.
Gallstones An abnormal formation of gravel or stones, composed of cholesterol and bile salts and sometimes bile pigments, in the gallbladder; they result when substances that normally dissolve in bile precipitate out.
Gastritis Inflammation of the stomach.
Glucagon A hormone produced by the pancreas that works to increase blood glucose concentration.
Glucose A six-carbon monosaccharide found in sucrose, honey, and many fruits and vegetables; the major carbohydrate found in the body.
Glucose tolerance factor (GTF) A hormone-like substance containing chromium, niacin, and protein that helps the body to use glucose.
Glyceride A simple lipid composed of fatty acids and glycerol.

Glycogen The storage form of carbohydrates in the body; composed of glucose molecules.
Goiter Enlargement of the thyroid gland as a result of iodine deficiency.
Goitrogens Substances that induce goiter, often by interfering with the body's utilization of iodine.

Heme A complex iron-containing compound that is a component of hemoglobin.
Hemicellulose Any of various indigestible plant polysaccharides.
Hemochromatosis A disorder of iron metabolism.
Hemoglobin The iron-containing protein in red blood cells that carries oxygen to the tissues.
High-density lipoprotein (HDL) A lipoprotein that acts as a cholesterol carrier in the blood; referred to as "good" cholesterol because relatively high levels of it appear to protect against atherosclerosis.
Hormones Compounds secreted by the endocrine glands that influence the functioning of various organs.
Humectants Substances added to foods to help them maintain moistness.
Hydrogenation The chemical process by which hydrogen is added to unsaturated fatty acids, which saturates them and converts them from a liquid to a solid form.
Hydrolyze To split a chemical compound into smaller molecules by adding water.
Hydroxyapatite The hard mineral portion (the major constituent) of bone, composed of calcium and phosphate.
Hypercalcemia A high level of calcium in the blood.
Hyperglycemia A high level of "sugar" (glucose) in the blood.
Hypocalcemia A low level of calcium in the blood.
Hypoglycemia A low level of "sugar" (glucose) in the blood.

Incomplete protein A protein lacking or deficient in one or more of the essential amino acids.
Inorganic Describes a substance not containing carbon.
Insensible loss Fluid loss, through the skin and from the lungs, that an individual is unaware of.
Insulin A hormone produced by the pancreas that regulates the body's use of glucose.
Intrinsic factor A protein produced by the stomach that makes absorption of B_{12} possible; lack of this protein results in pernicious anemia.

Joule A unit of energy preferred by some professionals instead of the heat energy measurements of the calorie system for calculating food energy; sometimes referred to as "kilojoule."

Keratinization Formation of a protein called keratin, which, in vitamin A deficiency, occurs instead of mucus formation; leads to a drying and hardening of epithelial tissue.
Ketogenic Describes substances that can be converted to ketone bodies during metabolism, such as fatty acids and some amino acids.
Ketone bodies The three chemicals—acetone, acetoacetic acid, and betahydroxybutyrie—that are normally involved in lipid metabolism and accumulate in blood and urine in abnormal amounts in conditions of impaired metabolism (such as diabetes).
Ketosis A condition resulting when fats are the major source of energy and are incompletely oxidized, causing ketone bodies to build up in the bloodstream.
Kilocalorie One thousand calories, or the energy required to raise the temperature of one kilogram of water one degree Celsius; the preferred unit of measurement for food energy.
Kilojoule See Joule.
Kwashiorkor A form of malnutrition resulting from a diet severely deficient in protein but high in carbohydrates.

Lactase A digestive enzyme produced by the small intestine that breaks down lactose.
Lactation Milk production/secretion.
Lacto-ovo-vegetarian A person who does not eat meat, poultry, or fish but does eat milk products and eggs.
Lactose A disaccharide composed of glucose and galactose and found in milk.
Lactose intolerance The inability to digest lactose due to a lack of the enzyme lactase in the intestine.
Lacto-vegetarian A person who does not eat meat, poultry, fish, or eggs but does drink milk and eat milk products.
Laxatives Food or drugs that stimulate bowel movements.
Lignins Certain forms of indigestible carbohydrate in plant foods.
Linoleic acid An essential polyunsaturated fatty acid.
Lipase An enzyme that digests fats.
Lipid Any of various substances in the body or in food that are insoluble in water; a fat or fat-like substance.
Lipoprotein Compound composed of a lipid (fat) and a protein that transports both in the bloodstream.
Low-density lipoprotein (LDL) A lipoprotein that acts as a cholesterol carrier in the blood; referred to as "bad" cholesterol because relatively high levels of it appear to enhance atherosclerosis.

Macrocytic anemia A form of anemia characterized by the presence of abnormally large blood cells.
Macroelements (also macronutrient elements) Those elements present in the body in amounts exceeding 0.005 percent of body weight and required in the diet in amounts exceeding 100 mg/day; include sodium, potassium, calcium, and phosphorus.
Malnutrition A poor state of health resulting from a lack, excess, or imbalance of the nutrients needed by the body.
Maltose A disaccharide whose units are each composed of two glucose molecules, produced by the digestion of starch.
Marasmus Condition resulting from a deficiency of calories and nearly all essential nutrients.
Melanin A dark pigment in the skin, hair, and eyes.
Metabolism The sum of all chemical reactions that take place within the body.
Microelements (also micronutrient elements; trace elements) Those elements present in the body in amounts under 0.005 percent of body weight and required in the diet in amounts under 100 mg/day.
Monoglyceride A lipid containing glycerol and only one fatty acid.
Monosaccharide A single sugar molecule, the simplest form of carbohydrate; examples are glucose, fructose, and galactose.
Monosodium glutamate (MSG) An amino acid used in flavoring foods, which causes allergic reactions in some people.
Monounsaturated fatty acid A fatty acid containing one double bond.
Mutagen A mutation-causing agent.

Negative nitrogen balance Nitrogen output exceeds nitrogen intake.
Niacin (nicotinic acid) One of the B vitamins.
Nitrogen equilibrium (zero nitrogen balance) Nitrogen output equals nitrogen intake.
Nonessential amino acid Any of the 13 amino acids that the body can manufacture in adequate amounts, but which are nonetheless required in the diet in an amount relative to the amount of essential amino acids.
Nutrients Nourishing substances in food that can be digested, absorbed, and metabolized by the body; needed for growth, maintenance, and reproduction.
Nutrition (1) The sum of the processes by which an organism obtains, assimilates, and utilizes food. (2) The scientific study of these processes.

Obesity Condition of being 15 to 20 percent above one's ideal body weight.
Oleic acid A monounsaturated fatty acid.

Organic foods Those foods, especially fruits and vegetables, grown without the use of pesticides, synthetic fertilizers, etc.

Osmosis Passage of a solvent through a semipermeable membrane from an area of higher concentration to an area of lower concentration until the concentration is equal on both sides of the membrane.

Osteomalacia Condition in which a loss of bone mineral leads to a softening of the bones; adult counterpart of rickets.

Osteoporosis Disorder in which the bones degenerate due to a loss of bone mineral, producing porosity and fragility; normally found in older women.

Overweight Body weight exceeding an accepted norm by 10 or 15 percent.

Ovo-vegetarian A person who does not eat meat, poultry, fish, milk, or milk products but does eat eggs.

Oxidation The process by which a substrate takes up oxygen or loses hydrogen; the loss of electrons.

Palmitic acid A saturated fatty acid.

Pantothenic acid One of the B vitamins.

Pellagra Niacin deficiency syndrome, characterized by dementia, diarrhea, and dermatitis.

Pepsin A protein-digesting enzyme produced by the stomach.

Peptic ulcer An open sore or erosion in the lining of the digestive tract, especially in the stomach and duodenum.

Peptide A compound composed of amino acids that are joined together.

Peristalsis Motions of the digestive tract that propel food through the tract.

Pernicious anemia One form of anemia caused by an inability to absorb vitamin B_{12}, owing to the absence of intrinsic factor.

pH A measure of the acidity of a solution, based on a scale from 0 to 14: a pH of 7 is neutral; greater than 7 is alkaline; less than 7 is acidic.

Phenylketonuria (PKU) A genetic disease in which phenylalanine, an essential amino acid, is not properly metabolized, thus accumulating in the blood and causing early brain damage.

Phospholipid A fat containing phosphorus, glycerol, two fatty acids, and any of several other chemical substances.

Polypeptide A molecular chain of amino acids.

Polysaccharide A carbohydrate containing many monosaccharide subunits.

Polyunsaturated fatty acids A fatty acid in which two or more carbon atoms have formed double bonds, with each holding only one hydrogen atom.

Positive nitrogen balance Condition in which nitrogen intake exceeds nitrogen output in the body.

Protein Any of the organic compounds composed of amino acids and containing nitrogen; found in the cells of all living organisms.

Provitamins Precursors of vitamins that can be converted to vitamins in the body (e.g., beta-carotene, from which the body can make vitamin A).

Pyridoxine One of the B vitamins (B_6).

Pull date Date after which food should no longer be sold but still may be edible for several days.

Recommended Daily Allowances (RDAs) Standards for daily intake of specific nutrients established by the Food and Nutrition Board of the National Academy of Sciences; they are the levels thought to be adequate to maintain the good health of most people.

Rhodopsin The visual pigment in the retinal rods of the eyes which allows one to see at night; its formation requires vitamin A.

Riboflavin One of the B vitamins (B_2).

Ribosome The cellular structure in which protein synthesis occurs.

Rickets The vitamin D deficiency disease in children characterized by bone softening and deformities.

Saliva Fluid produced in the mouth that helps food digestion.

Salmonella A bacterium that can cause food poisoning.

Saturated fatty acid A fatty acid in which carbon is joined with four other atoms; i.e., all carbon atoms are bound to the maximum possible number of hydrogen atoms.

Scurvy A disease characterized by bleeding gums, pain in joints, lethargy, and other problems; caused by a deficiency of vitamin C (ascorbic acid).

Standard of identity A list of specifications for the manufacture of certain foods that stipulates their required contents.

Starch A polysaccharide composed of glucose molecules; the major form in which energy is stored in plants.

Stearic acid A saturated fatty acid.

Sucrose A disaccharide composed of glucose and fructose, often called "table sugar."

Sulfites Agents used as preservatives in foods to eliminate bacteria, preserve freshness, prevent browning, and increase storage life; can cause acute asthma attacks, and even death, in people who are sensitive to them.

Teratogen An agent with the potential of causing birth defects.

Thiamin One of the B vitamins (B_1).

Thyroxine Hormone containing iodine that is secreted by the thyroid gland.

Toxemia A complication of pregnancy characterized by high blood pressure, edema, vomiting, presence of protein in the urine, and other symptoms.

Transferrin A protein compound, the form in which iron is transported in the blood.

Triglyceride A lipid containing glycerol and three fatty acids.

Trypsin A digestive enzyme, produced in the pancreas, that breaks down protein.

Underweight Body weight below an accepted norm by more than 10 percent.

United States Recommended Daily Allowance (USRDA) The highest level of recommended intakes for population groups (except pregnant and lactating women); derived from the RDAs and used in food labeling.

Urea The main nitrogenous component of urine, resulting from the breakdown of amino acids.

Uremia A disease in which urea accumulates in the blood.

Vegan A person who eats nothing derived from an animal; the strictest type of vegetarian.

Vitamin Organic substance required by the body in small amounts to perform numerous functions.

Vitamin B complex All known water-soluble vitamins except C; includes thiamin (B_1), riboflavin (B_2), pyridoxine (B_6), niacin, folic acid, cobalamin (B_{12}), pantothenic acid, and biotin.

Xerophthalmia A disease of the eye resulting from vitamin A deficiency.

Index

A

Acesulfame-K, 30–31, 45
Adequate Intake (AI), 14
adolescence, physical activity levels and, 99–100. *See also* children
Africa, starvation syndrome and, 214–215
alcohol, 104–105; supposed benefit of, 77
algae, 195
allergies, myths and, 86–89; vs. food intolerances, 87
alternative medicine, 182–185
America, food insecurity and hunger in, 217–221
American Heart Association (AHA): Mediterranean diet and, 78–79; obesity and, 109; vitamin E and, 53
anorexia nervosa, 131–137; effect of starvation and, 133–137
antibiotics, use of in animals, 200–201
aspartame, 30, 45
Audits International. *See* Home Food Safety Survey

B

Benecol margarine, 25
binge eating, 131, 134, 135
biotechnology, 8
Blackburn, George, and research into fat and cholesterol connection, 38–39
blood clots, fiber and, 62
blood pressure, fiber and, 62. *See also* hypertension
body fat, BMI and, 119–121
body mass index (BMI), 122; children and, 94; debate over health and, 119–121; NIH guidelines and, 115–116; obesity and, 109; undernourishment and, 216
body weight, 9; nutritional status and, 216
bone development, 57, 93–94
bovine spongiform encephalopathy, 8
breast cancer; alcohol and, 104–105; fat intake and, 91; fiber and, 62–63; olive oil and, 76; vitamin D and, 50. *See also* cancer; estrogen
bulimia, 131–133

C

caffeine, dehydration and, 196
calcium: bone development and, 57, 58; children and, 93; dietary sources of, 58; NAS recommendations, 56–60; supplements, 58
Campylobacter jejuni, 8, 155–157, 164; chicken and, 155–156; resistance to antibiotics and, 156; vaccine and, 156–157
cancer: diet and, 90–91; fruits and vegetables and, 19, 76; green or black tea and, 77; physical activity and, 101; vitamin C and, 48. *See also* breast cancer; colon cancer; Dietary Guidelines for Americans
carbohydrates, diabetes and, 43–44; syndrome X and, 40–42;
cataracts, vitamin C and, 48
cavities, dietary sugar and, 19, 93
Centers for Disease Control (CDC), aspartame and, 30; hemochromatosis and, 54
Child and Adult Care Feeding Program (CACFP), 219
children: consumption of recommended foods and, 93–94; diet and, 92–96; obesity in, 94; parental role in diet and, 95; physical activity and, 99–100
cholesterol, 122; alcohol and, 105; fat intake and, 38–39; fiber and, 61–62; insulin resistance and, 43–44; Mediterranean diet and, 78–79; soy and, 83; syndrome X and, 40–42
clinical trials, 179–180
Clinton, Bill, genetically modified crops and, 28
colds, vitamin C and, 49
colon cancer, fiber and, 62–63
Community Childhood Hunger Identification Project (CCHIP), 217, 218
Continuing Survey of Food Intakes by Individuals (CSFII), 92, 93; elderly and, 97–98
Council for Agricultural Science and Technology (CAST), nitrites and, 11
Council for Responsible Nutrition (CRN), 203–204
creatine, 195
cross-contamination, 150–153; avoidance of, 151–152. *See also* thermometers

D

dehydration, 196
diabetes, 43, 122; adult onset correlation with physical activity and, 101; medication instead of weight loss and, 124
dietary carcinogens, 9
dietary fats, 38–39; cancer and, 90–91; children and, 93; Mediterranean diet and, 78–79; obesity and, 109–110; syndrome X and, 40–42
Dietary Guidelines for Americans, 97; dietary supplements and, 67; tips for cancer prevention and, 91
dietary reference intake (DRI), 13–15; appropriate uses of, 14; definition of terms, 14; of calcium, 56–57
dietary supplements, 9, 66–73, 195–196; health food stores and, 201; pharmacists' unethical behavior and, 203–204; quacks and, 174–175
diets: limited effectiveness of, 128–130; problems with fad diets, 125–127. *See also* eating disorders; weight loss
double-blind study, 181

E

eating disorders, 131–132, 133–137; signs of, 132
elderly, nutrition and, 97–98
epidemiologic studies, 180
Escheria coli (E:coli) bacteria, 8, 158–159, 163–164, 167–168
Estimated Average Requirements (EAR). *See* dietary reference intakes
estrogen, soy and, 84, 85
Expanded Food and Nutrition Education Program, the (EFNEP), 219

F

fats. *See* fats; polyunsaturated fats; saturated fats
fertilizers, 10
fiber, 61–65; cancer and, 90; children and, 94; content in selected foods, 64; heart disease and, 19, 61–62; Mediterranean diet and, 79; other benefits of, 62–64
fish, supposed benefit of, 77
fluoride, quacks and, 173
folate: heart disease and, 81; neural tube birth defects and, 19
Food and Agriculture Organization (FAO): developing countries and food security and, 212–213; measurement of malnutrition through BMI and, 216; report on poverty and hunger, 208–211
Food and Drug Administration (FDA), 16–19, 23–25, 29, 160; advisory on alfalfa sprouts and, 167; alternative medicine and, 184; egg refrigeration rules and, 160; genetically modified organisms and, 29; health claims and, 16–19; herbal weight loss teas and, 193–194; low-calorie sweeteners and, 30–31; Modernization Act and, 17; olestra and, 32; radiation to kill *E: coli* bacteria and, 163–164. *See also* health claims
food assistance programs, 217–221. *See also* Special Programme for Food Security (SPFS)
Food Guide Pyramid, children and, 92–94

food insecurity, 212–213; Americans, hunger and, 217–221; ways to reduce, 220–221. *See also* undernourishment
food intolerances, myths and, 86–89
food irradiation, 10, 162–166, 169
food poisoning: bacteria that cause, 157; *Campylobacter* and, 155–157; *Escheria coli (E:coli)* and, 8, 158–159; *Salmonella* and, 160–161; sprouts and, 167–169. *See also Campylobacter*; cross-contamination; *Escheria coli (E:coli)*; food irradiation' food safety; *Salmonella*, thermometers
food safety, 8, 11, 143–149; common household violations of, 145–146; myths regarding, 140–142; nitrites and, 11; survey of, 143–149. *See also* cross-contamination; food poisoning
Food Safety and Inspection Service (FSIS), eggs and, 160–161
Food Stamp Program, the. *See* food assistance programs
fruits: cancer and, 90; nutrition and, 20, 76; organically grown, 200
functional foods, 23–26. *See also* health claims; herbal remedies

G

genetic heritage: dietary supplements and, 67; obesity and, 109
genetically modified organisms (GMOs), 27–29; European response to, 28–29; safety and, 28

H

health claims, 16–19, 23; authorized examples of, 18–19; capitalization and, 23; definition of, 16–17; food manufacturers and, 23–26; public confidence in, 17. *See also* herbal remedies; Kellogg's
health food stores, versus traditional supermarkets, 200–202
health scares, Internet and, 186–188. *See also* study results
Healthy Eating Index (HEI), elderly and, 98–98
heart disease: alcohol and, 77, 104–105; fiber and, 19, 61; fish and, 77; garlic and, 76; green or black tea and, 77; homocysteine and, 80–82; Mediterranean diet and, 78–79; nuts and, 76; oat bran and, 76; olive oil and, 76; physical activity and, 100; soy and, 77, 83–84; vitamin C and, 47; vitamin E and, 52–53
herbal remedies, 183–184; adverse reactions with traditional medicine and, 190; health claims and, 26; myths and, 189–191; risks of, 190; weight loss and, 122–124, 192–194
hereditary hemochromatosis, iron and, 54–55
Home Food Safety Survey, 143–149; definition of terms used in, 148–149
homocysteine, heart disease and, 80–82
Homocysteine Revolution, The (McCully), 80
hunger. *See* food insecurity; undernourishment
hyperactivity, sugar and, 46, 93
hypertension, 122; medication instead of weight loss and, 123–124; physical activity and, 100

I

Institute of Food Science and Technology, the, and research into cross-contamination, 150–153
insulin: fiber and, 62; resistance to, 43–44; syndrome X and, 40, 42. *See also* sugar
iron: deficiency in children in, 94, 218; overload of, 54–55
irradiation. *See* food irradiation
Internet, 12; health scares and, 186–188; Web sites for accurate nutritional information, 188

K

Kellogg's, Ensemble product line, health claims and, 24
Keys, Ancel, and research into effects of starvation, 133–137

L

Laci Le Beau Super Dieter's Tea, 192, 193
lactose intolerance, 87–88; products to aid, 196
laxatives, herbal weight loss teas and, 193
liquid meal replacements, 195–196
low income food-deficit countries (LIFDCs), 212–213
low-calorie sweeteners, 30–31, 45; weight loss and, 31

M

macular degeneration, vitamin C and, 48
malnutrition. *See* undernourishment
margarine, medicinal claims and, 24–26
marketing ploys: food packaging and, 33–35; color and, 33–34; grocery store signs and, 34–35; package shape and, 34

medical food, 25
medical information, American sources of, 187
Mediterranean diet, 78–79
menopause, soy and, 77, 85
Mongolia, benefits of Special Programme for Food Security and, 213
monosodium glutamate (MSG) intolerance, 88
monounsaturated fats, 38–39
Mountain People, The (Turnbull), 214

N

National Academy of Sciences: calcium recommendations and, 56–60; dietary supplements report and, 67
National Cholesterol Education Program (NCEP), 78–79
National Health and Nutrition Survey (NHANES) III, 94
National Institutes of Health (NIH): evaluation of diets and, 129; evaluation of guidelines of, 115–118; Office of Alternative Medicine and, 182; vitamin C and, 47
National School Lunch Program, 219
neural tube defects, folate and, 19
nitrites, 11
nutraceuticals. *See* functional foods
Nutrition Labeling and Education Act, 16, 17
Nutritional Research Council (NRC), nitrites and, 11
nutritional information, American sources of, 187
Nutritional Insight, elderly and, 97
nuts, supposed benefit of, 76

O

oat bran, supposed benefit of, 76
obesity: causes of, 109; children and, 94, 113–114; consequences of, 109; epidemic of, 108–109; National Institutes of Heath guidelines and, 115–118; prevention of, 111; racial differences in, 113–114. *See also* overweight; weight control
olestra, 32
olive oil, supposed benefit of, 76
omega 3 fatty acids: fish and, 77; Mediterranean diet and, 78–79
organic foods, 200–201
Organization for Economic Cooperation and Development, genetically modified crops and, 28
Ornish, Dean, 41
osteoporosis: calcium and, 56–60; children and, 93–94; physical activity and, 101; soy and, 84–85
overweight: adults and, 100; children and, 92, 99–100. *See also* obesity; weight control

oxidation, vitamin C and, 48

P

Partnership for Healthy Weight Management, 125
Personal Responsibility and Work Opportunity Reconciliation Act of 1996, the, 219
pharmacists, unethical behavior by and supplements, 203–205
phosphorous, bone development and, 57–58
physical activity, 99–103; adults and, 100–101; benefits of, 99; children and, 99–100; disease(s) and, 100–101; later adult years and, 101–102; weight control and, 111, 116
placebo-controlled study, 181
polyunsaturated fats, 38–39
population-based intervention trials, 180
poverty, American hunger and, 217–221; world hunger and, 208–211;
prospective study, 181
protein, bone development and, 57–58
public health nutrition, 11
Pure Food and Drug Law, Delaney amendment, 9
pyruvate, unsubstantiated claims regarding, 197–199

Q

quackery, spotting of, 172–178

R

race, obesity and, 113–114
Recommended Dietary Allowance (RDA): dietary supplements and, 67; history of, 13; quacks and, 173–174
revision of, 13–14, 68
retrospective study, 181
rheumatoid arthritis, fish and, 77

S

saccharin, 30–31, 45
salmonella bacteria, 8, 164, 167–168; eggs and, 160–161
saturated fat, 38–39; margarine and, 24

Schaefer, Ernst, and research into carbohydrates and syndrome X, 41
School Lunch Program, 219
selenium, 9
socioeconomic status, obesity and, 113–114
soil depletion, nutrition in foods and, 20; quacks and, 173
sorbitol, 45
soy, 83–85; cancer and, 84; cholesterol reduction and, 83; heart disease and, 83–84; menopause and, 85; osteoporosis and, 84; supposed benefit of, 77
Special Programme for Food Security (SPFS), 212–213
Special Supplemental Program for Women, Infants and Children, the (WIC), 219
sprouts, food-borne disease and, 167–169
starvation: behavior of African people undergoing, 214–215; binge eating and, 134–135; cognitive and physical changes and, 136; emotional and personality changes and, 135; preoccupation with food and, 133–134; social and sexual changes and, 135–136. See also undernourishment
State of Food Agriculture 1998, the (SOFA 98) report, 208–211
strawberries, irradiation and, 164, 165
stress, quacks and nutrition and, 174
study results, questions to ask, 179–181
sucralose, 30–31, 45
sugar, 43–46; cavities and, 19, 45; children and, 93; insulin resistance and, 43–44; weight gain and, 44; white versus natural, 44
Summer Food Service Program, 219
supplements. See dietary supplements
syndrome X, 40–42
synthetic fat. See olestra

T

Take Control margarine, 25
thermometers, food poisoning and, 153–154
Tolerable Upper Intake Level (UL), 14
tomatoes, supposed benefit of, 76
trans fat, 38–39; cholesterol and, 38; margarine and, 24–25
tofu. See soy

Turnbull, Colin, and research into effects of starvation on Africans, 214–215

U

undernourishment: BMI and, 216; developing countries and, 209–210; effects on children and, 217–218; food insecurity and, 212–213; poverty and, 208–211, 217–221. See also starvation

V

vegetables, 20, 21–22; cancer and, 90; freshness and, 21–22; nutrition and, 20, 76; organic, 200–201; protection of frozen and, 22
vitamin B6, heart disease and, 81
vitamin B12, heart disease and, 81
vitamin C, 47–49; bone development and, 57–58
vitamin D, 50–51; bone development and, 57–58
vitamin E, 52–53
vitamin K, bone development and, 57–58

W

Web sites, accurate nutrition information and, 187–188
weight control, 108–112. See also obesity; overweight; weight gain; weight loss
weight gain, sugar and, 44
weight loss, 122–124, 125–127, 128–130; approaches for, 110, 120, 126–127; argument against correlation between health and, 122–124; behavioral modifications and, 111; body mass index (BMI) and, 119–121; combined therapy for, 111; diet therapy, 102; effectiveness of dieting and, 128–130; fiber and, 62; harmful effects of, 124; herbal teas and, 192–194; NIH guidelines and, 116; physical activity and, 111; problems with fad diets and, 125–127; pyruvate and, 197–199; quackery and, 175. See also eating disorders

AE Article Review Form

We encourage you to photocopy and use this page as a tool to assess how the articles in **Annual Editions** expand on the information in your textbook. By reflecting on the articles you will gain enhanced text information. You can also access this useful form on a product's book support Web site at **http://www.dushkin.com/online/**.

NAME: DATE:

TITLE AND NUMBER OF ARTICLE:

BRIEFLY STATE THE MAIN IDEA OF THIS ARTICLE:

LIST THREE IMPORTANT FACTS THAT THE AUTHOR USES TO SUPPORT THE MAIN IDEA:

WHAT INFORMATION OR IDEAS DISCUSSED IN THIS ARTICLE ARE ALSO DISCUSSED IN YOUR TEXTBOOK OR OTHER READINGS THAT YOU HAVE DONE? LIST THE TEXTBOOK CHAPTERS AND PAGE NUMBERS:

LIST ANY EXAMPLES OF BIAS OR FAULTY REASONING THAT YOU FOUND IN THE ARTICLE:

LIST ANY NEW TERMS/CONCEPTS THAT WERE DISCUSSED IN THE ARTICLE, AND WRITE A SHORT DEFINITION:

We Want Your Advice

ANNUAL EDITIONS revisions depend on two major opinion sources: one is our Advisory Board, listed in the front of this volume, which works with us in scanning the thousands of articles published in the public press each year; the other is you—the person actually using the book. Please help us and the users of the next edition by completing the prepaid article rating form on this page and returning it to us. Thank you for your help!

ANNUAL EDITIONS: Nutrition 00/01

ARTICLE RATING FORM

Here is an opportunity for you to have direct input into the next revision of this volume. We would like you to rate each of the 63 articles listed below, using the following scale:

1. **Excellent: should definitely be retained**
2. **Above average: should probably be retained**
3. **Below average: should probably be deleted**
4. **Poor: should definitely be deleted**

Your ratings will play a vital part in the next revision. So please mail this prepaid form to us just as soon as you complete it. Thanks for your help!

RATING	ARTICLE
	1. Millennium: Food and Nutrition
	2. Nutrient Requirements Get a Makeover: The Evolution of the Recommended Dietary Allowances
	3. Staking a Claim to Good Health
	4. Are Fruits and Vegetables Less Nutritious Today?
	5. The Freshness Fallacy
	6. The New Foods: Functional or Dysfunctional?
	7. The Curse of Frankenfood: Genetically Modified Crops Stir Up Controversy at Home and Abroad
	8. Low-Calorie Sweeteners
	9. It's Crunch Time for P&G's Olestra
	10. Supermarket Psych-Out
	11. Fats: The Good, the Bad, the Trans
	12. Should You Be Eating *More* Fat and *Fewer* Carbohydrates?
	13. Sugar: What's the Harm?
	14. Vitamin C: Foods Yes, Pills No
	15. The Best D-Fense
	16. Can Vitamin E Prevent Heart Disease?
	17. A Disease of Too Much Iron
	18. National Academy of Sciences Introduces New Calcium Recommendations
	19. Fiber: Strands of Protection
	20. Food for Thought about Dietary Supplements
	21. Disease-Fighting Foods? (Many Are Overhyped. But All Offer Important Lessons about Good Nutrition)
	22. "Mediterranean Diet" Reduces Risk of Second Heart Attack
	23. Homocysteine: "The New Cholesterol"?
	24. Soy: Cause for Joy?
	25. False Alarms about Food
	26. Questions and Answers about Cancer, Diet and Fats
	27. How to Grow a Healthy Child
	28. A Focus on Nutrition for the Elderly: It's Time to Take a Closer Look
	29. Physical Activity and Nutrition: A Winning Combination for Health
	30. Alcohol and Health: Straight Talk on the Medical Headlines
	31. Weight Control: Challenges and Solutions

RATING	ARTICLE
	32. Childhood Obesity and Family SES Racial Differences
	33. NIH Guidelines: An Evaluation
	34. The Great Weight Debate
	35. Exploding the Myth: Weight Loss Makes You Healthier
	36. Simplifying the Advice for Slimming Down
	37. The History of Dieting and Its Effectiveness
	38. Dieting Disorder
	39. The Effects of Starvation on Behavior: Implications for Dieting and Eating Disorders
	40. Food Safety: Don't Get Burned
	41. Audits International's Home Food Safety Survey
	42. Avoiding Cross-Contamination in the Home
	43. Why You Need a Kitchen Thermometer
	44. Campylobacter: Low-Profile Bug Is Food Poisoning Leader
	45. *E. Coli* 0157:H7—How Dangerous Has It Become?
	46. A Crackdown on Bad Eggs
	47. Irradiation: A Safe Measure for Safer Food
	48. Questions Keep Sprouting about Sprouts
	49. Twenty-Five Ways to Spot Quacks and Vitamin Pushers
	50. Yet Another Study—Should You Pay Attention?
	51. Alternative Medicine—The Risks of Untested and Unregulated Remedies
	52. The Mouse That Roared: Health Scares on the Internet
	53. Uprooting Herbal Myths
	54. Herbal Weight Loss Tea: Beware the Unknown Brew
	55. 5 Nutrition Topics That Are Not All They're Cracked Up to Be
	56. Pyruvate: Just the Facts
	57. Are Health Food Stores Better Bets than Traditional Supermarkets?
	58. The Unethical Behavior of Pharmacists
	59. FAO Releases Annual State of Food and Agriculture Report Showing Worldwide Number of Hungry People Rising Slightly
	60. Special Programme for Food Security at the Food and Agriculture Organization
	61. Starvation Syndrome in Africa
	62. How to Measure Malnutrition
	63. Hunger and Food Insecurity

(Continued on next page)

ANNUAL EDITIONS: NUTRITION 00/01

BUSINESS REPLY MAIL
FIRST-CLASS MAIL   PERMIT NO. 84   GUILFORD CT
POSTAGE WILL BE PAID BY ADDRESSEE

Dushkin/McGraw-Hill
Sluice Dock
Guilford, CT 06437-9989

ABOUT YOU

Name _____ Date _____

Are you a teacher? ☐   A student? ☐
Your school's name

_____

Department

_____

Address _____ City _____ State _____ Zip _____

School telephone # _____

YOUR COMMENTS ARE IMPORTANT TO US!

Please fill in the following information:
For which course did you use this book?
_____

Did you use a text with this *ANNUAL EDITION*? ☐ yes ☐ no
What was the title of the text?
_____

What are your general reactions to the *Annual Editions* concept?
_____

Have you read any particular articles recently that you think should be included in the next edition?
_____

Are there any articles you feel should be replaced in the next edition? Why?
_____

Are there any World Wide Web sites you feel should be included in the next edition? Please annotate.
_____

May we contact you for editorial input? ☐ yes ☐ no
May we quote your comments? ☐ yes ☐ no
_____